Making Sense of Echocardiography

Echocardiography is one of the most useful and powerful diagnostic tools in the assessment of cardiac structure and function. It remains a rapidly expanding modality, with new techniques constantly developing and maturing. Building on the success of the second edition, the third edition of *Making Sense of Echocardiography: A Hands-on Guide* provides a timely overview for those learning echocardiography for the first time as well as an accessible handbook that experienced sonographers can refer to. The strong clinical focus and concentration on real-life scenarios make this book relevant in day-to-day practice. Key updates for this edition include the latest guidelines for the evaluation of diastolic function and pulmonary hypertension and fully updated reference intervals throughout.

Key Features

- Covers not only the fundamentals of echocardiography, including ultrasound physics, but also new technologies such as 3D echocardiography
- Provides a comprehensive approach for the echo trainee, and serves as a useful reference for more seasoned echocardiographers
- Incorporates current guidelines and reference intervals throughout

Making Sense of Echocardiography
About the Series

The Making Sense series covers a variety of medical topics and subjects allied to medicine. Some of them are practical and technique-based, some provide professional advice, and some relate to professional development. All titles are easy to navigate for quick reference and include plenty of features such as 'summary boxes', 'pearls of wisdom', and 'clinical considerations'. Easy to understand, written in a jargon-free style, and convenient for carrying around, the Making Sense series provides hands-on guidance to be referred to often in both clinical and reference contexts.

Making Sense of the ECG: A Hands-on Guide, 5th Edition
Andrew R. Houghton

Making Sense of Fluids and Electrolytes: A Hands-on Guide, 1st Edition
Zoja Milovanovic, Abisola Adeleye

Making Sense of Exercise Testing, 1st Edition
Robert B. Schoene, H. Thomas Robertson

Making Sense of Clinical Teaching: A Hands-on Guide to Success, 1st Edition
Samy A Azer

Making Sense of Clinical Examination of the Adult Patient: A Hands-on Guide, 1st Edition
Douglas Model

Making Sense of Critical Appraisal, 1st Edition
Olajide Ajetunmobi

Making Sense of Sleep Medicine: A Hands-on Guide
Karuna Datta and Deepak Shrivastava

Making Sense of Echocardiography: A Hands-on Guide, 3rd Edition
Andrew R. Houghton

Making Sense of Echocardiography
A Hands-on Guide

Third Edition

Andrew R Houghton

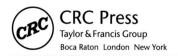

CRC Press
Taylor & Francis Group
Boca Raton London New York

CRC Press is an imprint of the
Taylor & Francis Group, an **informa** business

Designed cover image: Shutterstock

Third edition published 2024
by CRC Press
6000 Broken Sound Parkway NW, Suite 300, Boca Raton, FL 33487-2742

and by CRC Press
4 Park Square, Milton Park, Abingdon, Oxon, OX14 4RN

CRC Press is an imprint of Taylor & Francis Group, LLC

© 2024 Andrew R Houghton

First edition published by Hodder Arnold 2009
Second edition published by Taylor & Francis 2014

ISBN: 9781032303574 (hbk)
ISBN: 9781032303543 (pbk)
ISBN: 9781003304654 (ebk)

DOI: 10.1201/9781003304654

Typeset in Minion Pro
by KnowledgeWorks Global Ltd.

Dedication

This book is dedicated to the British Society of Echocardiography for their leading role in promoting best practice and high standards of professional competence in echocardiography, and the advancement of education, training and research.

Contents

Preface

Since the publication of the second edition of *Making Sense of Echocardiography*, there have been many advancements in the field of echo. The quality and sophistication of echo technology continues to improve, and techniques such as 3D/4D echo and speckle tracking are now firmly incorporated into clinical practice.

There have also been major updates of many of the key echo guidelines, and these updates have been incorporated throughout the text. Updated key references for further reading are provided for each chapter, and these reflect the latest guidelines and papers in each field. Several new figures have been included, and several chapters have been restructured to provide even greater clarity to the text.

The primary aim of this third edition of *Making Sense of Echocardiography* remains the same as that of its predecessors – to provide the echo trainee with a comprehensive yet readable introduction to echo and to provide more experienced sonographers with an accessible handbook for reference when required. Information not just on performing echo but also on the supporting topics of ultrasound physics, anatomy, physiology and clinical cardiology is interwoven throughout the book.

The approach to echo studies taken in this book is based on guidelines published by national echo societies, principally the British Society of Echocardiography (BSE), and I am particularly grateful to the BSE for granting permission to use their recommended reference intervals throughout the book. I am also grateful to everyone who has taken the time to comment on draft copies of the text and to all those who have provided echo images for this book. Finally, I would like to thank all the staff at CRC Press/Taylor & Francis who have contributed to the success of the *Making Sense…* series of books.

Andrew R Houghton

Acknowledgements

I would like to thank everyone who provided suggestions and constructive criticism while I prepared the third edition of *Making Sense of Echocardiography*.

I would like to thank Cara Mercer, Stephanie Baker, Nigel Dewey and Sophie Beech in the Cardiology Department at Grantham & District Hospital for their invaluable help in the preparation of this book. I am also grateful to the following colleagues for assisting me in acquiring the images that illustrate this book:

Mookhter Ajij
Denise Archer
Mark Philip Cassar
Tina Dale
Paul Gibson
Catherine Goult

Lawrence Green
Prathap Kanagala
Jane Kemm
Jeffrey Khoo
David O'Brien
Heidi Pleasance

Prashanth Raju
Nimit Shah
Kay Tay
Upul Wijayawardhana
Bernadette Williamson

I am indebted to Jo Sopala at the British Society of Echocardiography (BSE) for permission to quote the society's recommended echo reference intervals which, where applicable, form the basis of the reference intervals used in this book.

I am grateful to Dr Grant Heatlie at the University Hospital of North Staffordshire in Stoke on Trent and to Dr Thomas Mathew at the Trent Cardiac Centre in Nottingham for their contributions to the previous edition of this book, and for the images which have been carried forward to this new edition.

I would like to thank my wife, Kathryn Ann Houghton, for her support and patience during the preparation of this book.

Finally, I would also like to express my gratitude to everyone at CRC Press/Taylor & Francis for their guidance and support.

Author

Dr Andrew R Houghton studied medicine at the University of Oxford and undertook postgraduate training in Nottingham and Leicester. He was appointed as a consultant cardiologist at Grantham & District Hospital in Lincolnshire, UK, in 2002. His subspecialty interest is in non-invasive cardiac imaging, in particular echocardiography and cardiovascular MRI. He has been a member of the British Society of Echocardiography's departmental accreditation committee and a lecturer at BSE annual congresses.

Dr Houghton has co-authored a number of textbooks, including *Making Sense of the ECG* (now in its fifth edition) and its companion volume *Making Sense of the ECG: Cases for Self-Assessment*, and is also a faculty member at the Medmastery online medical education website. *Making Sense of the ECG* has won several awards, including the Royal Society of Medicine's Richard Asher prize and the British Medical Association's Student Textbook Award, while *Making Sense of Echocardiography* was highly commended at the BMA Medical Book Awards.

Acronyms and Abbreviations

2D	two-dimensional
3D	three-dimensional
4D	four-dimensional
a′	atrial contraction velocity on tissue Doppler imaging of mitral annulus
A	peak A wave velocity
ACE	angiotensin-converting enzyme
A$_{dur}$	duration of atrial reversal in pulmonary vein flow
AF	atrial fibrillation
Ao	aorta
AR	aortic regurgitation
ARVC	arrhythmogenic right ventricular cardiomyopathy
AS	aortic stenosis
ASD	atrial septal defect
ASE	American Society of Echocardiography
AV	aortic valve *or* atrioventricular
BCS	British Cardiovascular Society
BSA	body surface area
BSE	British Society of Echocardiography
CI	cardiac index
CO	cardiac output
CRT	cardiac resynchronization therapy
CSA	cross-sectional area
CTRCD	cancer therapy–related cardiac dysfunction
CW	continuous wave (Doppler)
Cx	circumflex (coronary) artery
DCM	dilated cardiomyopathy
e′	early myocardial velocity on tissue Doppler imaging of mitral annulus
E	peak E wave velocity
EACVI	European Association of Cardiovascular Imaging
ECG	electrocardiogram
EDV	end-diastolic volume
EF	ejection fraction
ESC	European Society of Cardiology
ESV	end-systolic volume
ET	ejection time
FS	fractional shortening
HCM	hypertrophic cardiomyopathy
HFmrEF	heart failure with mildly reduced ejection fraction
HFpEF	heart failure with preserved ejection fraction
HFrEF	heart failure with reduced ejection fraction
HID	half-intensity depth
HOCM	hypertrophic obstructive cardiomyopathy
HR	heart rate
ICD	implantable cardioverter defibrillator
ICt	isovolumic contraction time

INR	international normalized ratio
IRT or IVRT	isovolumic relaxation time
IV	intravenous
IVC	inferior vena cava
IVNC	isolated ventricular non-compaction
IVS	interventricular septum
IVSd	interventricular septal thickness in diastole
IVSs	interventricular septal thickness in systole
JVP	jugular venous pressure
LA	left atrium
LAA	left atrial appendage
LAD	left anterior descending (coronary artery)
LCA	left coronary artery
LCC	left coronary cusp
LLPV	left lower pulmonary vein
LMS	left main stem
LUPV	left upper pulmonary vein
LV	left ventricle
LVEDV	left ventricular end-diastolic volume
LVEDVi	left ventricular end-diastolic volume (indexed)
LVEF	left ventricular ejection fraction
LVESV	left ventricular end-systolic volume
LVESVi	left ventricular end-systolic volume (indexed)
LVH	left ventricular hypertrophy
LVIDd	left ventricular internal diameter in diastole
LVIDs	left ventricular internal diameter in systole
LVOT	left ventricular outflow tract
LVMi	left ventricular mass (indexed)
LVPW	left ventricular posterior wall
LVPWd	left ventricular posterior wall thickness in diastole
LVPWs	left ventricular posterior wall thickness in systole
MCE	myocardial contrast echo
MI	mechanical index *or* myocardial infarction
MPSE	myocardial perfusion stress echo
MR	mitral regurgitation
MS	mitral stenosis
MV	mitral valve
NCC	non-coronary cusp
NSTEMI	non-ST elevation myocardial infarction
NT-pro-BNP	N-terminal-pro-B-type natriuretic peptide
OM	obtuse marginal (coronary artery)
P½T	pressure half-time
PA	pulmonary artery
PADP	pulmonary artery diastolic pressure
PASP	pulmonary artery systolic pressure
PBMV	percutaneous balloon mitral valvuloplasty
PDA	persistent ductus arteriosus *or* posterior descending artery
PFO	patent foramen ovale
PG	pressure gradient
PISA	proximal isovelocity surface area
$\mathbf{P_{max}}$	peak pressure
$\mathbf{P_{mean}}$	mean pressure
PR	pulmonary regurgitation

PRF	pulse repetition frequency
PS	pulmonary stenosis
PV	pulmonary valve *or* pulmonary vein
PV$_a$	peak atrial reversal ('A' wave) velocity in pulmonary vein
PV$_D$	peak diastolic ('D' wave) velocity in pulmonary vein
PV$_S$	peak systolic ('S' wave) velocity in pulmonary vein
PW	pulsed-wave (Doppler)
RA	right atrium
RAP	right atrial pressure
RCA	right coronary artery
RF	regurgitant fraction
RIMP	right ventricular index of myocardial performance
RLPV	right lower pulmonary vein
RT3D	real-time three-dimensional
RT3DFV	real-time three-dimensional full volume
RUPV	right upper pulmonary vein
RV	regurgitant volume *or* right ventricle
RVDP	right ventricular diastolic pressure
RVOT	right ventricular outflow tract
RVSP	right ventricular systolic pressure
RWT	relative wall thickness
S′	systolic myocardial velocity on tissue Doppler imaging of mitral annulus
SD	stroke distance
SV	stroke volume
SVi	stroke volume index
STEMI	ST elevation myocardial infarction
SVC	superior vena cava
SVI	stroke volume index
TAVI	transcatheter aortic valve implantation
TDI	tissue Doppler imaging
TGC	time-gain compensation
TIA	transient ischaemic attack
TOE	transoesophageal echo
ToF	tetralogy of Fallot
TR	tricuspid regurgitation
TS	tricuspid stenosis
TTE	transthoracic echo
UEA	ultrasound enhancing agent
V$_{max}$	peak velocity
V$_{mean}$	mean velocity
VSD	ventricular septal defect
VTI	velocity time integral
WHO	World Health Organization
Zva	valvular–arterial impedance

PART I: ESSENTIAL PRINCIPLES

CHAPTER 1

History of echocardiography

The first application of diagnostic ultrasound in medicine was in the late 1930s, when Karl Dussik, an Austrian psychiatrist and neurologist, became interested in the potential use of ultrasound for brain imaging. Ultrasound was already in use at that time by mariners for underwater imaging and also by engineers for flaw detection in metals. The piezoelectric effect was already well known, having been discovered more than half a century earlier, and the concept of using a piezoelectric crystal to both transmit and receive ultrasound was described in 1917.

Dussik's brain imaging technique was different to today's ultrasound, in that it was based on the transmission of ultrasound waves *through* an object, rather than detecting waves *reflected from* an object. His technique, which he called hyperphonography, involved placing a transmitter on one side of the head and a receiver on the other, and using this apparatus, he was able to produce images of the ventricles of the brain. Echo transmission was also the first ultrasound technique used for cardiac imaging, by the German physiologist Wolf-Dieter Keidel, in order to make measurements of the heart and thorax.

Echo reflection was first used by Inge Edler and Carl Hellmuth Hertz in Sweden. One weekend in 1953, they borrowed an industrial device, used to detect flaws in metals by the Kockum shipyard in Malmö, to conduct their work on human subjects. By a fortunate coincidence, the frequency of the echo transducer happened to be one that was suitable for cardiac imaging. The image of the heart they produced was known as an amplitude mode (A-mode) scan and it was thought to show the posterior wall of the left ventricle (LV). They were soon granted an ultrasound machine of their own and began to produce motion mode (M-mode) scans, with which they were able to examine the mitral valve and also detect atrial thrombus, myxoma and pericardial effusion.

Nonetheless, it was not until the early 1960s that the potential value of cardiac ultrasound became more widely recognized. The first dedicated cardiac ultrasound machine, developed by Jack Reed and Claude Joyner, appeared and the term 'echocardiography' was coined for the first time.

Real-time 2D echo followed in the 1960s, spurred on by advances in electronics, and by the early 1970s, mechanical transducers were available that could produce 2D images by steering the transducer back and forth, sweeping the ultrasound beam across the heart. Phased-array transducers soon followed, in which the mechanical beam-steering mechanism was replaced by solid-state electronics.

The 1970s also saw rapid developments in the use of Doppler techniques, and by the early 1980s, colour Doppler imaging was becoming a common feature of echo studies. During the 1980s, the technique of transoesophageal echo started to enter clinical practice, initially with monoplane probes but later with biplane probes, multiplane probes and, ultimately, the use of 3D transoesophageal imaging.

DOI: 10.1201/9781003304654-1

The 1990s saw a gradual change in archiving methods, with a move away from recording studies on videotape towards more versatile digitally based archiving. There were also refinements in the quality of echo, with the introduction of harmonic imaging and the growing use of echo contrast agents to enhance endocardial border definition. Tissue Doppler imaging entered mainstream practice towards the end of the 1990s, adding a new modality that has proven particularly valuable in the assessment of LV diastolic function.

The new millennium saw the increasing adoption of 3D/4D echo, in both transthoracic and transoesophageal studies. The use of speckle-tracking echo provided valuable insights into myocardial mechanics and soon moved from the research setting into routine clinical practice. Meanwhile, echo machines have gradually shrunk, initially to the size of laptop computers and subsequently to the size of handheld devices, greatly increasing the portability and availability of echo technology.

The growing use of echo has reinforced the need for professional regulation, and the past few years have seen the publication of many key national and international guidelines that set clear quality standards for the performance of echo in the years ahead.

Further reading

Coman IM. Christian Andreas Doppler: the man and his legacy. *European Journal of Echocardiography* (2005). PMID 157449.

Edler I et al. The use of ultrasonic reflectoscope for the continuous recording of the movements of heart walls. *Kungliga Fysiografiska Sällskapets i Lund Förhandlingar* (1954). PMID 15165281.

Fraser AG et al. A concise history of echocardiography: timeline, pioneers, and landmark publications. *European Heart Journal – Cardiovascular Imaging* (2022). PMID 35762885.

Iskander J et al. Advanced echocardiography techniques: the future stethoscope of systemic diseases. *Current Problems in Cardiology* (2022). PMID 33992429.

Roelandt JRTC. Seeing the invisible: a short history of cardiac ultrasound. *European Journal of Echocardiography* (2000). PMID 11916580.

CHAPTER 2

Cardiac anatomy and physiology

The heart lies within the thorax, to the left of the midline, protected by the rib cage and lying in close proximity to the lungs and, underneath, the diaphragm (**Figure 2.1**). The ribs and lungs can pose a challenge to the sonographer trying to obtain clear images of the heart, as ultrasound does not penetrate bone or aerated lung well.

The heart consists of four main chambers (left and right atria and left and right ventricles) and four valves (aortic, mitral, pulmonary, and tricuspid). Venous blood returns to the right atrium (RA) via the superior and inferior venae cavae and leaves the right ventricle (RV) for the lungs via the pulmonary artery. Oxygenated blood from the lungs returns to the left atrium (LA) via the four pulmonary veins and leaves the left ventricle (LV) via the aorta (**Figure 2.2**).

CARDIAC CHAMBERS AND VALVES

The aortic valve

The aortic valve lies between the left ventricular outflow tract (LVOT) and aortic root (**Figure 2.3**) and has three cusps, which open widely during systole. In diastole, the valve closes and in the parasternal short-axis view (aortic valve level), it has a Y-shaped appearance (sometimes referred to as resembling a 'Mercedes-Benz badge'; **Figure 7.5**, p. 47).

Upstream of the aortic valve are the sinuses of Valsalva, an expanded region of the aortic root, from which the coronary arteries originate. Each of the sinuses and aortic valve cusps is named according to its relationship to these coronary arteries: Hence the right coronary cusp lies adjacent to the sinus giving rise to the right coronary artery (RCA), and the left coronary cusp lies adjacent to the sinus giving rise to the left coronary artery (LCA). The third sinus does not have a coronary artery, and the adjacent cusp is named the non-coronary cusp.

Where the valve cusps attach to the aortic root is often termed the aortic valve annulus, although the annulus is not a discrete structure (unlike the mitral valve annulus). The point where adjacent cusps meet is called the commissure. Each cusp has a small nodule at its centre, called the nodule of Arantius, which is more prominent in older patients. The ventricular surface of a cusp sometimes carries small mobile filaments, called Lambl's excrescences, arising from the edge of the cusp. Lambl's excrescences are of no clinical significance but should not be mistaken for vegetations (Chapter 28) or papillary fibroelastoma (Chapter 32).

Below the aortic valve lies the LVOT, which includes the membranous part of the interventricular septum (IVS) and the anterior mitral valve leaflet. The fibrous tissue of the aortic root is continuous with the anterior mitral valve leaflet.

DOI: 10.1201/9781003304654-2

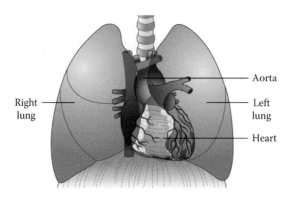

Figure 2.1   The heart and its relation to the rest of the thorax.

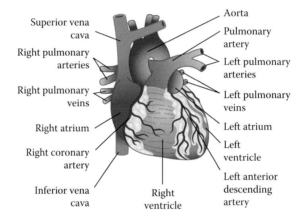

Figure 2.2   The heart and major vessels.

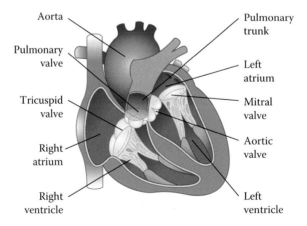

Figure 2.3   The heart valves and chambers.

The left ventricle

The normal LV is an approximately symmetrical structure, which is cylindrical at its base (the mitral annulus) and tapers towards its apex. It is the main pumping chamber of the heart, and its wall is thicker (and myocardial mass greater), although less trabeculated, than that of the RV. The LV myocardium is conventionally subdivided into 16 or 17 segments, the function of each of which should be assessed individually (Chapter 17).

The mitral valve

The mitral valve lies between the LA and LV and has two leaflets that open during diastole and close in systole to prevent regurgitation of blood from the LV back into the LA. The mitral valve needs to be thought of as more than just two leaflets, however, because the mitral annulus, papillary muscles and chordae tendineae are all essential to the valve's structure and function (**Figure 2.4**).

The mitral leaflets are termed anterior and posterior and attach around their base to the fibrous mitral annulus, an elliptical ring separating the LA and LV. The anterior mitral leaflet is longer (from base to tip) than the posterior leaflet, but the length of its attachment to the annulus is shorter and so the surface area of both leaflets is almost equal. Each leaflet is divided into three segments, or scallops, which are named A1, A2 and A3 (anterior leaflet) and P1, P2 and P3 (posterior leaflet), with the numbering running from the anterolateral commissure (A1/P1) to the posteromedial commissure (A3/P3) (**Figure 21.2**, p. 156).

There are two papillary muscles, named anterolateral and posteromedial (after the location of their attachment to the LV), which are attached to the mitral leaflets via the chordae tendineae. Although there are two leaflets and two papillary muscles, each papillary muscle supplies chordae to *both* leaflets – it is not a 1:1 relationship. Chordae from the medial aspects of both leaflets attach to the posteromedial papillary muscle and from the lateral aspects to the anterolateral papillary muscle.

The chordae keep the mitral leaflets under tension during systole, preventing prolapse of the leaflets back into the LA. They are categorized into three groups:

- first-order or marginal chordae, which attach to the free edges of the mitral leaflets
- second-order or strut chordae, which attach to the ventricular surface of the leaflets (away from the free edges)
- third-order or basal chordae, which run directly from the ventricular wall (rather than the papillary muscles) to the ventricular surface of the posterior leaflet, usually near the annulus

The mitral leaflets are normally thin and open widely during diastole, with the anterior leaflet almost touching the IVS. As the leaflets close (coapt), they overlap at their tips by several millimetres (apposition). A reduced degree of apposition results in poor coaptation and can cause mitral regurgitation.

The left atrium

The LA is situated at the back of the heart, in front of the oesophagus (and it is therefore the chamber immediately adjacent to the probe in the mid-oesophageal transoesophageal echo view). The LA is a relatively smooth-walled structure but does have an appendage which can act as a focus for thrombus formation. It is entered by four pulmonary veins carrying oxygenated blood from the lungs – two from the right lung and two from the left lung.

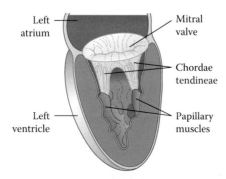

Figure 2.4   Mitral valve anatomy.

The LA is not just a passive conduit between the pulmonary veins and the LV, but rather it contracts during atrial systole (immediately after the onset of the P wave) to provide additional diastolic filling of the LV (the 'atrial kick'). This is particularly important when diastolic filling is impaired, in the presence of elevated LV filling pressures.

The LA is separated from the RA by the interatrial septum, but there can be a communication between the two in the form of a patent foramen ovale or atrial septal defect (ASD) (Chapter 33).

The pulmonary valve

The pulmonary valve lies between the right ventricular outflow tract (RVOT) and pulmonary artery, opening during systole to allow blood to pass from the ventricle into the pulmonary circulation and closing in diastole to prevent regurgitation (a small amount of 'physiological' pulmonary regurgitation is normal). The valve itself is structurally similar to the aortic valve, having three cusps (called anterior, left and right), although the pulmonary valve cusps are thinner than the aortic valve cusps (owing to the lower pressures in the right heart).

The right ventricle

The RV is more complex to assess by echo than the LV, forming a crescent-shaped structure around the LV. It is more heavily trabeculated, but thinner-walled than the LV, and contains a moderator band that stretches between the free wall and the septum. The RVOT is not trabeculated and leads to the pulmonary valve. The RV acts as the pumping chamber for deoxygenated blood returning from the body en route to the lungs.

The tricuspid valve

The tricuspid valve lies between the RA and RV, opening during diastole to allow blood to pass from the atrium to the ventricle, and closing in systole to prevent regurgitation (although a small amount of 'physiological' tricuspid regurgitation is commonly seen in normal individuals).

As its name suggests, the tricuspid valve has three cusps – in order of decreasing size, these are called the anterior, posterior, and septal cusps. There are also three papillary muscles, which, in a similar way to the mitral valve, are attached to the cusps via chordae tendineae. The orifice area of the tricuspid valve is greater than that of the mitral valve, normally 7–9 cm^2.

The right atrium

The RA receives blood returning to the heart via the superior and inferior venae cavae. It also receives blood draining from the myocardium via the coronary sinus, which enters the RA posteriorly, just superior to the tricuspid valve. The coronary sinus is often visible on echo, particularly when it is dilated (**Figure 32.4**, p. 261).

The Eustachian valve, an embryological remnant, may be seen in the RA near the junction with the inferior vena cava.

The coronary arteries

The coronary circulation normally arises as two separate vessels from the sinuses of Valsalva – the LCA from the left coronary sinus, and the RCA from the right coronary sinus (**Figure 2.5**).

The initial portion of the LCA is the left main stem, which soon divides into the left anterior descending (LAD) and circumflex (Cx) arteries. The LAD artery runs down the anterior interventricular groove giving rise to diagonal branches, which course towards the lateral wall of the LV, and septal perforators that supply the IVS. The Cx artery runs in the left atrioventricular groove, giving rise to obtuse marginal branches which extend across the lateral surface of the LV.

The RCA runs in the right atrioventricular groove, and in most people gives rise to the posterior descending artery, which runs down the posterior interventricular groove. This defines

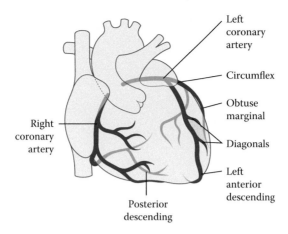

Figure 2.5   The coronary circulation.

'dominance' – most people, therefore, have a 'dominant' RCA, but in some people the Cx gives rise to the posterior descending artery, and they are said to have a 'dominant' Cx.

The pericardium

The pericardium is a sac-like structure that surrounds most of the heart. There is an outer fibrous layer – the *fibrous pericardium* – which blends with the diaphragm inferiorly, and an inner layer – the *serous pericardium* – which itself has two layers (the parietal pericardium, continuous with the fibrous outer layer, and the visceral pericardium, which is the epicardium of the heart).

The pericardium contains 'gaps' where vessels enter and leave the heart, and the pericardium forms a small sleeve around these vessels. As a result, there is a small pocket of pericardium around the aorta/pulmonary artery (transverse sinus) and between the four pulmonary veins (oblique sinus).

The pericardial cavity is a potential space between the parietal and visceral layers, and normally it contains less than 50 mL of fluid. Inflammation of the pericardium (pericarditis) can lead to the accumulation of a larger volume of fluid – a pericardial effusion. If this affects the normal functioning of the heart, cardiac tamponade can result. In the longer term, inflammation of the pericardium can lead to thickening of the pericardium and pericardial constriction.

THE CARDIAC CYCLE

The events that occur during each heartbeat are termed the cardiac cycle, commonly represented in a diagrammatic form (**Figure 2.6**). The cardiac cycle has four phases:

1. Isovolumic contraction
2. Ventricular ejection
3. Isovolumic relaxation
4. Ventricular filling

These phases apply to both left and right heart, but we will focus on the left heart here for clarity. Phases 1 and 2 correspond with ventricular systole and phases 3 and 4 with ventricular diastole.

Isovolumic contraction begins with closure of the mitral valve, caused by the rising LV pressure at the start of ventricular systole. After the mitral valve has closed, pressure within the LV continues to rise but the LV volume remains constant (hence 'isovolumic') until the point when the aortic valve opens.

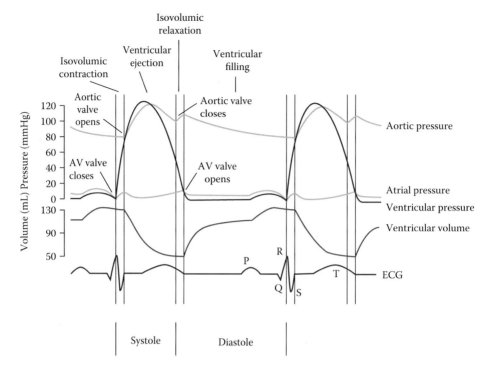

Figure 2.6   The cardiac cycle. *Abbreviations:* AV: Atrioventricular, ECG: Electrocardiogram.

Ventricular ejection commences when the aortic valve opens, and blood is ejected from the LV into the aorta. The LV volume falls during the ejection phase, as blood is expelled from the LV, but pressure continues to rise until it peaks and then starts to fall.

Isovolumic relaxation commences with closure of the aortic valve. Pressure within the LV falls during this phase (but volume remains constant), until the LV pressure falls below the LA pressure. At this point, the pressure difference between LA and LV causes the mitral valve to open and the isovolumic relaxation ends.

Ventricular filling begins as the mitral valve opens and blood flows into the LV from the LA. This phase ends when the mitral valve closes at the start of ventricular systole. Towards the end of the ventricular filling phase, atrial systole (contraction) occurs, coinciding with the P wave on the ECG, and this augments ventricular filling.

As shown in **Figure 2.6**, the pressures within the cardiac chambers vary throughout the cardiac cycle. **Table 2.1** lists the typical pressures found within each chamber. A pressure difference between two chambers causes the valve between them to open or close. For example, when the LA pressure exceeds the LV pressure, the mitral valve opens; and when the LV pressure exceeds the LA pressure, the mitral valve closes.

Table 2.1   Normal intracardiac pressures

	Pressure (mmHg)
Right atrium	Mean 0–5
Right ventricle	Systolic 15–25/Diastolic 0–5
Pulmonary artery	Systolic 15–25/Diastolic 5–12
Left atrium	Mean 5–12
Left ventricle	Systolic 100–140/Diastolic 5–12
Aorta	Systolic 100–140/Diastolic 60–90

Closure of the mitral and tricuspid valves can be heard with a stethoscope as the first heart sound (S_1). Closure of the aortic and pulmonary valves causes the second heart sound (S_2). During expiration, S_2 occurs as a single sound; but during inspiration, the return of venous blood to the right heart makes the pulmonary valve close slightly later than the aortic valve, causing normal physiological splitting of S_2 with the pulmonary component (P_2) occurring just after the aortic component (A_2). The presence of an ASD removes this respiratory variation in S_2, so that the slight gap between A_2 and P_2 is there all the time ('fixed splitting').

Further reading

Anderson RH et al. Anatomic basis of cross-sectional echocardiography. *Heart* (2001). PMID 11359762.

Anderson RH et al. Development of the heart: (2) septation of the atriums and ventricles. *Heart* (2003). PMID 12860885.

Anderson RH et al. Development of the heart: (3) formation of the ventricular outflow tracts, arterial valves, and intrapericardial arterial trunks. *Heart* (2003). PMID 12923046.

Moorman A et al. Development of the heart: (1) formation of the cardiac chambers and arterial trunks. *Heart* (2003). PMID 12807866.

Mori S et al. What is the real cardiac anatomy? *Clinical Anatomy* (2021). PMID 30675928.

CHAPTER 3

Physics and instrumentation

Echocardiography uses ultrasound to examine the structure and function of the heart. A firm understanding of the physics of ultrasound gives the sonographer:

- an understanding of the capabilities and limitations of their echo machine
- the confidence to adjust the machine's controls to optimize the images

ELEMENTARY PHYSICS

Sound travels as a longitudinal mechanical wave, and it can be thought of as a series of vibrating particles in a line. Unlike electromagnetic waves (e.g., light waves, radio waves), sound waves need the presence of particles to be transmitted – sound cannot travel through a vacuum but instead requires a medium such as air, water or a solid. When a sound wave travels through a medium, there are areas of compression (high pressure and density, where the particles are closer together) and rarefaction (low pressure and density, where they are farther apart). Sound can be represented as a sine wave, showing the variation in pressure through the medium (**Figure 3.1**).

The **amplitude** of a sound wave indicates its strength, measured as the difference between the peak pressure in the medium and the average pressure. The unit of measurement is decibels (dB), using a logarithmic scale such that a difference of 6 dB represents a doubling in amplitude. Amplitude can be adjusted by the sonographer by changing the echo machine's power output (transmit power).

The **wavelength** of a sound wave is the distance between two successive waves – we normally measure this between the peak (or trough) of one wave and the identical point on the next wave. Wavelength is measured in appropriate units of length, such as metres (m) or millimetres (mm).

The **frequency** of a sound wave is the number of wave cycles (or oscillations) per second, and this is measured in Hertz (Hz). A sound wave with 100 oscillations per second has a frequency of 100 Hz. For high frequencies, the units of kilohertz (kHz = 10^3 Hz) or megahertz (MHz = 10^6 Hz) can be used.

Audible sound lies in the frequency range of 20–20,000 Hz (20 kHz). Sound with a frequency below 20 Hz is called infrasound, and sound with a frequency greater than 20 kHz is called ultrasound. Ultrasound used for echocardiography usually lies in the frequency range of 1.5–7 MHz.

The **propagation velocity** of a sound wave refers to the speed at which the wave propagates through the medium. This varies from one medium to another, depending on both the density and the stiffness of the medium. Propagation velocities for different body tissues are listed in **Table 3.1**. The average propagation velocity for the heart (and for soft tissues in general) is 1540 m/s.

DOI: 10.1201/9781003304654-3

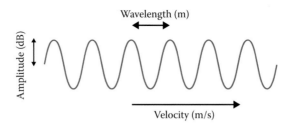

Figure 3.1   An ultrasound wave.

Wavelength, frequency and velocity are linked by the following equation:

$$\text{Propagation velocity} = \text{Frequency} \times \text{Wavelength}$$

For the heart, the propagation velocity of sound waves is fixed at approximately 1540 m/s – this cannot be altered by the sonographer. The sonographer can, however, choose the frequency of the sound waves being transmitted towards the heart. Choosing different frequencies will therefore influence the wavelength of the sound waves as they are transmitted through the heart (and the surrounding tissues). If, for instance, the sonographer was to choose a frequency of just 5 kHz, then the wavelength of the sound waves would be as follows:

$$\text{Wavelength} = \frac{\text{Propagation velocity}}{\text{Frequency}}$$

$$\text{Wavelength} = \frac{1540 \text{ m/s}}{500 \text{ Hz}}$$

$$\text{Wavelength} = 0.308 \text{ m}$$

Such a long wavelength, of just over 30 cm, would give very little spatial resolution and would be of little use for cardiac imaging. The higher the frequency chosen, the shorter the wavelength. As shorter wavelengths provide better resolution (see later), higher frequencies of 1.5–7 MHz are used for echo imaging.

So why not use even higher frequencies and get even better image resolution? One reason is that there is a trade-off between resolution and penetration – the higher the ultrasound frequency, the better the resolution, but the poorer the penetration of the ultrasound into the body. The ultrasound frequencies used for echo offer a good balance between resolution and penetration. Paediatric echo uses higher frequencies (typically 5–10 MHz) than adult echo, as the patient's smaller body size means that less penetration is required. Similarly, in intravascular ultrasound (p. 99), where high resolution but little penetration is required, frequencies of 20–50 MHz are used.

Table 3.1   Propagation velocities in various body tissues

Medium	Speed (m/s)
Air	330
Fat	1,450
Soft tissue (average)	1,540
Blood	1,570
Muscle	1,580
Bone	3,500

ULTRASOUND PROPAGATION

As an ultrasound pulse is transmitted from a transducer into the body, it will encounter a number of different tissues, each of which having a different **acoustic impedance** ('resistance' to ultrasound transmission). These differences in acoustic impedance are particularly important at the boundaries between tissues. When an ultrasound pulse crosses a boundary between two tissues with very different acoustic impedances, a large proportion of the energy within the pulse will be **reflected** back towards the transducer.

This effect is most marked at the boundary between the air and the skin, where almost all of the ultrasound energy will be reflected back to the transducer and less than 1% will enter the body. This would be a major drawback to performing medical ultrasound; thus, to get around this problem, sonographers use gel to bridge the gap between the transducer and the skin. By excluding the air between the transducer and the skin, the gel reduces the impedance mismatch and allows much more of the ultrasound energy to enter the body. Similarly, echo can be challenging in patients with hyperinflated lungs (e.g., emphysema), where views of the heart can be obscured by air-filled lung tissue causing a large impedance mismatch.

As the ultrasound pulse is transmitted through the body, it will meet further boundaries where different degrees of reflection occur. There are two types of reflections (**Figure 3.2**):

● specular reflection
● backscatter

Specular ('mirror-like') reflection occurs at tissue boundaries where the reflector is relatively large (at least two wavelengths in diameter) and smooth – structures such as the heart valves and the walls of the heart chambers and major vessels are examples of specular reflectors. The proportion of ultrasound energy reflected by a specular reflector is highly dependent on the angle of incidence of the incoming ultrasound beam – in order to maximize the amount of energy reflected, the incoming beam should be as perpendicular (i.e., as close to 90°) to the reflector as possible.

Backscatter occurs with small and/or rough-surfaced structures, where the reflected ultrasound will scatter in many different directions. The returning signal will be weaker than that from a specular reflector, but will not be dependent on the angle of incidence of the (incoming) ultrasound beam. An example of a scatter reflector is the tissue within the myocardium. Red blood cells also cause scatter, and as this scatter is equal in all directions. they are referred to as a special group known as **Rayleigh scatterers**.

As an ultrasound pulse travels through tissue, it will gradually lose energy, a process known as **attenuation**. Attenuation results from reflection and backscatter, and also from the absorption of energy by the tissues themselves (where the sound energy is converted into heat). This loss of energy can be quantified in decibels, and in soft tissues a change of −3 dB equates to a fall in signal intensity of 50%. The **half-intensity depth** (HID) is the depth (in cm) in soft tissue in which the intensity

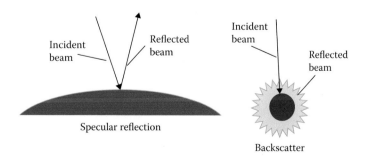

Figure 3.2   Specular reflection and backscatter.

of the ultrasound is reduced by 50%, and it depends upon the frequency (f) of the ultrasound emitted by the transducer, measured in MHz:

$$\text{HID (Soft tissue)} = \frac{6}{f}$$

Thus, the ultrasound emitted by a 4-MHz transducer would lose 50% of its intensity after travelling through just 6/4 = 1.5 cm of soft tissue. Attenuation is therefore greater at higher frequencies.

Refraction is the change in direction of an ultrasound pulse as it passes across a boundary between two tissues (or materials) of different acoustic impedance. Although refraction can be useful (for instance, refraction is used to focus the ultrasound beam with an acoustic lens), it can also be a source of artifact (p. 19).

ULTRASOUND TRANSDUCERS

In transthoracic echo, ultrasound is generated by a transducer (commonly called a probe) which is held on the patient's chest. For other imaging techniques (e.g., transoesophageal echo [TOE], intravascular ultrasound), the transducer may be passed into the oesophagus or even into the heart itself. The transducer is both a transmitter and a receiver – it transmits ultrasound into the chest, and also detects the return of the reflected ultrasound back to the probe.

Ultrasound transducers work using the **piezoelectric effect**. Piezoelectric crystals change shape when an electrical voltage is applied, and so an alternating voltage can make them oscillate rapidly, thereby generating ultrasound. In addition, if the crystals are themselves caused to oscillate by a *returning* ultrasound wave, they *generate* an electrical voltage which can be detected as a signal. Thus, the crystals both generate and detect ultrasound.

Contemporary **phased-array transducers** consist of an array of piezoelectric elements (typically 128 for a 2D echo probe, several thousand for a 3D probe). The ultrasound beam can be 'steered' and focused electronically by altering the timing of activation (or 'phasing') of the individual elements. Older mechanical transducers used a motor within the transducer to move the piezoelectric elements but had limited Doppler capabilities, and were prone to mechanical failure.

The key components of a transducer are shown in **Figure 3.3**. The **piezoelectric elements** are mounted on a **backing layer**, which has high impedance and is designed to absorb ultrasound and

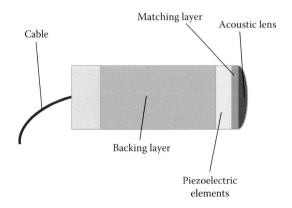

Figure 3.3   Structure of an ultrasound transducer.

'damp down' reverberation ('ringing') of the piezoelectric elements. In front of the elements is a **matching layer**, which improves the impedance matching between the elements and the body.

A transducer will transmit short bursts of ultrasound (lasting just a few microseconds) and then wait for a few hundred microseconds for the reflected ultrasound to return before transmitting the next bursts of ultrasound. A small amount of the ultrasound energy will be reflected back to the transducer each time the ultrasound pulse reaches an interface, and as the transducer detects these returning pulses, it measures the time taken between the pulse being emitted and returning to the transducer ('round trip time'). From this, and from a knowledge of the propagation velocity of ultrasound in soft tissue, the echo machine can calculate the distance between the transducer and the reflector.

The transducer can also determine the intensity of the returning signal, and use this information in building up the image display. Other features of the returning signal, such as its frequency and any frequency shift compared to the transmitted signal, are discussed in relation to Doppler principles in Chapter 4.

The ultrasound beam slightly converges after it leaves the transducer (the **near field** or Fresnel zone), before reaching the **focal point** (where lateral resolution is greatest), and then diverges (the **far field** or Fraunhofer zone). Imaging quality is best within the near field, and maximizing the depth of the near field (i.e., the distance travelled by the ultrasound beam before it diverges) is important for image optimization. The length of the near field is greater at higher transducer frequencies and wider transducer diameters.

Focusing the ultrasound beam does *not* affect the length of the near field, but it does produce a narrower beam (and higher resolution) within the near field, albeit at the expense of making the beam wider in the far field (**Figure 3.4**).

A plastic **acoustic lens** at the front of the transducer helps to focus the ultrasound beam. A phased-array transducer also offers electronic focusing, which allows the sonographer to control the depth at which the ultrasound beam is most tightly focused. Electronic focusing utilizes **transmit focusing** (which adds a time delay to the triggering of the piezoelectric elements, with the outer elements triggering before the central elements) and **dynamic receive focusing** (which introduces electronic delays to the returning signals to compensate for the greater time taken for echoes to return to the outermost elements) to optimize resolution.

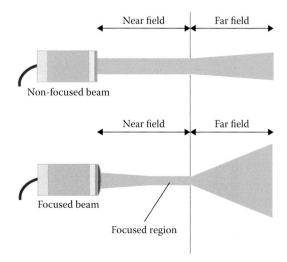

Figure 3.4 Effect of focusing on near and far field.

> **SECOND HARMONIC IMAGING**
>
> The reflected echo signal that returns to the transducer contains not just ultrasound at the original (fundamental) frequency of the transmitted signal, but also harmonics (multiples of the original frequency). These harmonics originate mainly from the central portion of the beam and also from deeper structures. Second harmonic imaging filters the returning signal to remove the fundamental frequency and build up an image using the second harmonic components of the signal. In so doing, the image resolution improves (because of the higher frequency), particularly for far field structures. Disadvantages of second harmonic imaging are that it requires a higher power output, and it does slightly alter the appearance of myocardial texture and also the apparent thickness of structures such as valve leaflets compared with fundamental imaging.

IMAGING MODALITIES

The earliest echo modality was amplitude mode (A-mode) imaging, which simply plotted the amplitude of the reflected ultrasound (as a 'spike' with a certain amplitude) versus the distance of the reflected signal from the transducer. Brightness mode (B-mode) imaging was similar in principle, but rather than plotting the returning signals as a row of spikes of varying sizes, it represented the amplitude of the returning signal by the brightness of a dot. A-mode and B-mode imaging have been superseded by motion mode (M-mode) and 2D imaging.

M-mode imaging

M-mode imaging records motion along a single 'line of sight', selected by careful positioning of the on-screen cursor across a region of interest (**Figure 3.5**). Once the cursor is in place, activation of M-mode imaging produces a scrolling display of movement (along the vertical y-axis), as it occurs along the cursor line, plotted against time (along the horizontal x-axis). A typical M-mode trace for a normal mitral valve is shown in **Figure 3.6**.

The very narrow field of view of M-mode imaging – essentially a single scan line, represented by the on-screen cursor – means that a very high pulse repetition frequency can be used, giving a sampling rate of around 1800 times per second. This is very useful in visualizing rapid motion, such as the movement of valve leaflets, and permits accurate timing of events as well as measurement of cardiac dimensions.

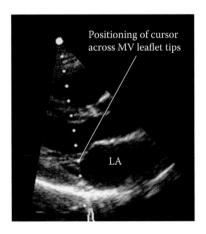

Figure 3.5   Positioning of the cursor for an M-mode study of the mitral valve. *Abbreviations:* LA: Left atrium, MV: Mitral valve.

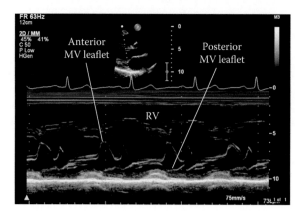

Figure 3.6   M-mode study of the mitral valve. *Abbreviations:* MV: Mitral valve, RV: Right ventricle.

2D imaging

Whereas in M-mode imaging the heart is imaged along just a single scan line, in 2D imaging a picture of the heart is built up from a series of scan lines side by side. In 2D imaging, the ultrasound probe sweeps a beam across the heart around 20–30 times per second, creating a series of scan lines (usually around 120) each time it makes a sweep, in order to build up a 2D image (**Figure 3.7**).

The probe has to transmit and receive an ultrasound pulse for each scan line of the image, and there is, therefore, a limit on how many image 'frames' can be generated each second, determined by the number of scan lines that make up the image (the sector width) and the depth of the image. Reducing the sector width and/or depth will reduce the time taken to generate an image frame, increasing the number of image frames that can be generated each second ('frame rate'). It is, therefore, important to optimize image quality by narrowing down the size of the image sector to cover just the key area of interest.

ECHO MACHINE INSTRUMENTATION

At first sight, the number of controls on an echo machine can appear daunting. In reality, the controls are relatively simple to understand and to use, and it is important to know how to optimize their settings to obtain the best possible image quality. In this section, the controls that affect M-mode and 2D imaging will be discussed. Controls for the spectral and colour Doppler modalities are discussed in Chapter 4.

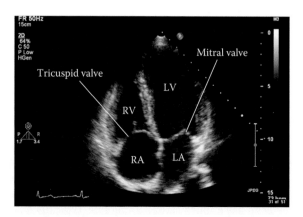

Figure 3.7   Normal 2D echo. *Abbreviations:* LA: Left atrium, LV: Left ventricle, RA: Right atrium, RV: Right ventricle.

Transmit power controls the amount of ultrasound energy delivered to the patient, and to minimize the risk of adverse mechanical or thermal effects, it is important to use the lowest setting possible (p. 20).

Gain refers to the amplification of the received signal to increase the brightness of the displayed images. Gain can be adjusted for the whole image (overall gain) or for part of the image (see time-gain compensation [TGC] below). While a high gain setting can be useful for detecting weaker signals that might otherwise not be visible, it reduces lateral resolution and also increases noise.

Depth setting determines how far the ultrasound beam 'looks' into the patient and is an important determinant of frame rate. The greater the depth setting, the longer the transducer will have to wait for the ultrasound pulse to make its round trip before repeating the pulse, and so the lower the frame rate. Select a depth setting so that the whole area of interest can be seen, but not so deep that it includes irrelevant structures beyond the region of interest.

Sector width determines the field of view across which the ultrasound beam sweeps. As with depth, sector width is an important determinant of frame rate and should be optimized for each view to include the region of interest but no more.

Focus can be fine-tuned with phased-array transducers and should be adjusted for each view so that the beam is focused on the region of interest.

TGC is also known as depth compensation and corrects for the attenuation of the ultrasound signal that occurs with increasing distance from the transducer. TGC boosts the gain of the signals returning from the far field to ensure an even 'echo brightness' across the whole depth of the image. The TGC controls can be fine-tuned by the sonographer using slider bars.

Greyscale compression (dynamic range) adjusts the number of shades of grey that are displayed in the image. This allows the sonographer to choose the degree of contrast in the image.

RESOLUTION

Resolution refers to the ability to discriminate between two objects that are close together in space (spatial resolution) or two events that occur close together in time (temporal resolution). Spatial resolution has two components:

- axial resolution
- lateral resolution

Axial resolution relates to objects that lie along the axis of the ultrasound beam and is mainly determined by transducer frequency (Higher frequency = Better axial resolution) and pulse length (Shorter pulse length = Better axial resolution). Axial resolution is typically around 3 mm.

Lateral resolution, also known as azimuthal resolution, relates to objects that lie side by side, perpendicular to the ultrasound beam, and varies according to how far the objects lie from the transducer. The narrower the beam, the better the lateral resolution. The width of the beam can be optimized by focusing it on the region of interest (see **Figure 3.4**). Lateral resolution is also affected by gain settings – the higher the gain, the worse the lateral resolution. Lateral resolution is typically around 1 mm.

Temporal resolution, or frame rate, is important in trying to distinguish events that occur close together in time. Frame rate depends upon the time taken to collect all the data required to create one image, which in turn depends upon the sector width and depth. M-mode imaging offers very high sampling rates, typically 1800 times per second, because of the very narrow field of view (see above). Two-dimensional echo has a much slower frame rate, typically 40–80 frames per second, because of the much greater amount of ultrasound data that must be collected to create a single frame.

IMAGING ARTIFACTS

Imaging artifacts occur when 'structures' and/or distortions are seen on the echo image that are not actually present in the heart (or, at least, not at the apparent location), or when structures that *are* present seem to be absent on the image.

Acoustic shadowing occurs when a highly echo-reflective structure (e.g., a mechanical replacement valve) blocks ultrasound from penetrating any further, causing echo dropout in the far field. This can pose a particular problem when assessing the structure and function of replacement valves.

Reverberation occurs when ultrasound rebounds several times between two strong specular reflectors before returning to the transducer. The time spent 'rebounding' delays the return of the signal to the transducer, and so the processing software misinterprets the returning signal as having originated farther away than it really has. This leads to 'ghost' images occurring in the far field, which can be recognized because they move in tandem with the structure that caused the reverberation.

Refraction artifact arises when an object is falsely duplicated behind a structure that refracts the ultrasound beam, acting like a lens (hence the alternative name of 'lens artifact'). This causes a double image of the object in question. This form of artifact is most commonly encountered in the parasternal and subcostal windows.

Beam width artifact arises because the ultrasound beam has a finite width (especially in the far field) and the machine is unable to discriminate whether a returning echo signal has arisen from the centre of the beam and/or the edge. Strong reflectors at the edge of the beam are therefore displayed by the echo machine as though they arise from the centre of the beam, 'smearing' the displayed echo. Beam width artifact can be reduced by focusing the ultrasound beam to minimize its diameter.

Side lobe artifact is similar in its mechanism to beam width artifact, but arises from unwanted but unavoidable 'side lobe' beams (which are additional beams surrounding the main ultrasound beam). Signals returning from the side lobe beams are interpreted by the echo machine as having arisen from the central beam, and can be displayed some distance away from the true location of the structure in question.

DISPLAY AND RECORDING METHODS

The returning echo signal at the transducer undergoes a series of initial processing steps which include amplification, TGC and filtering. The video signal is then sent to a scan converter, which converts the signal into a 'rectangular' format suitable for display. The resulting data undergo further processing ('post-processing') and can then be stored in a digital format and/or can undergo digital-to-analogue conversion to create a video signal for display on a monitor (and/or archiving onto videotape). This process occurs so rapidly that the acquired data can be displayed on a monitor almost in 'real time'.

Digital archiving is the contemporary standard for the storage of imaging data, using hard drives or optical discs. The quantity of digital data generated by an echo study can be considerable, so high-volume storage media (and 'lossless' data compression techniques) are required if large numbers of studies are to be archived.

SAFETY OF ULTRASOUND

Ultrasound involves the delivery of external energy to body tissues, and so it is important to consider the potential adverse biological effects that this could entail. The intensity of exposure to ultrasound is expressed as power per unit of area (W/cm^2) expressed as the maximum intensity within the ultrasound beam (the spatial peak) averaged over the duration of exposure (temporal average), the **spatial peak temporal average** (SPTA). There are two main biological effects of exposure to ultrasound energy – thermal (heating) and mechanical (e.g., cavitation).

Thermal effects are caused by conversion of the mechanical energy of the ultrasound into heat energy as it passes through the tissues. The amount of heating is hard to predict but relates to several factors, including transducer frequency, transmit power, focus and depth. Thermal effects are most relevant to TOE where the probe may remain stationary in the oesophagus for long periods, particularly during intraoperative studies. Heat may be generated not just by the ultrasound but also directly by the probe itself. It is prudent to keep imaging time to a minimum and to ensure that the TOE probe is repositioned regularly and to monitor the temperature of the probe.

Mechanical effects include cavitation, in which gas bubbles are created as ultrasound passes through the tissues. It is not thought to be a problem during standard transthoracic studies, but it is important when bubble contrast agents are used as it can cause resonance and even disruption of the bubbles (p. 79). Mechanical effects of ultrasound can also be measured by **mechanical index** (MI), which is the peak negative (rarefactional) pressure divided by the square root of the transducer frequency. An MI of <1 is considered safe.

Although echo has an excellent safety record, it is nevertheless prudent to minimize risk by

- only performing echo for appropriate clinical indications
- keeping the power output as low as possible
- keeping the exposure time to a minimum

M-mode and 2D echo have the lowest ultrasound intensity, and pulsed-wave Doppler has the highest intensity (with colour Doppler having an intermediate value).

Ensuring safety also requires an awareness of more general hazards such as

- risk of electrical shock from damaged or poorly maintained equipment
- risk of injury from trips and falls, particularly when transferring onto the examination couch
- risk of infection from inadequate infection control measures

Echo departments should have appropriate risk assessment tools and protocols in place to minimize risks to patients and staff.

Further reading

Bertrand PB et al. Fact or artifact in two-dimensional echocardiography: avoiding misdiagnosis and missed diagnosis. *Journal of the American Society of Echocardiography* (2016). PMID 26969139.

Edelman SK. *Understanding ultrasound physics*. 4th edition (ESP Ultrasound, 2012).

Gibbs V et al. *Ultrasound physics and technology: how, why and when* (Churchill Livingstone, 2009).

Le HT et al. Imaging artifacts in echocardiography. *Anesthesia and Analgesia* (2016). PMID 26891389.

CHAPTER 4

Doppler physics

Echo can be used to examine not just the heart's anatomical structure but also the flow of blood through the heart. This in turn provides valuable information about valvular function, intracardiac shunts and so forth. The study of the heart's fluid dynamics is made possible by the Doppler principle, discussed in this chapter. Besides allowing the assessment of blood flow, the Doppler principle can also be applied to the study of myocardial mechanics (Tissue Doppler Imaging [TDI]).

DOPPLER PRINCIPLES

The Doppler effect describes how an observer perceives a change in the wavelength or frequency of a sound (or light) wave if the source is moving relative to them. A classic example is that of a moving ambulance sounding its siren – as the ambulance approaches an observer, its siren sounds higher pitched than when it is moving away. **Figure 4.1** shows how sound waves from a source, moving towards observer A, shorten in wavelength (and therefore increase in frequency) in the direction of movement. Observer A would therefore hear a higher pitch, and observer B a lower pitch, than if the source was stationary.

The same phenomenon occurs with ultrasound waves when they are reflected from moving red blood cells. The frequency of the returning ultrasound is increased if the red blood cells are moving towards the ultrasound transducer, or decreased if they are moving away. This change in frequency between the transmitted and returning ultrasound signal is the Doppler shift, from which the velocity (V) of the red blood cells can be calculated:

$$V = \frac{c \times f_d}{2 \times f_t \times Cos\theta}$$

where c is the speed of sound in blood, f_d is the Doppler shift in frequency between transmitted and returning signals, f_t is the frequency of the transmitted signal and θ is the angle between the ultrasound beam and the direction of blood flow.

It follows from this equation that a large angle between the direction of blood flow and the ultrasound beam will lead to an underestimation of flow velocity, and this is particularly marked for angles >20°. For this reason, when undertaking echo Doppler studies, it is important to align the ultrasound beam with the direction of blood flow as closely as possible.

SPECTRAL DOPPLER

When the ultrasound beam returns to the transducer, the difference in frequency between the transmitted and returning beams is compared to calculate the Doppler shift. This is a complex

DOI: 10.1201/9781003304654-4

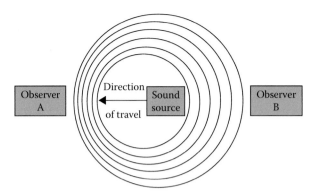

Figure 4.1 The Doppler effect.

process as the returning signal contains a spectrum of frequencies, and a mathematical technique called a fast Fourier transform is used to undertake the necessary spectral analysis.

A spectral Doppler display can then be produced (**Figure 4.2**). These displays conventionally plot frequency shifts (shown as velocities) on the vertical axis against time on the horizontal axis. A zero line is shown, and the flow towards the transducer is plotted above the line (and the flow away from the transducer, as shown in **Figure 4.2**, is plotted below the line). For each time point, the grey pixels show the blood flow velocity detected, and the density of the signal (i.e., the shade of grey plotted at each point in the spectrum) represents the amplitude of the signal at that particular velocity (i.e., the proportion of red blood cells moving at that particular velocity). The overall brightness of the greyscale display can also be adjusted by the sonographer using the Doppler gain setting. Such spectral displays form the basis of continuous wave (CW) and pulsed-wave (PW) Doppler techniques (see **Figure 4.2**).

Spectral (CW and PW) Doppler controls on an echo machine include the following:

- *Transmit power*: this controls the amount of ultrasound energy delivered to the patient
- *Gain*: this amplifies the received signal to increase the brightness of the displayed spectral trace High gain settings amplify weaker signals that might otherwise not be visible, but increase noise
- *Baseline shift*: this shifts the 'zero point' of the display up or down
- *Velocity range*: it alters the vertical velocity scale to a higher or lower range

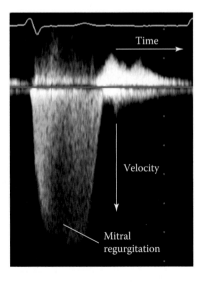

Figure 4.2 Spectral Doppler display (showing mitral regurgitation).

The frequency range seen with Doppler shift (−10 to +10 kHz) falls within the audible range of the human ear, so it is possible to listen the blood flow via the loudspeaker on the echo machine, adjusting the volume as appropriate, and to use the audible 'quality' of the sound to guide fine adjustments in the alignment of the ultrasound beam with the blood flow, in order to obtain the best possible signal.

Continuous wave Doppler

CW Doppler uses *continuous* transmission and receiving of ultrasound (unlike the intermittent pulses used in 2D imaging). Two crystals in the transducer are used – one to transmit an ultrasound signal and the other to receive the returning signal. A dedicated CW Doppler probe ('pencil probe') can also be used; this contains two crystals specifically for performing CW Doppler.

A typical CW Doppler display, obtained by interrogating flow across the mitral valve in the apical 4-chamber view, is shown in **Figure 4.3**. This shows a positive spectral trace above the zero line which corresponds to forward flow across the valve during diastole, and a negative trace below the line corresponding to regurgitant flow during systole. The 2D image/colour Doppler image in the upper part of the figure shows the positioning of the cursor to align the ultrasound beam with the mitral valve flow.

It is important to appreciate that in CW Doppler, the echo machine obtains signals along the *entire length* of the ultrasound beam (or cursor line) – the resulting spectral trace, therefore, reflects the direction and velocity of movement of red blood cells at every point along the beam, and so CW Doppler is unable to assess flow at any one specific point in the heart. The spectral display reflects the full range of red blood cell velocities detected along the beam at any particular time point, usually ranging from zero up to the peak velocity demarcated by the edge of the spectral trace.

Although the inability to discriminate flow velocity at any specific point puts CW Doppler at a disadvantage in comparison to the specific sampling ability of PW Doppler, CW Doppler has the advantage of being able to measure higher velocities without aliasing (see below).

Pulsed-wave Doppler

PW Doppler measures blood flow velocity at a specific location, which the sonographer chooses by placing a **sample volume** (indicated by two parallel lines perpendicular to the main cursor line) at the point of interest (**Figure 4.4**). The length of the sample volume can be adjusted by the sonographer – typically a length of 3 mm is used.

In order to measure Doppler shift (and hence flow velocity) within the boundaries of the sample volume, the transducer cannot use continuous transmission/reception of ultrasound. Instead, the

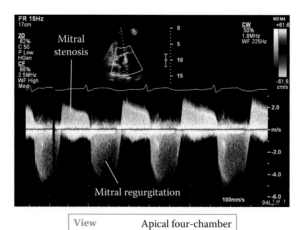

View	Apical four-chamber
Modality	CW Doppler

Figure 4.3   Continuous wave Doppler imaging, showing mitral stenosis and regurgitation.

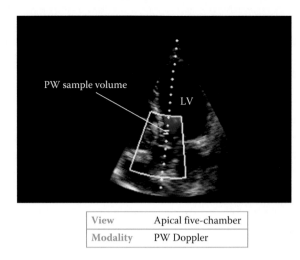

View	Apical five-chamber
Modality	PW Doppler

Figure 4.4   Pulsed-wave (PW) Doppler imaging, showing sample volume. *Abbreviation:* LV: Left ventricle.

transducer transmits an ultrasound pulse and then only samples the reflected signal as it returns from the point of interest – the machine can calculate how long the signal will take to make the return journey between the transducer and the sample volume, and 'listens out' for the returning signal at that time point. In doing so, the machine 'ignores' the returning ultrasound from all other points along the beam.

The fact that the echo machine has to transmit a pulse and then wait for it to return places a limit on how rapidly it can send out consecutive pulses – the **pulse repetition frequency** (PRF). The farther away the sample volume from the transducer, the longer the 'round trip time' of the ultrasound pulse and so the lower the PRF. This gives rise to the phenomenon known as aliasing, which is one of the main limitations to the usefulness of PW Doppler.

An example of a PW Doppler spectral display is shown in **Figure 4.5**, with the sample volume placed in the left ventricular outflow tract (LVOT). Note that a PW Doppler spectral display

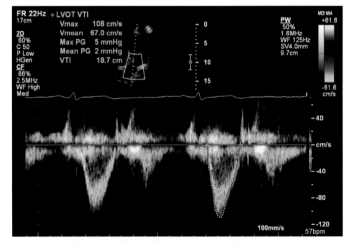

View	Apical five-chamber
Modality	PW Doppler

Figure 4.5   Pulsed-wave Doppler imaging in the left ventricular outflow tract.

ALIASING

The concept of aliasing is traditionally explained in terms of a movie film of a rotating spoked wheel. If the wheel is rotating 30 times per second, and the film is running at 30 frames per second, then every time the wheel is captured (or 'sampled') on a movie frame, it will have made one full rotation and will have returned to the same orientation. When the film is played back, the wheel will look as though it is stationary.

In order to capture the rotation of the wheel, the movie frame rate (or 'sampling rate') needs to be higher – with regard to sampling ultrasound, in order to unambiguously measure wavelength, a waveform must be sampled at least twice in each cycle (**Nyquist's theorem**). This places an upper limit on the Doppler shift that can be measured using PW Doppler (**Nyquist limit**), which equals half the PRF. Once the blood velocity exceeds this limit, the spectral trace will appear with the top of the waveform 'missing' (in fact, transposed to the opposite side of the baseline).

Shifting the baseline can help reduce the problem of aliasing to some extent, but the phenomenon nevertheless places a significant limitation on the maximum velocity that can be assessed with PW Doppler. Aliasing can also be reduced by

- adjusting the Doppler velocity scale (as far as possible)
- sampling at the lowest possible distance from the transducer
- decreasing the transmitted frequency
- increasing the angle of incidence

Ultimately it may prove necessary to switch to CW Doppler instead, where possible. One further alternative is to use high-PRF PW Doppler, in which a higher PRF is used, which means that sampling now occurs at two or more distinct sites along the ultrasound beam but a higher velocity can be measured before aliasing occurs. Careful placement of the sample volumes so that one lies in the region of interest and all the others lie in low-velocity regions means that high-PRF PW Doppler can sometimes be a useful way round the aliasing problem.

typically has a more distinct 'border' to the spectral envelope, with less 'filling in' within the lower-velocity regions of the envelope, compared with CW Doppler. This is because the limited sample volume of PW Doppler means that the red blood cells sampled have a narrower range of velocities than those sampled along the whole length of the ultrasound beam with CW Doppler.

FLUID DYNAMICS

Normal intracardiac blood flow is described as laminar, in which a column of blood flows in parallel (or concentric) streams, each having a uniform flow velocity. Turbulent flow occurs when this breaks down, for instance, when passing through an area of stenosis, causing blood to flow in multiple directions and at different velocities (**Figure 4.6**).

The point at which laminar flow along a vessel becomes turbulent is described by the Reynolds equation, in which turbulent flow is more likely when blood with high density and low viscosity flows at high velocity through a wide-calibre vessel.

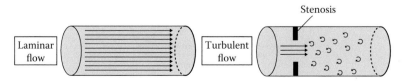

Figure 4.6   Laminar and turbulent flow.

Blood flow is pulsatile, increasing (and then decreasing) in velocity with time during each cardiac cycle. A number of velocity measurements can be made from a spectral Doppler display. The outermost edge of the spectral trace represents the **peak velocity** at any particular time point. The brightest portion of the spectral display represents the velocity of the majority of the red blood cells (**modal velocity**). The average velocity of the red blood cells is expressed as the **mean velocity**.

STROKE DISTANCE AND VOLUME

Measurement of flow volume in a tube, *for a constant flow rate*, can be calculated by simply multiplying the cross-sectional area (CSA) of the tube by the flow velocity. However, blood flow is pulsatile, not constant; so to calculate flow volume (mL per heartbeat), it is necessary to measure both the CSA of the region of interest and the **velocity time integral** (VTI) of flow in that region. VTI is measured by integrating the area under the spectral envelope – this can easily be achieved by tracing the outline of the spectral Doppler envelope and allowing the echo machine software to calculate the VTI. VTI is measured in cm and represents the **stroke distance** – the distance travelled by a column of blood in the region of interest during one flow period (**Figure 4.7**). To measure the CSA, measure the diameter of the region where the spectral Doppler trace was obtained:

$$CSA = 0.785 \times (Diameter)^2$$

Flow volume, in mL per flow period, can now be calculated:

$$Flow\ volume = CSA \times VTI$$

This method is commonly used to calculate **stroke volume** using CSA and VTI measurements taken in the LVOT.

Continuity equation

The law of conservation of mass states that volume flow through the cardiovascular system is constant (assuming that blood is incompressible and that the chamber or vessel carrying the blood is not elastic). Thus, the flow rate in one area is equal to the flow rate in another, assuming a closed circuit (i.e., no loss of blood between the two regions of measurement):

$$Flow\ volume\ in\ region\ A = Flow\ volume\ in\ region\ B$$

$$CSA_A \times VTI_A = CSA_B \times VTI_B$$

This means that if the CSA and VTI can be measured in region A, and the VTI measured in region B, then the CSA of region B can be calculated:

$$CSA_B = CSA_A \times \frac{VTI_A}{VTI_B}$$

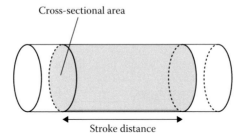

Figure 4.7   Calculation of blood flow volume.

This is the **continuity equation**. If a particular CSA (e.g., the orifice of a stenosed aortic valve) is difficult to measure directly, then the continuity equation can be used to calculate it by measuring the VTI in that area together with the VTI and CSA of a different area (where CSA is easier to measure).

A typical example is the measurement of CSA and VTI (using PW Doppler) in the LVOT, and VTI (using CW Doppler) through the aortic valve (AV), and using these data to calculate aortic valve orifice area:

$$CSA_{AV} = CSA_{LVOT} \times \frac{VTI_{LVOT}}{VTI_{AV}}$$

Pressure gradient

Doppler measurements of blood flow velocity can be used to calculate pressure gradients between two regions, for instance, the pressure gradient between left ventricle (LV) and aorta in aortic stenosis. The relationship between the pressure gradient and velocity is expressed by the Bernoulli equation:

$$\Delta P = 4 \times (V_2^2 - V_1^2)$$

where ΔP is the pressure gradient between the two regions, V_1 is the velocity proximal to the stenosis and V_2 is the velocity distal to the stenosis.

If V_2 is significantly greater than V_1, then V_1 can be ignored and an even simpler version (the simplified Bernoulli equation) can be used:

$$\Delta P = 4 \times V^2$$

where V is the peak velocity of the jet flowing between the two regions. A typical example is the calculation of aortic valve gradient in aortic stenosis – if the peak velocity of flow through the aortic valve is 4 m/s, measured using CW Doppler, then the peak pressure gradient across the valve is as follows:

$$\Delta P = 4 \times V^2$$
$$\Delta P = 4 \times 4^2$$
$$\Delta P = 64 \text{ mmHg}$$

COLOUR DOPPLER

Colour flow mapping, or colour Doppler, is based upon the principle of PW Doppler. However, rather than measuring blood flow at just a single sample volume, in colour Doppler the blood flow is assessed at multiple points within a preselected area. The sonographer chooses the area in which to display the colour Doppler data by overlaying a 'box' on the 2D image. The size and position of this box can be adjusted so that it covers the region of interest (**Figure 4.8**).

A colour Doppler display colour-codes blood flow according to its direction and the *mean* velocity within each sample volume. The flow away from the transducer is traditionally shown as blue, and towards the transducer is shown as red (BART: Blue Away, Red Towards). Turbulent flow, in which there are rapid changes in the flow velocity (high 'variance') in a particular region, is colour-coded green.

At the edge of the display is a velocity scale, correlating the shade of colour with the measured flow velocity. As it is based upon PW Doppler, colour Doppler suffers the same limitation of aliasing and so once the flow exceeds the upper measurable limit, it will be coded in the 'opposite' colour. The

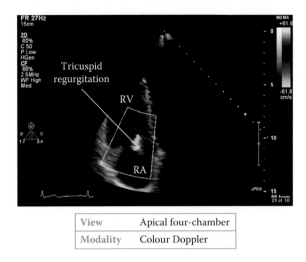

View	Apical four-chamber
Modality	Colour Doppler

Figure 4.8 Colour Doppler imaging, showing tricuspid regurgitation. *Abbreviations:* RA: Right atrium, RV: Right ventricle.

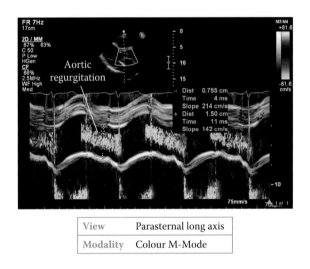

View	Parasternal long axis
Modality	Colour M-Mode

Figure 4.9 Colour Doppler M-mode imaging, showing aortic regurgitation.

numbers at the top and bottom of the velocity scale indicate the maximum velocities towards/away from the transducer that can be measured before aliasing occurs (Nyquist limit). To optimize the image by maximizing frame rates, keep the size of the colour Doppler 'box' as small as possible.

Colour Doppler M-mode

Colour Doppler M-mode uses the same principles as colour Doppler, but instead of overlaying the colour data on a 2D display, it overlays it on an M-mode display (**Figure 4.9**). It can be useful for precisely timing the occurrence of colour jets, and is commonly used for measuring the width of a jet of aortic regurgitation in relation to the diameter of the LVOT (p. 148).

TISSUE DOPPLER IMAGING

For many years, the Doppler techniques described in this chapter were simply used to assess the movement of blood in the heart and great vessels. Although other structures, including the myocardium, move as well, filtering techniques were used to remove the Doppler signals returning from myocardium in order to optimize the signals relating to blood flow.

However, beginning in the 1990s, there was growing interest in Doppler assessment of the myocardium. The Doppler signals returning from the myocardium are distinct from signals from the blood (myocardial motion generates a stronger but lower-velocity signal) and so can be selected with appropriate filtering. The resulting signals can be displayed as spectral PW Doppler traces to assess the motion in specific myocardial regions or as colour Doppler images to visualize myocardial motion more generally.

TDI measures myocardial **velocity**. When measuring myocardial velocity using TDI, it is important to remember that PW TDI measures **peak** myocardial velocity, whereas colour TDI measures **mean** myocardial velocity. Thus, the myocardial velocity values generated from colour Doppler are generally around 25% lower than that from PW Doppler.

The role of TDI in assessing the myocardial mechanics is discussed in more detail in Chapter 5, and the clinical applications of TDI are discussed in Chapter 11.

Further reading

Edelman SK. *Understanding ultrasound physics*. 4th ed. (ESP Ultrasound, 2012).

Gibbs V et al. *Ultrasound physics and technology: how, why and when* (Churchill Livingstone, 2009).

Myocardial mechanics

This chapter considers the essential principles of myocardial mechanics, which can be assessed using the techniques of tissue Doppler imaging (TDI) and speckle tracking. The practical applications of TDI are discussed in more detail in Chapter 11 and of speckle tracking in Chapter 12.

Much of the assessment of the function of the left ventricle (LV) is focused on the quantitative and qualitative evaluation of contractility, through the calculation of global measures of systolic function such as ejection fraction (Chapter 16) and the description of regional wall motion (Chapter 17). Myocardial deformation imaging provides another means for assessing both the global and regional myocardial mechanics.

During systole, the myocardium shortens along the long axis of the LV (longitudinal plane) and also around its circumference (circumferential plane), while simultaneously thickening across the short axis of the LV (radial plane), as shown in **Figure 5.1**. Myocardial deformation imaging lets us quantify this myocardial shortening and thickening through the parameters of myocardial **strain** and **strain rate**.

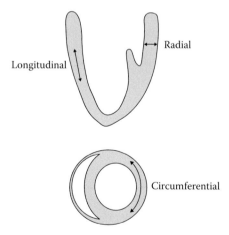

Figure 5.1   Longitudinal, radial and circumferential planes of the left ventricle.

Strain is the deformation produced by stress. Think of pulling on a spring, where the force (stress) you apply to the spring causes it to lengthen (strain). If you can measure this deformation (strain), and the time taken for it to occur (strain rate), then this will tell you something about the force (stress) that caused it.

This same can be applied to the myocardium. If you can measure myocardial strain and strain rate, then this will give you useful information about myocardial contractility. Such measures are less

DOI: 10.1201/9781003304654-5

load-dependent than measures such as ejection fraction, and in some conditions, they offer the prospect of detecting abnormalities of myocardial contractility at an earlier (preclinical) stage in the disease process.

Myocardial strain is simply the percentage change in length of the myocardium. If you imagine a strip of myocardium that is 4 cm long and it then stretches to 5 cm, the change in length is

$$5 - 4 = 1 \text{ cm}$$

Strain is defined as the change in length divided by the original length, multiplied by 100 to express the result as a percentage:

$$\text{Strain} = \frac{\text{Final length} - \text{Original length}}{\text{Original length}} \times 100$$

$$\text{Strain} = \frac{5 - 4}{4} \times 100$$

$$\text{Strain} = \frac{1}{4} \times 100$$

$$\text{Strain} = 0.25 \times 100$$

$$\text{Strain} = 25\%$$

A positive strain represents expansion (lengthening) and a negative strain represents contraction (shortening). For example, if the strip of myocardium starts with a length of 4 cm and contracts to a length of 2 cm, the strain is as follows:

$$\text{Strain} = \frac{\text{Final length} - \text{Original length}}{\text{Original length}} \times 100$$

$$\text{Strain} = \frac{2 - 4}{4} \times 100$$

$$\text{Strain} = \frac{-2}{4} \times 100$$

$$\text{Strain} = -0.5 \times 100$$

$$\text{Strain} = -50\%$$

The use of negative numbers is a common source of confusion, particularly when comparing serial results and trying to decide whether a change from −20% to −30% represents an improvement or a deterioration in strain. It is important to visualize what the numbers represent and to explain in your reports what a result actually means.

Strain rate is how quickly the strain occurs. Average strain rate is calculated by dividing strain by time taken. For example, if the strain of −50% took 2 seconds to occur, then the (average) strain rate is as follows:

$$\text{Average strain rate} = \frac{\text{Strain}}{\text{Time taken}}$$

$$\text{Average strain rate} = \frac{-50}{2}$$

$$\text{Average strain rate} = -25\% \text{ per second}$$

In contrast with strain, strain rate is not dimensionless, and its units are per second.

In principle, these concepts can be applied to any chosen segment of heart muscle and their strain and strain rates calculated. This then allows a detailed analysis of the regional myocardial mechanics within the heart. These descriptors can be derived from either TDI or speckle tracking techniques.

TISSUE DOPPLER IMAGING

As we saw in the previous chapter, Doppler principles can be used to examine movement of the myocardium as well as of blood in the heart and great vessels. TDI uses filtering to select the Doppler signals returning from myocardium and can display these either as spectral pulsed-wave Doppler traces to assess the motion in specific myocardial regions or as colour Doppler images to visualize the myocardial motion more generally.

TDI measures myocardial **velocity**. If the velocities at two points in the myocardium are known, then the difference between these velocities gives a measure of strain rate (i.e., the rate at which these two regions are moving closer together or farther apart). If you want to measure strain itself using TDI, then you need to integrate strain rate over time to obtain a value for strain.

Although widely available, TDI has several limitations in the assessment of myocardial deformation, not least its angle dependency. TDI can only assess the deformation that occurs parallel to the ultrasound beam, and therefore directed towards (or away from) the ultrasound probe. The technique of TDI and its clinical applications are discussed in more detail in Chapter 11.

SPECKLE TRACKING

Strain and strain rate can also be measured using speckle tracking, which is sometimes referred to as 'feature tracking'. On a greyscale echo image of the heart, there is a fixed pattern of speckles within the myocardium. Sophisticated imaging software can follow the position of these speckles from one image frame to the next and can thereby track the movement of a selected region of interest in the myocardium.

Using this information, it is possible to measure the **displacement** of the region of interest over time, and from this information both regional and global myocardial strains can be measured. Speckle tracking offers advantages over TDI for the assessment of myocardial deformation, most notably its independence from the angle of the ultrasound beam. The technique of speckle tracking and its clinical applications are discussed in more detail in Chapter 12.

Further reading

Moharram MA et al. Myocardial tissue characterisation using echocardiographic deformation imaging. *Cardiovascular Ultrasound* (2019). PMID 31730467.

Mor-Avi V et al. Current and evolving echocardiographic techniques for the quantitative evaluation of cardiac mechanics: ASE/EAE consensus statement on methodology and indications endorsed by the Japanese Society of Echocardiography. *European Journal of Echocardiography* (2011). PMID 21385887.

Shah AM et al. Myocardial deformation imaging: current status and future directions. *Circulation* (2012). PMID 22249531.

Waggoner AD et al. Tissue Doppler imaging: a useful echocardiographic method for the cardiac sonographer to assess systolic and diastolic ventricular function. *Journal of the American Society of Echocardiography* (2001). PMID 11734780.

CHAPTER 6

Service provision

In addition to the technicalities of performing and reporting an echo study, there are wider issues to consider in relation to providing an echo service. This chapter looks at service provision in terms of the departmental and staffing issues involved and also examines the question of quality control.

DEPARTMENTAL ISSUES

The British Society of Echocardiography (BSE) sets out standards for departmental accreditation in the UK, which include (but are not limited to) the following:

1. An echo department should have a designated head of department, and there should be a defined medical lead, healthcare scientist lead and quality assurance lead.
2. The department should have agreed indications and minimum standards for echo studies and a system for the review of uncertain studies.
3. Studies should be triaged according to urgency and systems should be in place to alert clinicians to important abnormalities.
4. Studies should be reported on the day they are performed and should be archived for future reference.
5. A database of echo reports should be maintained.
6. Echo rooms should be of adequate size (at least 20 m² if used for inpatient studies).
7. Equipment maintenance must be carried out regularly, with echo machines being replaced (or having a major upgrade) at least every 5 years.
8. A minimum period of 40 minutes should be allowed for routine transthoracic studies and up to 1 hour for complex studies.
9. A patient information leaflet should be available.
10. Chaperones should be available.

STAFFING ISSUES

Training and accreditation

Echo trainees should have at least one protected half-day tutorial session each week and have access to appropriate training materials (books, journals) and echo meetings. Sonographers who undertake and report echo studies unsupervised should have appropriate seniority and accreditation.

Undertaking a recognized accreditation programme provides the sonographer with a structured means of attaining a minimum standard in echo. Although gaining accreditation does not in itself guarantee competence, it nonetheless provides a foundation on which to build one's knowledge and skills. The process of learning about echo does not end with accreditation but must continue to develop with continuing professional education and ongoing experience in performing echo studies, and by seeking reaccreditation at regular intervals.

Several national societies provide accreditation programmes. The BSE offers accreditation in

- adult transthoracic echo (TTE)
- transoesophageal echo (TOE)
- level 1 echo
- critical care echo
- stress echo
- congenital echo

The European Association of Cardiovascular Imaging (EACVI) offers accreditation in

- adult TTE
- adult TOE
- congenital heart disease echo

Further details can be obtained from the relevant society's website: BSE – www.bsecho.org; EACVI – www.escardio.org/Sub-specialty-communities/European-Association-of-Cardiovascular-Imaging-(EACVI).

Workforce requirements

Echocardiography is a high-volume service, with 1.6 million echo studies performed annually in the UK and activity rising by 5.7% per annum. With such heavy demands, there are considerable challenges for providing timely access to echo services. At the end of April 2021, during the COVID-19 pandemic, it was estimated that 37% of patients were waiting more than 6 weeks for an echo in England, and in Northern Ireland more than one third of patients had waited longer than 12 months.

More than 90% of echo studies in the UK are performed by cardiac physiologists, and so there is a pressing need to increase staff recruitment and retention to help meet demands for echo services, and to explore new ways of working that may help to reduce the burden on hard-pressed services.

Echo departments need to pay careful attention to health and safety, particularly regarding musculoskeletal and eye problems, liaising with local occupational health and risk management departments as appropriate. Sonographers should ideally perform no more than 2,000 echo studies per year.

QUALITY ASSURANCE

It should be the aim of every sonographer and every echo department to provide a high-quality echo service. This chapter has already covered the key staffing and departmental issues that have to be addressed in order to lay the foundations of a high-quality service, However, ensuring that all the foundations are in place is only half the story – it's also essential to monitor whether the echo service is performing as well as it should with an ongoing audit assurance programme.

With this in mind, the BSE has set out an Echocardiography Quality Framework (EQF) to form the foundation of a department's quality assurance programme. The EQF focuses on four domains:

- echo quality
- reproducibility and consistency

- education and training
- customer and staff satisfaction

Within each domain, departments are encouraged to gather data to demonstrate how they are applying quality standard and reviewing their performance. For instance, about echo quality, echo teams should be regularly reviewing and improving the quality of their echo images and reports. To this end, there should be quarterly departmental quality review meetings with documented evidence of feedback, quality improvement and reassessment, with evidence that the whole team is engaged in the process.

Assessment of reproducibility and consistency needs to assess the degree of variability between studies (through re-reporting) and audits of performance against established quality standards. Audit is a systematic way of assessing the quality of healthcare and is often described in terms of an 'audit cycle'. The cycle begins with the selection of a topic or 'question' to be looked at (see the box **Audit Topics**). Next, an appropriate 'gold standard' must be chosen, against which the department's performance will be compared (e.g., national standards on the minimum dataset for an echo report). A method of collecting the data is then chosen, and then the necessary data are collected and analysed. The results are then presented and discussed, comparing the department's performance against the agreed standard. Any deficiencies should be identified (while at the same time recognizing areas of good performance) and a mechanism agreed by which improvements can be made. Any changes should then be implemented, and, after an appropriate timescale, the audit cycle should be repeated to see whether the changes have led to the expected improvements.

AUDIT TOPICS

Whatever topic you choose to audit, it's important to have an agreed guideline or standard to compare against. Possible audit topics include:

- appropriateness of echo requests (compared against published appropriateness criteria)
- waiting times for inpatient/outpatient echo studies (compared against your agreed departmental target)
- time taken to issue echo reports (compared against the BSE's recommendation that studies be reported on the day they are performed)
- accuracy of assessment of valvular disease on TTE (compared against TOE findings)
- accuracy of assessment of myocardial ischaemia on stress echo (compared against findings at coronary angiography)

Education and training focuses on the education of all service providers by looking at the implementation of a structured training programme, participation in relevant educational meetings (at a local, regional and national level) and success achieved in training outcomes (such as accreditation).

Customer and staff satisfaction looks at gaining feedback from service users and providers on a regular 'rolling' basis, to identify areas to focus on for service improvement. Feedback can be gained via questionnaires or interviews, and action plans should be drawn up once common themes have been identified and areas of improvement identified.

Further reading

Ingram TE. A patient-centred model to quality assure outputs from an echocardiography department: consensus guidance from the British Society of Echocardiography. *Echo Research & Practice* (2018). PMID 30400064.

Masani N. The Echocardiography Quality Framework: a comprehensive, patient-centred approach to quality assurance and continuous service improvement. *Echo Research & Practice* (2018). PMID 30400065.

NHS England. (2020). https://www.england.nhs.uk/wp-content/uploads/2020/11/diagnostics-recovery-and-renewal-independent-review-of-diagnostic-services-for-nhs-england-2.pdf

Ritzmann S. British Society of Echocardiography departmental accreditation standards 2019 with input from the Intensive Care Society. *Echo Research & Practice* (2020). PMID 32190342.

PART II: CARDIAC IMAGING TECHNIQUES

CHAPTER 7

The standard transthoracic echo study

INDICATIONS FOR TRANSTHORACIC ECHO

The versatility of transthoracic echo (TTE) means that it can play a useful role in a diverse range of clinical situations. The British Society of Echocardiography (BSE) has published guidance on the appropriate clinical indications for TTE (see 'Further Reading'). The American College of Cardiology Foundation has also produced guidance (jointly with a number of other societies). The two sets of guidelines are broadly similar and describe echo as being an appropriate investigation in the assessment of patients with

- symptoms, signs or previous tests that indicate possible structural heart disease
- heart murmurs when associated with symptoms or when structural heart disease is suspected, and the follow-up of those with known significant valvular stenosis or regurgitation
- replacement valves (except asymptomatic patients with mechanical valves or those in whom no further intervention would be undertaken)
- suspected or proven infective endocarditis
- known or suspected ischaemic heart disease (e.g., diagnostic stress echo, assessment following myocardial infarction)
- known or suspected cardiomyopathy
- suspected pericarditis, pericardial effusion, cardiac tamponade or pericardial constriction, and follow-up of patients with known moderate or large pericardial effusions (or small effusions if there has been a clinical change)
- suspected or possible cardiac masses (and follow-up of patients following surgical excision of a cardiac mass)
- pulmonary disease (with cardiac involvement)
- pulmonary hypertension
- thromboembolism
- neurological disorders (with cardiac involvement)
- arrhythmia, palpitations and syncope (with suspected/possible structural heart disease)
- prior cardioversion (unless the patient is on long-term anticoagulants at a therapeutic level and there is no suspicion of structural heart disease)
- hypertension (if left ventricular hypertrophy [LVH]/dysfunction or coarctation of the aorta are suspected)
- aortic disease (e.g., monitoring of aortic root dimensions in Marfan syndrome)

DOI: 10.1201/9781003304654-7

- known or suspected congenital heart disease

Transthoracic echo is also indicated for preoperative assessment in patients awaiting elective or semi-urgent surgery if they have

- known ischaemic heart disease with a reduced functional capacity
- unexplained breathlessness (with an abnormal electrocardiogram and/or chest X-ray)
- a murmur (with suspected structural heart disease or in the presence of cardiac or respiratory symptoms)

It is essential that echo requests contain adequate clinical data both to judge the appropriateness of the request and to allow the sonographer to place the echo findings into an appropriate clinical context (see the box **Sensitivity, Specificity and Bayesian Analysis**). Echo requests must therefore carry appropriate clinical details and contain information about known cardiac diagnoses or previous cardiac interventions/surgery (e.g., replacement valves). Clinicians requesting echo studies should be encouraged to include specific questions with their request (e.g., 'Does this patient have pulmonary hypertension?'), as this provides a clear focus for the echo study and ensures that the sonographer can address the specific concerns of the clinician.

SENSITIVITY, SPECIFICITY AND BAYESIAN ANALYSIS

A perfect diagnostic test would always detect an abnormality when present ('true positive') or rule out an abnormality when absent ('true negative'). However, as with virtually every clinical test, echo has its limitations and can sometimes produce an erroneous result. Detecting an abnormality when in fact none is present is called a 'false positive', and missing an abnormality that is present is a 'false negative'. The terms 'sensitivity' and 'specificity' are often used to describe the accuracy of a test:

- *Sensitivity*: It is the degree to which a test will identify all those who have a particular disease – if 100 people with disease 'X' undergoes a test with 90% sensitivity, the test will detect the disease in 90 of them (but will produce a false negative in 10)
- *Specificity*: It is the degree to which a test will identify all those without a particular disease – if 100 people without disease 'X' undergoes a test with 90% specificity, the test will be normal in 90 of them (but will produce a false positive in 10)

The number of people who receive false positive/negative results is determined not only by the sensitivity and specificity of the test, but also by the population prevalence of the disease in question. Screening a large number of normal individuals for a rare disease using a test with imperfect specificity will produce a relatively large number of false positive results.

The technique of **Bayesian analysis** takes this into account by considering how likely it is that the patient has the disease in question (the pretest probability) in order to predict how likely it is that a positive or negative test result is genuinely positive or negative. In general terms, a positive test result for disease 'X' is more likely to be a true positive if the patient already had a high probability of having disease 'X' before the test was done – it is therefore important to know a patient's full clinical details before performing a test such as an echo in order to judge the likely significance of any abnormalities that you find.

Triage of inpatient echo requests

The BSE has produced a series of posters outlining recommendations on the triage of echo requests in the outpatient setting, in the emergency inpatient and critical care setting and (specifically) for patients with heart valve disease.

These guidelines categorize outpatient referrals into those where echo is **urgent** and needs to be prioritized, those where echo is **indicated** and can be performed routinely and those where echo is

not indicated as it is unlikely to routinely provide useful information. For example, a heart murmur in the presence of class 3 or class 4 heart failure symptoms or syncope requires an urgent echo, whereas an unchanged murmur in an asymptomatic individual with a previous normal echo would be regarded as not indicated.

For those in the emergency inpatient and critical care setting, the guidelines categorize referrals as follows:

- Emergency echo (within 60 minutes)
  - e.g., chest pain with haemodynamic instability
- Urgent echo (within 24 hours)
  - e.g., murmur following a recent myocardial infarction
- Indicated as an inpatient, but not urgent
  - e.g., following confirmed acute myocardial infarction to assess the infarct size, left ventricular function and complications
- Not indicated as an inpatient
  - e.g., evaluation of cardiac chest pain with a normal ECG, no murmur and negative cardiac biomarkers

---

GUIDELINES FOR FOCUSED ECHOCARDIOGRAPHY

In the emergency situation, it is sometimes necessary to perform a focused echo study to rapidly identify serious pathology. Several focused protocols have been developed, including Focused Echocardiography in Emergency Life support (FEEL) and Focused Intensive Care Echocardiography (FICE). The BSE offers accreditation in the rapid bedside echo assessment of the acutely unwell patient, termed Level 1 accreditation. This utilizes a dataset of 17 images to allow the detection (or ruling out) of gross hypovolaemia, severe LV dysfunction, RV dilatation/failure, aortic valve (AV) dysfunction/disruption, mitral valve dysfunction/disruption and abnormal pericardial fluid volume.

Emergency TTE is indicated where a clinician of sufficient seniority suspects

- acute circulatory failure due to life-threatening hypovolaemia
- acute systolic or diastolic heart failure
- acute or severe valve pathology
- acute right heart failure due to pulmonary embolism
- cardiac tamponade

PATIENT PREPARATION

Patients attending for an echo study may feel anxious, not only about having the test itself but also about any abnormalities that it may reveal. To help reduce anxiety, describe the test to patients in clear and reassuring terms – explain to patients why they are having an echo, whether any special preparation is needed before they attend, what happens during the scan and how long it is likely to take. Reassure patients that having an echo is safe and painless. Patients can eat and drink normally before attending for a standard TTE and they can take their medication as usual.

It is good practice to offer patients an information leaflet before they attend (and to make available large-print/Braille and translated versions as appropriate). The patient information leaflet and/or appointment letter can also invite the patient to bring a friend or relative if they wish to have someone accompany them during the echo. If a friend or relative does not accompany the patient when they attend, offer the patient a chaperone in line with hospital policy.

Prior to performing the echo study, gain the patient's verbal consent to having the scan performed. Record the patient's height and weight, as this will allow the indexing of echo measurements. You should also record the patient's heart rate (and rhythm) and blood pressure.

Once you have checked that the patient understands the test that is about to be performed, ask the patient to undress to the waist for the echo study. Always offer patients a gown to wear during the echo. Ask the patient to sit on the echo couch and recline at 45°, rolling on to their left side. The patient should then raise their left arm and place their left hand behind their head. Be sure to check if the patient has any physical limitations that may make it difficult or uncomfortable for them to adopt this position. If so, you may need to adapt the patient's position until they are comfortable. Sonographers who prefer to scan left-handed will also need to adapt the patient's positioning accordingly.

When the patient is in a comfortable position, apply the ECG electrodes and ensure that a clear ECG tracing is visible on the screen of the echo machine. You may need to adjust the electrodes and/or the ECG gain setting to obtain a good trace. Ensure that the correct patient identification and clinical details are entered into the echo machine, and then perform and report the study as described in the sections that follow. At the end of the study, explain to the patient that you will be writing a report which will be sent to the referring clinician.

STANDARD WINDOWS AND VIEWS

The BSE has produced a guidance document, entitled *A practical guideline for performing a comprehensive transthoracic echocardiogram in adults*, which provides a framework for performing a comprehensive transthoracic echo study. This document forms the basis of the approach outlined in this chapter, and identifies *minimum requirements* and *recommendations* (in terms of views and measurements).

A comprehensive echo study should include not only the minimum requirements but also the recommendations, and this is particularly important in individuals who are being scanned for the first time. Moreover, if pathology is found, then additional views/measurements (over and above the minimum requirements and recommendations) may be appropriate. However, it is also acknowledged that some echo studies (for instance, follow-up studies or focused/targeted studies) will not necessarily need to include all of the minimum requirements described here.

There are five TTE windows (**Figure 7.1**), each providing one or more views of the heart. The right parasternal window is optional and can be used when other views are suboptimal or when additional information is needed:

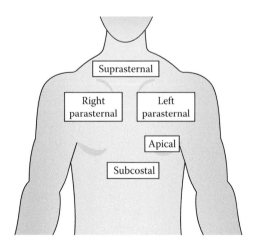

Figure 7.1   Transthoracic echo windows.

- Left parasternal window
  - parasternal long-axis view
  - parasternal right ventricular (RV) inflow view
  - parasternal RV outflow view
  - parasternal short-axis view (AV, base, mid-cavity, apex)
- Right parasternal window
- Apical window
  - apical four-chamber view
  - apical five-chamber view
  - apical two-chamber view
  - apical three-chamber (long-axis) view
  - RV-focused apical view (to assess the right heart)
- Subcostal window
  - subcostal long-axis view
  - subcostal short-axis view
- Suprasternal window
  - aorta view

TIMING OF ECHO MEASUREMENTS

It is important to make echo measurements at an appropriate point in the cardiac cycle, and this will depend upon which structure is being assessed. Most measurements are made at ventricular end-systole and/or at end-diastole, although for some measurements the optimal time may be different (e.g., left ventricular outflow tract [LVOT] diameter, which is optimally made in early to mid-systole when the outflow tract is most circular).

End-systole is defined as the frame where the AV closes and this coincides with a closure 'click' on the Doppler tracing of AV flow. Where the AV is not seen, such as when using the apical two- or four-chamber views, end-systole is taken as the frame prior to mitral valve opening. Other alternatives include the nadir of the volume curve or the global longitudinal strain curve.

End-diastole is defined as the frame before the mitral valve closes. If the mitral valve cannot be seen, alternatives include the frame with the greatest left ventricular cavity size, the start of the QRS complex of the ECG, or the peak of the global longitudinal strain curve.

Left parasternal window

The left parasternal window is located to the left of the sternum, usually in the third or fourth intercostal space, but in some patients you may need to adjust the position to optimize the image by moving the probe up/down a rib space or farther towards/away from the sternum. From the left parasternal window, a number of views can be obtained.

Parasternal long-axis view

The parasternal long-axis (LAX) view is shown in **Figure 7.2**. To obtain the view with the probe in the left parasternal window, rotate the probe so that the probe's 'reference point' (sometimes a 'dot') is pointing towards the patient's right shoulder.

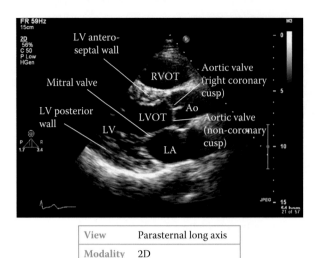

View	Parasternal long axis
Modality	2D

Figure 7.2 *Normal parasternal long-axis view. Abbreviations:* Ao: Aorta, LA: Left atrium, LV: Left ventricle, LVOT: Left ventricular outflow tract, RVOT: Right ventricular outflow tract.

For an optimal view, aim to position the probe so that the view cuts through the centre of the mitral and AVs, without foreshortening the left ventricle (LV) or ascending aorta. In this view, use the following:

- Use 2D to
  - measure the LV cavity size and wall thickness at end-systole and end-diastole
  - assess the LV radial function (thickening and motion of the basal and mid-anteroseptal and inferolateral walls)
  - inspect the appearance of the left atrium (LA) and measure its size at end-systole
  - assess the structure and mobility of the mitral valve
    - in the standard PLAX view, the A2 and P2 segments are visible
    - medial tilt of the probe brings the A3 and P3 segments into view
    - lateral tilt of the probe brings the A1 and P1 segments into view
  - assess the structure and mobility of the AV. The right coronary cusp is seen anteriorly, and either the non-coronary or left coronary cusp is visible posteriorly. The cusps normally have a central closure line – an eccentric closure line suggests bicuspid AV
  - inspect the appearance of the LVOT and measure its diameter in early to mid-systole (as close to the AV annulus as possible)
  - measure the diameter of the right ventricular outflow tract (RVOT) in end-diastole
  - inspect the aortic root and measure its diameter
    - at the sinuses of Valsalva and sinotubular junction in end-diastole
    - at the proximal ascending aorta (1 cm above the sinotubular junction) in end-diastole
    - at the aortic annulus in mid-systole
  - look at the descending aorta as it runs behind the LA – this is a useful landmark for assessing a pericardial/pleural effusion
  - assess the pericardium and check for any pericardial (or pleural) effusion
- For M-mode
  - with the cursor placed at the level of the mitral valve leaflet tips to assess the leaflet motion and measure the mitral valve E point septal separation (the distance between the E point of the anterior mitral leaflet and the septum, p. 155)

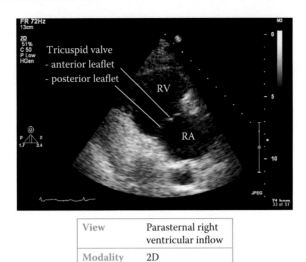

View	Parasternal right ventricular inflow
Modality	2D

Figure 7.3   Normal right ventricular inflow view. *Abbreviations:* RA: Right atrium, RV: Right ventricle.

- Use colour Doppler to
  - assess the AV for stenosis or regurgitation (if regurgitation is present, measure the vena contracta and the width of the jet in relation to the diameter of the LVOT)
  - assess the mitral valve for stenosis or regurgitation (if regurgitation is present, measure the vena contracta)
  - check for flow acceleration in the LVOT in association with septal hypertrophy
  - check the integrity of the interventricular septum (IVS)

Parasternal right ventricular inflow view

This view is obtained from the left parasternal window by tilting the probe inferiorly/medially (towards the patient's right hip). This brings the liver and diaphragm into view, along with the right atrium (RA), tricuspid valve and RV into view (**Figure 7.3**).

- Use 2D to
  - assess the size and function of the RV
  - inspect the structure of the RA. In this view, it may be possible to see the coronary sinus and the inferior and superior venae cavae as they join the RA. There may be a prominent Eustachian valve at the junction with the inferior vena cava (IVC)
  - assess the structure and mobility of the tricuspid valve (the leaflet seen to the right of the image sector is the anterior leaflet; the one to the left may be the septal or posterior leaflet)
- Use colour Doppler to
  - examine tricuspid valve inflow and check for regurgitation
- Use continuous wave (CW) Doppler to
  - assess the tricuspid valve function. If tricuspid regurgitation is present, measure the peak velocity of the regurgitant jet

Parasternal right ventricular outflow view

This view is obtained from the left parasternal window by tilting the probe superiorly/laterally so that it points towards the patient's left shoulder, bringing the RVOT, pulmonary valve and pulmonary artery into view (**Figure 7.4**). It may be possible to see the pulmonary artery bifurcation.

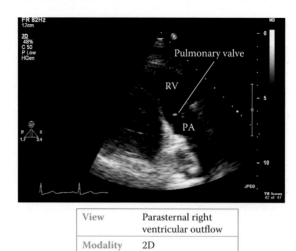

View	Parasternal right ventricular outflow
Modality	2D

Figure 7.4 Normal right ventricular outflow view. *Abbreviations:* PA: Pulmonary artery, RV: Right ventricle.

- Use 2D to
  - assess the structure of the RVOT and main pulmonary artery; check for the presence of thrombus (pulmonary embolus)
  - assess the structure and mobility of the pulmonary valve

Doppler assessments can be made in the parasternal RVOT view as an alternative to the parasternal short-axis (SAX) view:

- Use colour Doppler to
  - examine flow in the RVOT and pulmonary artery and to assess the pulmonary valve for stenosis or regurgitation

It may be possible to detect the abnormal jet of a persistent ductus arteriosus by examining the pulmonary artery with colour Doppler in this view.

- Use PW Doppler to
  - assess the RVOT flow, just below the pulmonary valve cusps, at end-expiration in order to measure the pulmonary acceleration time
- Use CW Doppler to
  - assess the pulmonary stenosis or regurgitation

Parasternal short-axis view

To obtain the parasternal SAX view, keep the probe in the left parasternal window and rotate it so that the 'dot' is pointing towards the patient's left shoulder. There are actually four SAX views, obtained by sweeping the probe along the axis of the heart from the level of the AV down to the apex. The standard SAX views are

- AV level (sometimes called the RV 'outflow' level)
- mitral valve level (also known as the 'base')
- mid-LV level (also known as the 'papillary muscle level')
- apical level

At the **AV level (Figure 7.5)**:

- Use 2D to
  - assess the structure and mobility of the AV; all three cusps should be visible

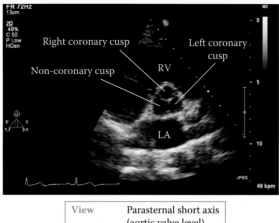

View	Parasternal short axis (aortic valve level)
Modality	2D

Figure 7.5   Normal parasternal short-axis view (at the aortic valve level). *Abbreviations:* LA: Left atrium, RV: Right ventricle.

- assess the structure and mobility of the tricuspid valve (the two leaflets seen are the septal and anterior leaflets)
- assess the structure and mobility of the pulmonary valve
- assess the structure and function of the RVOT
- measure the RVOT diameter at the AV level (known as RVOT1) and at the pulmonary valve annulus level (known as RVOT2) at end-diastole
- assess the morphology of the main pulmonary artery up to its bifurcation and measure its diameter (known as PA1) at end-diastole
- inspect the LA and RA and interatrial septum

You may be able to inspect the origins of the left main stem and right coronary artery arising just above the AV cusps.

- Use colour Doppler to
  - examine the AV for regurgitation
  - check the integrity of the interatrial septum
  - examine tricuspid valve inflow and check for regurgitation
  - examine the pulmonary valve for stenosis or regurgitation

It may be possible to detect the abnormal jet of a ventricular septal defect (VSD) or a persistent ductus arteriosus with colour Doppler in this view.

- Use PW Doppler to
  - assess the flow in the RVOT, just proximal to the pulmonary valve
- Use CW Doppler to
  - assess the pulmonary valve for stenosis or regurgitation. If pulmonary regurgitation is present, assess the pulmonary artery diastolic pressure
  - assess the tricuspid valve function. If tricuspid regurgitation is present, assess the RV systolic pressure

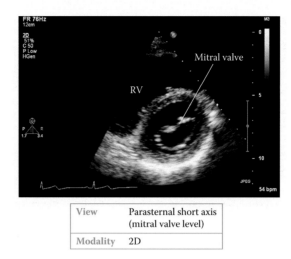

View	Parasternal short axis (mitral valve level)
Modality	2D

Figure 7.6   Normal parasternal short-axis view (at the mitral valve level). *Abbreviation:* RV: Right ventricle.

At the **mitral valve level** (**Figure 7.6**):

● Use 2D to

- inspect the MV leaflets, mitral annulus and subvalvular apparatus. The anterior and posterior leaflets are visible as is the classical mitral valve orifice, which can be planimetered to measure the orifice area
- assess the mobility of the mitral valve leaflets
- assess the LV radial function and look for any regional wall motion abnormalities at the basal level
- assess the RV size and function

● Use colour Doppler to

- examine mitral valve inflow
- check for mitral regurgitation and identify precisely where it occurs in relation to the leaflet scallops
- check the integrity of the IVS

At the **mid-LV level** (**Figure 7.7**):

● Use 2D to

- assess the structure of the posteromedial and anterolateral papillary muscles
- measure the LV wall thickness
- assess the LV radial function and look for any regional wall motion abnormalities at the mid-ventricle level
- measure the RV wall thickness
- assess the RV size and function

● Use colour Doppler to

- check the integrity of the IVS

Finally, sweep the probe down towards the **apical level**.

● Use 2D to

- assess the LV radial function and look for any regional wall motion abnormalities at the apical level
- assess the RV size and function

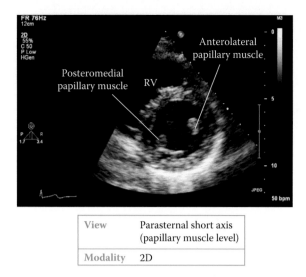

View	Parasternal short axis (papillary muscle level)
Modality	2D

Figure 7.7   Normal parasternal short-axis view (at the mid-LV level). *Abbreviation:* RV: Right ventricle.

- Use colour Doppler to
  - check the integrity of the IVS

Right parasternal window

The right parasternal window is 'optional' but can be useful for assessing the flow in the ascending aorta. With the patient lying on their right-hand side, place the probe to the right of the sternum in the third intercostal space (some adjustment may be required, as with the left parasternal window) and angle the probe downwards and pointing towards the heart. It is a challenging view, but it may be possible to visualize the ascending aorta and assess the colour Doppler within it. This view is most useful for undertaking the CW Doppler assessment of the AV, particularly with a stand-alone pencil probe.

Apical window

The apical window is located at the LV apex. This is normally in the mid-clavicular line and the fifth intercostal space, but may be displaced downwards and to the left if the heart is enlarged. From the apical window, a number of views can be obtained.

Apical four-chamber view

To obtain this view, place the probe in the apical position with the 'dot' pointing towards the patient's left. For an optimal view, aim to position the probe exactly at the apex to avoid distortion or foreshortening of the cardiac structures. The interatrial and interventricular septa should be in line with the probe and lie vertically on the screen (**Figure 7.8**). In this view, use the following:

- Use 2D to
  - measure the RV/LV basal diameter ratio at end-diastole
  - assess the LV radial and longitudinal function, looking carefully for any regional wall motion abnormalities (inferoseptal and anterolateral wall)
  - measure the LV cavity size at end-diastole and end-systole
  - measure the global longitudinal strain where image quality permits
  - assess the structure and mobility of the mitral valve – in this view, the P1, A2 and A3 segments are visible
  - inspect the appearance of the LA and measure its dimensions at end-systole

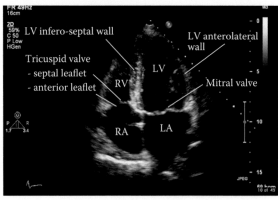

View	Apical four-chamber
Modality	2D

Figure 7.8   Normal apical four-chamber view. *Abbreviations:* LA: Left atrium, LV: Left ventricle, RA: Right atrium, RV: Right ventricle.

- ○ assess the atrial septal mobility
- ○ assess the pericardium and check for any pericardial (or pleural) effusion
- ● For M-mode
  - ○ with the cursor placed at the lateral tricuspid annulus to measure tricuspid annular plane systolic excursion (TAPSE)
  - ○ with the cursor placed at the lateral mitral annulus to measure mitral annular plane systolic excursion (MAPSE)
- ● Use colour Doppler to
  - ○ assess the mitral valve for stenosis or regurgitation
  - ○ assess the flow in the pulmonary veins (the right upper pulmonary vein is usually the easiest to locate)
  - ○ check the integrity of the interatrial and ventricular septa
- ● Use PW Doppler to
  - ○ assess the LV inflow at the level of the mitral valve tips
  - ○ assess the RV inflow at the level of the tricuspid valve tips
  - ○ assess the flow in the pulmonary veins
- ● Use CW Doppler to
  - ○ assess the mitral stenosis or regurgitation
  - ○ check if the mitral regurgitation is present, and then assess the LV systolic function by measuring dP/dt (p. 118)
- ● Use tissue Doppler imaging to
  - ○ assess the LV diastolic function at end-expiration
  - ○ measure the RV S' in systole

It should be noted that 3D assessment of the LV volumes and LV ejection fraction is superior to the 2D assessment, and is recommended in all cases where image quality permits.

Apical five-chamber view

From the apical four-chamber view, maintain the same window but angle the probe anteriorly so that the AV and aortic root (the 'fifth chamber') come into view (**Figure 7.9**). This view is used

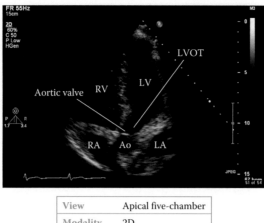

View	Apical five-chamber
Modality	2D

Figure 7.9   Normal apical five-chamber view. *Abbreviations:* Ao: Aorta, LA: Left atrium, LV: Left ventricle, LVOT: Left ventricular outflow tract, RA: Right atrium, RV: Right ventricle.

principally to assess the LVOT and AV, and it is important to align these with the ultrasound beam so that reliable Doppler traces can be obtained.

- Use 2D to
  - inspect the LVOT (any signs of asymmetrical hypertrophy?)
  - assess the structure and mobility of the AV
- Use colour Doppler to
  - check for flow acceleration in the LVOT in association with septal hypertrophy
  - assess the AV for regurgitation
  - check for a perimembranous VSD
- Use PW Doppler to
  - assess the flow in the LVOT
- Use CW Doppler to
  - assess the aortic stenosis or regurgitation
  - assess any subvalvular or supravalvular obstruction

Apical two-chamber view

Return to the apical four-chamber view and maintain the same window but rotate the probe about 60° anticlockwise so that the 'dot' points approximately towards the patient's left shoulder. Stop rotating the probe before the LVOT comes into view and ensure that the mitral valve is centred in the image (**Figure 7.10**).

- Use 2D to
  - assess the LV radial and longitudinal function, looking carefully for any regional wall motion abnormalities (anterior and inferior wall)
  - measure the LV cavity size at end-diastole and end-systole
  - measure the global longitudinal strain where image quality permits
  - assess the structure and mobility of the mitral valve – in this view, the P1, A2 and P3 segments are visible
  - inspect the appearance of the LA and measure its dimensions at end-systole (the LA appendage may be visible as a small 'pocket' to the right of the mitral valve, and the coronary sinus may be visible as a circular structure to the left of the mitral valve)

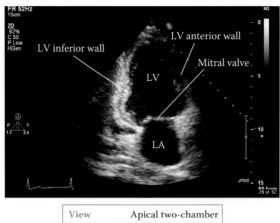

View	Apical two-chamber
Modality	2D

Figure 7.10   Transthoracic echo windows.

- Use colour Doppler to
  - assess the mitral valve for stenosis or regurgitation
- Use PW Doppler to
  - assess the LV inflow at the level of the mitral valve tips
- Use CW Doppler to
  - assess the mitral stenosis or regurgitation

Apical three-chamber (long-axis) view

From the apical two-chamber view, maintain the same window but rotate the probe a further 60° anticlockwise so that the 'dot' now points approximately towards the patient's right shoulder. Stop rotating the probe once the LVOT comes into view and ensure that the mitral and AV s are centred and not foreshortened (**Figure 7.11**). This view is the apical equivalent of the parasternal LAX view.

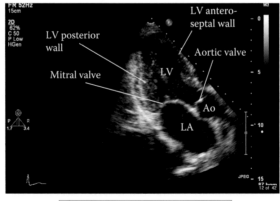

View	Apical three-chamber
Modality	2D

Figure 7.11   Normal apical three-chamber view. *Abbreviations:* Ao: Aorta, LA: Left atrium, LV: Left ventricle.

- Use 2D to
  - assess the LV radial and longitudinal function, looking carefully for any regional wall motion abnormalities (anteroseptal and inferolateral wall)
  - measure the global longitudinal strain where image quality permits
  - assess the appearance of the LVOT (any signs of asymmetrical hypertrophy?)
  - assess the structure and mobility of the AV
  - assess the structure and mobility of the mitral valve – in this view, the A2 and P2 segments are visible
  - inspect the appearance of the LA
- Use colour Doppler to
  - assess the mitral valve for stenosis or regurgitation
  - assess the AV for regurgitation
  - check for flow acceleration in the LVOT in association with septal hypertrophy
- Use PW Doppler to
  - assess the flow in the LVOT
- Use CW Doppler to
  - assess the aortic stenosis or regurgitation
  - assess any subvalvular or supravalvular obstruction

RV-focused apical view

To obtain an optimal view of the right heart, it is best to slightly adjust the standard apical four-chamber view to centre the right heart on the screen and to ensure that there is no foreshortening (**Figure 22.3**, p. 175). This is known as the 'RV-focused' or 'modified' apical view. Ensure that the LVOT is not seen. In this view, use the following:

- Use 2D to
  - measure the RV dimensions at end-diastole:
    - basal RV diameter (known as RVD1)
    - mid-RV diameter (RVD2)
    - RV length (RVD3)
  - assess the RV systolic function by measuring RV fractional area change
  - undertake the RV 3D volume and strain analysis, where available

Subcostal window

The subcostal window is obtained with the patient lying supine with their arms by their sides. It is important that the abdominal wall is relaxed, and asking the patient to lie with their knees bent can help this. Place the probe just below the xiphisternum and angle it up towards the heart, with the 'dot' to the patient's left. From the subcostal window, a number of views can be obtained.

Subcostal long-axis view

To optimize this view, ensure that the interatrial septum is perpendicular to the ultrasound beam (i.e., lies horizontally across the screen) with no foreshortening of the chambers (**Figure 7.12**).

- Use 2D to
  - assess the RV dimensions and function
  - assess the RA dimensions
  - assess the LV dimensions and function
  - assess the LA dimensions
  - assess the structure of the interatrial septum
  - assess the pericardium and check for any pericardial effusion

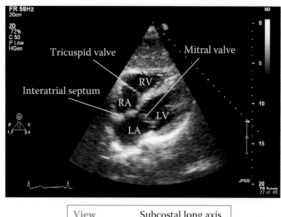

View	Subcostal long axis
Modality	2D

Figure 7.12   Normal subcostal long-axis view. *Abbreviations:* LA: Left atrium, LV: Left ventricle, RA: Right atrium, RV: Right ventricle.

- Use colour Doppler to
  - check the integrity of interatrial and interventricular septa
- Use CW and PW Doppler to
  - assess the flow across any septal defect

Subcostal short-axis view

Keeping the probe in the subcostal window, rotate the probe 90° to obtain a SAX view (**Figure 7.13**).

- Use 2D to
  - measure the IVC diameter at end-expiration
  - assess the IVS respiratory variation during a sharp 'sniff'
  - assess the hepatic veins (congested?)

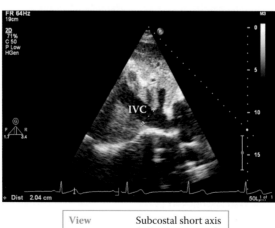

View	Subcostal short axis (inferior vena cava)
Modality	2D

Figure 7.13   Normal subcostal short-axis (inferior vena cava [IVC]) view.

- Optionally, you can also use 2D to
  - inspect the AV
  - inspect the interatrial septum
  - inspect the tricuspid valve
  - inspect the RVOT
  - inspect the pulmonary valve
  - inspect the pulmonary arteries
  - inspect the abdominal aorta (modified view).
- Use M-mode to
  - assess the IVC dimensions (check for respiratory variation by taking measurements in inspiration and expiration)
- Use colour Doppler to
  - assess the flow in the IVC and hepatic veins
  - check the integrity of the interatrial septum
- Optionally, you can use PW Doppler to
  - assess the flow in the hepatic veins
  - assess the flow in the descending aorta

Suprasternal window

The suprasternal window is located in the suprasternal notch. Ask the patient to lie supine and to raise their chin. Place the probe in the notch and angle it downwards into the chest. Be mindful that some patients find this uncomfortable. This view shows the aortic arch in LAX (**Figure 7.14**). A similar view can, if needed, be obtained from the right supraclavicular position.

Aorta view

- Use 2D to assess the appearances and dimensions of the aortic arch.
- Use colour Doppler to assess the flow in the aorta, looking in particular for evidence of coarctation or persistent ductus arteriosus.
- Use CW Doppler to assess the flow in the descending aorta in the presence of a coarctation (it may be better to use a non-imaging 'pencil' probe if alignment is difficult using an imaging probe).

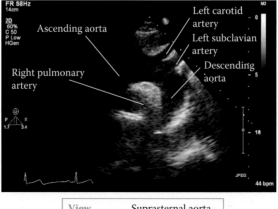

View	Suprasternal aorta
Modality	2D

Figure 7.14   Normal suprasternal aorta view.

THE TRANSTHORACIC ECHO REPORT

Once you've completed the echo study, ensure that the report is written up on the same day. Structure your echo report clearly and systematically, ensuring it contains

- patient's identifying and demographic information
- detailed findings
- study summary

Patient's identifying and demographic information

It is essential that the report contains adequate information to allow correct identification of the patient. Begin the report with the patient's name and a unique identifier (in the UK, this would be the patient's National Health Service [NHS] number). State the patient's age (or date of birth) and gender. The report must also identify the referring clinician and the sonographer and state the indication for the echo request and the date on which the study was performed.

It may also be appropriate to include the patient's location (e.g., outpatient or name of ward), where the study was performed (e.g., echo department, coronary care unit), when the echo was requested and whether it was performed as an emergency/urgent/routine study.

The report should include details of the patient's height, weight, heart rate and blood pressure (e.g., for indexing measurements to height or body surface area).

Detailed findings

The main body of your echo report should contain systematic descriptions of each of the main cardiac structures (chambers, valves, great vessels and pericardium). For each structure, you need to describe its appearance and also its function, grading any abnormalities as mild, moderate or severe where possible (and supporting these statements with measurements where appropriate).

It is usually easiest to set out your study findings by anatomical structure (e.g., mitral valve, LV, etc.) rather than by echo window or modality (which can make the report confusing and repetitive). You can simply describe the findings relating to each anatomical structure in turn, or you may prefer to adapt the list of findings so that the most significant abnormalities appear at the start. Any relevant measurements (M-mode, 2D and Doppler) and calculations can be included in the descriptive text of each anatomical structure, or if you prefer as a separate section.

It is important to use standardized terminology in your report to minimize variability between studies performed at different times and by different sonographers. The ASE reporting guidelines contain tables of recommended descriptive terms and diagnostic statements and it can be very helpful to use these guidelines as a reference when writing up your study findings.

Study summary

In the study summary, sum up the key findings of the echo study and place the findings in a clinical context with particular reference to the clinical question(s) posed by the referring clinician. The summary should not contain any information about the study that hasn't already been included in the detailed technical report, but it can include reference to previous studies performed on the same patient where a comparison is useful. Mention any technical limitations of the study (such as suboptimal imaging windows), and if any structures could not be adequately assessed, this must be highlighted so that the referring clinician can consider alternative imaging as necessary. Clinical advice should not normally be offered in the study summary.

Further reading

ACCF/ASE/AHA/ASNC/HFSA/HRS/SCAI/SCCM/SCCT/SCMR. Appropriate use criteria for echocardiography. *Journal of the American Society of Echocardiography* (2011). PMID 21338862.

Hindocha R et al. A minimum dataset for a Level 1 echocardiogram: a guideline protocol from the British Society of Echocardiography. *Echo Research and Practice* (2020). PMCID PMC7354713.

Mitchell C et al. Guidelines for performing a comprehensive transthoracic echocardiographic examination in adults: recommendations from the American Society of Echocardiography. *Journal of the American Society of Echocardiography* (2019). PMID 30282592.

Robinson S et al. A practical guideline for performing a comprehensive transthoracic echocardiogram in adults: the British Society of Echocardiography minimum dataset. *Echo Research and Practice* (2020). PMID 33112828.

Steeds RP et al. EACVI appropriateness criteria for the use of transthoracic echocardiography in adults: a report of literature and current practice review. *European Heart Journal – Cardiovascular Imaging* (2017). PMID 28329307.

The British Society of Echocardiography (www.bsecho.org) has published several useful documents relating to TTE:

- Clinical indications for echocardiography
- Clinical indications and triage of echocardiography:
    - Out-patient requests (excluding the follow-up of established valve disease)
    - Heart valve disease
    - Emergency inpatient and critical care
- Chaperones and echocardiography

The ASE has published Recommendations for a Standardized Report for Adult Transthoracic Echocardiography, which is available on its website (www.asecho.org).

CHAPTER 8

Transoesophageal echo

It is beyond the scope of this book to provide a comprehensive overview of transoesophageal echo (TOE), but for anyone performing transthoracic echo (TTE), it is important to know how it fits into the cardiac imaging armamentarium.

INDICATIONS FOR TRANSOESOPHAGEAL ECHO

The key difference between TTE and TOE is that for a TOE study, the echo probe views the heart from within the patient's oesophagus rather than via the chest wall (**Figure 8.1**). The advantage of this is that it allows for superior image quality – the proximity of the probe to the heart means that the ultrasound does not need to penetrate so deeply, and so higher ultrasound frequencies can be used (giving higher image resolution). The fact that the TOE probe lies behind the back of the heart also means that certain structures – such as the left atrial (LA) appendage and pulmonary veins – can be seen more clearly than with a transthoracic study.

The superior image quality of TOE means that it's generally indicated in situations where TTE is unable to deliver the image quality required to make a diagnosis. The commonest indications for a TOE study include the assessment of:

- cardiac source of emboli
- atrial fibrillation/flutter, to judge the thromboembolic risk (and thus guide decisions on antico-agulation and cardioversion)
- suspected or proven infective endocarditis
- regurgitant heart valves, to judge the suitability for surgical repair
- replacement heart valves (especially those in the mitral position)
- cardiac masses
- aortic diseases (e.g., aortic dissection/trauma)
- congenital heart disease and intracardiac shunts, e.g., atrial septal defect (ASD), patent foramen ovale (PFO)

TOE plays a major role in the cardiothoracic intraoperative setting, particularly in relation to valve repair and replacement, and also in the cardiac catheter laboratory for guiding certain interventional procedures (such as device closure of ASD or PFO, or during transcatheter aortic valve implantation). TOE is also useful in the intensive care unit, where the image quality of TTE is often limited in ventilated patients, and being a diagnostic tool, it can also help in haemodynamic monitoring.

DOI: 10.1201/9781003304654-8

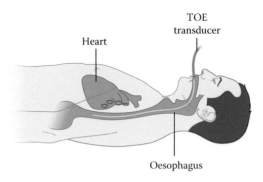

Figure 8.1   Transoesophageal echo (TOE).

CONTRAINDICATIONS TO A TOE STUDY

Any history of difficulty in swallowing should be investigated before a TOE study can be considered. A TOE study is contraindicated by

- patient refusal
- cervical spine instability
- any abnormality posing a risk of oesophageal or gastric perforation, e.g., oesophageal obstruction (e.g., stricture, tumour), oesophageal trauma, oesophageal fistula or diverticulum

Relative contraindications include the presence of clotting disorders, large hiatus hernia (apposition of the probe to the oesophageal wall can be difficult), oesophageal varices or upper gastrointestinal haemorrhage.

PATIENT PREPARATION

The British Society of Echocardiography (BSE) provides very helpful guidance on patient preparation for TOE (see 'Further Reading'). As with any investigation, patients should receive a clear explanation of what a TOE study entails and be offered an information leaflet (ideally at least 24 hours prior to the procedure). Inform the patient that a TOE study involves passing a probe into the oesophagus, in a similar manner to having an endoscopy for stomach ulcers, in order to obtain clear ultrasound pictures of the heart.

Inform the patient about the need for local anaesthetic throat spray and discuss with the patient whether or not conscious sedation is to be used (and the consequent need for an escort as appropriate). Conscious sedation is *optional* – the use of conscious sedation can improve tolerability of the TOE procedure, but does prolong the subsequent recovery period and carries a risk of side effects. Discuss the risks of the procedure. TOE is regarded as a low-risk procedure, but complications can occur and these include

- oropharyngeal trauma (e.g., chipped tooth, pharyngeal laceration)
- oesophageal trauma (e.g., laceration, perforation)
- laryngeal trauma (e.g., tracheal intubation, laryngospasm)
- gastric trauma (e.g., laceration, perforation)
- arrhythmias
- risks associated with sedation (e.g., respiratory depression)

The overall risk of a major TOE-related complication is reported as being 0.2%–0.5%. It has however been suggested that this is an underestimate, as many of the complications present a day or more after the procedure. The risk of death associated with TOE is estimated to be less than 1 in 10,000.

Ensure the patient is aware of the need to be nil by mouth on the day of the procedure, having nothing to eat for 6 hours (with clear liquids permitted up to 2 hours) prior to the test. In view of the need to be nil by mouth, patients with diabetes mellitus should receive appropriate advice about any adjustments that may be needed to their medication to avoid hypoglycaemia.

THE TRANSOESOPHAGEAL ECHO PROBE

The earliest TOE probes were **monoplane** probes, in which the echo transducer was fixed in a single plane at the end of the probe. To obtain views of different planes through the heart, the probe had to be advanced/withdrawn and/or rotated within the oesophagus, and the tip of the probe could be flexed to different angles. Nevertheless, monoplane probes could be challenging to use. The next generation were **biplane** probes, in which a second transducer, perpendicular to the first, was added to the tip of the probe. This allowed imaging in two planes at 90° to each other and made it easier to get certain views.

Multiplane TOE probes contain a transducer at the tip of the probe that can be rotated through an angle of 180° (using a control situated in the handle of the probe). Rotating the transducer changes the angle of the imaging plane so that a 'cut' through the heart can be obtained in just about any plane. Combining this with the ability to advance/withdraw the probe up and down the oesophagus (and stomach), to rotate the probe to the left or right and to flex the tip of the probe to the left/right and anteriorly/posteriorly, means that a comprehensive study can be undertaken utilizing a wide range of imaging planes.

> ### TOE PROBE DECONTAMINATION
>
> Data on the risk of cross-infection during a TOE study are lacking, but it is likely to be similar to the reported risk for upper gastrointestinal endoscopy (1 per 1.8 million studies). TOE probes do not need to be sterile, as they do not penetrate sterile areas of the body, but they do require decontamination between uses. This necessitates effective cleaning and disinfection. The TOE probe is a delicate instrument and care must be taken to maintain its integrity during the decontamination process, and to ensure that the manufacturer's warranty is not invalidated. It is also important, of course, to maintain the safety and welfare of staff undertaking the decontamination. The BSE has published detailed guidance on TOE probe decontamination (see 'Further Reading').

PERFORMING THE TRANSOESOPHAGEAL ECHO STUDY

A standard diagnostic TOE study is usually performed by a team of staff led by a primary operator who has overall responsibility for the procedure. The primary operator should hold appropriate accreditation (or equivalent) in TOE and be able to provide advanced life support (ALS). If the primary operator is a sonographer, a senior clinician should be available to provide immediate assistance if required.

The primary operator should be assisted by a second medically trained individual (a 'monitor') whose role is to monitor the patient throughout the procedure and to manage the patient's airway. The monitor should be trained in resuscitation to at least the level of immediate life support (ILS). It is also desirable for the primary operator to be supported by a second operator whose role is to control the echo machine, optimizing and acquiring the images.

The study is performed in a room containing a couch (with the facility for head-down tilt) for the patient, an echo machine and a TOE probe (with facilities for cleaning/disinfecting the probe between studies), a supply of oxygen, suction apparatus, a pulse oximeter, blood pressure monitoring, appropriate drugs for the procedure, a fully equipped resuscitation trolley, and an emergency alarm call and telephone for summoning help if required.

Prior to undertaking the TOE study, ensure that the patient confirms their identity and that they understand what is planned, and that they have completed a consent form. Review the patient's history and prior investigation findings.

The use of a written checklist is recommended, and the BSE has published a suggested safety checklist for this purpose (see 'Further Reading'). Specifically enquire about

- drug allergies
- previous problems with sedation
- relative contraindications
- whether the patient has fasted for the required period

Obtain intravenous access using a flexible cannula (not a butterfly needle). Attach the ECG electrodes of the echo machine and use these to monitor the patient's heart rate and rhythm during the study. Use an automated cuff to check blood pressure at regular intervals, and monitor arterial oxygen saturations continuously using pulse oximetry, providing the patient with inspired oxygen via nasal cannulae as appropriate. Oxygen should be available to all patients receiving intravenous sedation (usually 2 L/min), with caution in patients with chronic obstructive pulmonary disease who may be at risk of carbon dioxide retention. Oxygen should also be given to patients with significant comorbidities or to those aged >60 years who have not been given conscious sedation. Ensure medication (sedation/reversal agent) is available as appropriate, and check that the TOE probe is clean and ready to use. Check for (and remove) dentures.

Immediately before commencing the procedure, all team members should confirm their name and role and verbally confirm the patient and procedure. Any anticipated difficulties need to be flagged up at this stage: The TOE operator should highlight any sedation or patient issues, and the sonographer and nursing team should highlight any equipment issues.

Administer local anaesthetic throat spray and allow up to 5 minutes for it to take full effect. Before giving sedation (where necessary), ask the patient to lie on the couch on their left-hand side, facing towards the sonographer. Before giving sedation, check that appropriate transport/escort arrangements are in place for the patient's discharge after the procedure.

Sedation must be administered only by individuals who have had appropriate instruction and training. The most commonly used drug for providing conscious sedation is midazolam, administered intravenously in doses of 1 mg at a time allowing sufficient time (sometimes 3 minutes or more) between doses to assess the effect. Elderly patients, or those with significant comorbidities, may require doses of just 0.5 mg at a time. A total dose of 2 mg is commonly required (1 mg in those aged over 65 years), and it is unusual to require more than 5 mg.

The effects of midazolam can be reversed with flumazenil (which must be available for immediate use in case of respiratory depression). If required, an initial intravenous dose of 200 µg of flumazenil is given over 15 seconds, followed by further 100 µg doses every 60 seconds as required. Usually 300–600 µg are required, up to a maximum total dose of 1 mg. Bear in mind that flumazenil is shorter-acting than midazolam (which typically lasts for 20–80 minutes, albeit with individual variability), so the patient's conscious level may fall again later.

CONSCIOUS SEDATION

Where sedation is given, the aim is to achieve **conscious** sedation – the patient should still be able to respond to verbal instructions (such as 'open your eyes') from the primary operator. Oversedation to the point of unconsciousness carries a significant risk of complicamtions for the patient (and litigation for the primary operator!). If a patient can no longer maintain verbal responsiveness, they require the same level of care as someone who has had a general anaesthetic. Seek urgent support from an anaesthetist in that situation. Anaesthetic assistance should also be considered if a patient's oxygen saturations drop below 90% with no improvement after flumazenil.

When you are ready to begin the study, place a bite guard in the patient's mouth and flex their neck slightly, with the chin towards the chest. Flex the tip of the TOE probe and apply gel for lubrication. Next, pass the tip of the probe into the patient's mouth and, gently advancing it, ask the patient to swallow. Once the probe has passed round the back of the throat, start to straighten the tip of the probe and gently advance it to mid-oesophagus level, usually 30–40 cm (distances are marked along the side of the probe). **Never advance the probe against resistance.** When the patient has become used to the probe (some retching is common initially), commence the study while keeping a careful watch on their pulse, blood pressure and oxygen saturations.

THE 'STANDARD' TRANSOESOPHAGEAL ECHO STUDY

There is no fixed 'routine' to performing a TOE study and many operators will begin a study by assessing the most relevant pathology first. This is because the study may need to be cut short if the patient is unable to tolerate it or if there are arrhythmias and/or haemodynamic instability. Once the main aim of the study has been addressed, move on to look at the rest of the heart in a systematic manner, being sure not to overlook any coexistent pathology.

Mid-oesophageal views

With the probe in mid-oesophagus, a wide range of views can be obtained. Starting with the transducer at an angle of 40° (all angles quoted are approximate), the aortic valve is seen in short axis together with surrounding structures (**Figure 8.2**). Rotating a little farther to 60° brings the pulmonary and tricuspid valves into view, and then further rotation to 130° provides a long-axis view of the left heart with clear views of both the aortic and mitral valves (**Figure 8.3**).

Centring the image on the mitral valve, rotation of the transducer back to 90° provides a two-chamber view of the left heart (usually including a good view of the LA appendage), and rotating farther back to 60° reveals a bicommissural view of the mitral valve. Returning to a transducer angle of 90° and rotating the probe towards the patient's right produces the bicaval view, showing

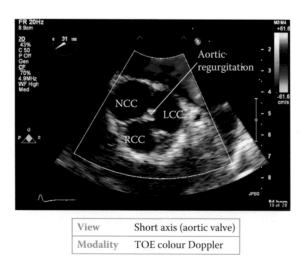

View	Short axis (aortic valve)
Modality	TOE colour Doppler

Figure 8.2   Transoesophageal echo short-axis view of aortic valve showing central jet of mild aortic regurgitation. *Abbreviations:* LCC: Left coronary cusp, NCC: Non-coronary cusp, RCC: Right coronary cusp.

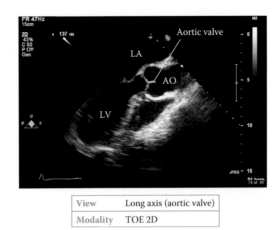

View	Long axis (aortic valve)
Modality	TOE 2D

Figure 8.3 Transoesophageal echo long-axis view of normal aortic valve. *Abbreviations:* Ao: Aorta, LA: Left atrium, LV: Left ventricle.

the interatrial septum, LA and right atrium (RA), and superior and inferior venae cavae (**Figure 8.4**).

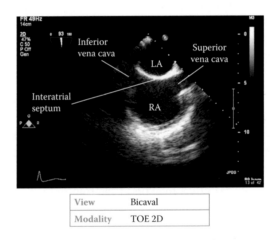

View	Bicaval
Modality	TOE 2D

Figure 8.4 Bicaval view. *Abbreviations:* LA: Left atrium, RA: Right atrium.

Advancing the probe slightly farther down the oesophagus, and maintaining a transducer angle of 0°, produces a four-chamber view (**Figure 8.5**).

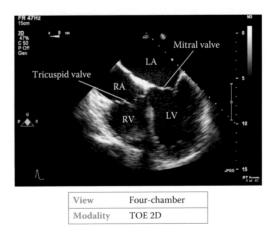

View	Four-chamber
Modality	TOE 2D

Figure 8.5 The four-chamber view. *Abbreviations:* LA: Left atrium, LV: Left ventricle, RA: Right atrium.

The ascending aorta can be inspected at the mid-oesophageal level, in both short axis (with the pulmonary artery looping around it) and long axis, and by rotating the entire probe by 180° (so that the transducer points posteriorly), the descending aorta can also be imaged in short and long axes.

Transgastric views

Advancing the probe into the stomach allows for a series of transgastric views. With the transducer set at 0°, you can obtain a short-axis view of the left ventricle (LV) at the level of the mitral valve and the papillary muscles (**Figure 8.6**). Rotating the transducer to 90° provides a two-chamber view with a particularly clear view of the papillary muscles and chordae tendineae. Further rotation of the transducer to 120° brings the left ventricular outflow tract and aortic valve into view. Remaining at an angle of 120° but rotating the probe towards the patient's right brings the right ventricle, tricuspid valve and RA into view.

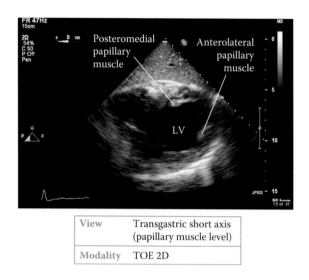

View	Transgastric short axis (papillary muscle level)
Modality	TOE 2D

Figure 8.6 Transgastric short-axis view (papillary muscle level). *Abbreviation:* LV: Left ventricle.

Advancing the probe further into the stomach, with the transducer angle at 0°, provides a **deep transgastric** view, with the transducer lying close to the apex of the LV. This view provides a good alignment with the aortic valve for Doppler studies.

Upper oesophageal views

With the probe facing posteriorly in the upper oesophagus, the aortic arch can be studied in long axis (transducer angle 0°) and short axis (transducer angle 90°).

AFTER THE TRANSOESOPHAGEAL ECHO STUDY

Once you have withdrawn the TOE probe, check it for any signs of bleeding (or for any damage) before sending it for cleaning and disinfection. Be sure too to check the patient's mouth for any trauma. Complete documentation of the procedure and ensure that all images have been acquired and stored. Check that the patient's post-procedure observations are satisfactory.

Once the patient has recovered from the procedure (and any sedation), discuss the results and management plan with them. Ensure they receive appropriate verbal and written instructions before going home, including

- to remain nil by mouth for an hour after the procedure (until the local anaesthetic throat spray wears off)
- not to drive, operate machinery or sign any legal documents for 24 hours following sedation
- to seek advice if they feel unwell or if a sore throat persists for more than 48 hours

Further reading

Hilberath JN et al. Safety of transesophageal echocardiography. *Journal of the American Society of Echocardiography* (2010). PMID 20864313.

Sharma V et al. A safety checklist for transoesophageal echocardiography from the British Society of Echocardiography and the Association of Cardiothoracic Anaesthetists. *Echo Research and Practice* (2015). PMID 26798486.

Wheeler R et al. A minimum dataset for a standard transoesophageal echocardiogram: a guideline protocol from the British Society of Echocardiography. *Echo Research and Practice* (2015). PMID 26798487.

The BSE (www.bsecho.org) has published several useful documents relating to transoesophageal echo:

- Recommendations for Safe Practice in Sedation during Transoesophageal Echocardiography
- Guidelines for Transoesophageal Echocardiography Probe Cleaning and Disinfection

CHAPTER 9

Stress echo

Stress echo is based upon the principle that an abnormality in myocardial perfusion leads to a change in myocardial function. Stress echo therefore plays a valuable role in the assessment of myocardial ischaemia and viability (and, therefore, of underlying coronary artery disease). It also can make an important contribution to the assessment of several other cardiovascular conditions, including valvular heart disease, cardiomyopathies and post-transplantation.

PRINCIPLES OF STRESS ECHO

The principal role of stress echo is in the detection of regional wall motion abnormalities – areas of left ventricular (LV) myocardium that show abnormal function at rest and/or during stress. Each region of the myocardium is supplied with blood (and therefore oxygen) by one of the coronary arteries (see Chapter 17), and an imbalance between supply and demand will cause myocardial ischaemia.

The impact of ischaemia upon myocardial physiology is often referred to as the 'ischaemic cascade', in which progressive ischaemia leads to a series of pathophysiological changes: Initially reduced perfusion, followed by diastolic dysfunction, then systolic dysfunction (manifesting as regional wall motion abnormalities), followed by abnormalities that manifest on the patient's electrocardiogram, before finally resulting in the clinical symptoms of angina.

Even a relatively severe stenosis in one of the major epicardial coronary arteries does not cause myocardial ischaemia at rest, as the myocardial vasculature compensates to maintain resting blood flow by dilating the arterioles downstream of the stenosis. However, this is inadequate to prevent ischaemia with stress, as the increase in myocardial oxygen demand exceeds the ability of the arterioles to dilate further. Thus, a patient with a significant coronary stenosis will usually have normal myocardial perfusion (and therefore contractility) at rest, but will develop myocardial ischaemia (and abnormal wall motion) with stress.

The myocardium can be 'stressed' by increasing myocardial oxygen demand, either with physical exercise or pharmacologically using an intravenous (IV) infusion of dobutamine. Alternatively, an IV infusion of a vasodilator (e.g., dipyridamole, adenosine, regadenoson) can be used as the stressor. Vasodilators work by redistributing coronary blood flow, causing dilatation of normal coronary arteries but not of abnormal ones. This increases blood flow down the normal arteries, but leads to a reduction in blood flow to areas supplied by stenosed coronaries, via a 'steal' mechanism, leading to ischaemia.

For the purposes of a stress echo study, the LV is subdivided into 16 or 17 myocardial segments, and the function of each segment is assessed at rest and with stress. Most commonly, the 16-segment model is used for stress echo. The 17-segment model includes the apical cap, and can be used if myocardial perfusion is being assessed (p. 79) or if you are comparing echo findings with a different imaging modality (Chapter 15).

A number of distinct patterns of response can be identified:

- a **normal** response is indicated by normal contractility (normokinetic) at rest, with normal or increased contractility (hyperkinetic) with stress
- an **ischaemic** response is indicated by normokinetic myocardium at rest, but worsening function on stress, shown by reduced (hypokinetic), absent (akinetic) or paradoxical (dyskinetic) contractility. This is usually due to a stenosis in the supplying coronary artery
- a **partial thickness infarction** is indicated by reduced contractility (hypokinetic) at rest which remains unchanged with stress
- a **non-viable (scar)** response is indicated by absent contractility (akinetic) at rest which remains akinetic or becomes dyskinetic with stress
- a **viability** response is indicated by abnormal contractility (akinetic, hypokinetic) at rest which improves with stress:
  - if the improvement is sustained throughout stress, the myocardium is said to be **stunned**. Stunned myocardium can result from a brief period of coronary occlusion and gradually improves with time
  - if the improvement only occurs at low-level stress, and the myocardium worsens again at higher levels of stress ('biphasic response'), it is said to be **hibernating**. Hibernating myocardium will not recover spontaneously but may improve following coronary revascularization

INDICATIONS FOR STRESS ECHO

Because it can provide valuable information about the presence and extent of coronary artery disease, the indications for a stress echo study include

- diagnosis of suspected coronary artery disease
- identification of viable myocardium prior to revascularization
- localization of myocardial ischaemia ('culprit coronary lesion' identification prior to revascularization)
- assessment of myocardial perfusion following revascularization
- risk assessment of patients with known coronary artery disease
- risk assessment prior to non-cardiac surgery

Stress echo is reported as having a sensitivity of 88% and a specificity of 83% in the detection of coronary artery disease (coronary stenosis >50%). This is similarly sensitive to, but more specific than, nuclear myocardial perfusion imaging (p. 101). Stress echo does not, however, involve exposure to ionizing radiation.

In addition to its role in the assessment of myocardial ischaemia and viability, stress echo can be useful in the evaluation of

- native valvular heart disease, e.g.:
  - asymptomatic severe aortic stenosis
  - low-gradient aortic stenosis with LV dysfunction
  - mitral stenosis where there is disparity between severity and symptoms
- aortic and mitral replacement valves
- non-ischaemic cardiomyopathy
- hypertrophic cardiomyopathy

- congenital heart disease
- heart transplantation
- pulmonary hypertension

CONTRAINDICATIONS TO A STRESS ECHO STUDY

For all forms of stress:

- acute myocardial infarction in the first 72 hours
- unstable angina
- known left main stem coronary artery stenosis
- decompensated heart failure
- haemodynamic instability (e.g., hypotension, hypoxia)
- severe systemic hypertension (systolic blood pressure >200 mmHg and/or diastolic blood pressure >110 mmHg)
- serious, uncontrolled arrhythmias
- severe symptomatic aortic stenosis
- haemodynamically significant left ventricular outflow tract obstruction
- left ventricular thrombus
- recent pulmonary embolism or infarction
- active endocarditis, myocarditis or pericarditis

For atropine:

- closed-angle glaucoma
- severe prostatic disease

For vasodilator (dipyridamole, adenosine, regadenoson) stress:

- pronounced active bronchospastic airway disease
- sick sinus syndrome, second- or third-degree atrioventricular block (unless a functioning pacemaker is present)
- hypotension (systolic blood pressure <90 mmHg)
- xanthine (e.g., caffeine, aminophylline) use in the last 12 hours or dipyridamole use in the last 24 hours

Vasodilator stress is relatively contraindicated by bradycardia of <40 beats/min, equivocal left main stem coronary artery stenosis, recent cerebral ischaemia or infarction.

PATIENT PREPARATION

Patients should receive a clear explanation of what a stress echo study entails and be offered an information leaflet. Ensure that patients taking beta-blockers are informed, where necessary, to omit the beta-blocker for 48 hours prior to the stress echo. Advise patients to bring a companion to drive them home.

A minimum of two personnel should be present throughout the stress echo study, one of whom should be trained in advanced life support and the other in basic life support. The sonographer should be experienced in stress echo, and a physician should be immediately available if not present during the study. Appropriate cardiopulmonary resuscitation equipment must be available.

Prior to undertaking the stress echo study, ensure that the patient understands what is planned and has given informed consent. Review the patient's history and prior investigation findings and check for contraindications or anything that may increase the risk of complications.

A 12-lead ECG must be recorded (and reviewed) at baseline and every minute during the stress study. Attach the ECG electrodes in their standard positions, although these may need to be modified slightly to allow access to the appropriate echo imaging windows. There must also be continuous ECG monitoring (usually via the ECG electrodes of the echo machine) to monitor for arrhythmias. Use an automated cuff to check blood pressure at baseline and again at each stress stage.

A baseline echo should be performed at the start of the study, to identify any relevant background pathology (unless such a study has been undertaken recently). The baseline echo needs to include an assessment of chamber dimensions and function, valve morphology and function and the aortic root.

ACQUIRING THE STRESS ECHO IMAGES

The key to a successful stress echo study is to obtain clear definition of the LV endocardial border. It is important to spend adequate time acquiring the rest images before starting the stress part of the study to ensure that image quality is **optimal** and that the imaging views will be **reproducible** when a set of images is acquired at each stage of the stress study – it is essential to compare 'like with like' at each stage.

Endocardial border definition can be enhanced using

- harmonic imaging (p. 16)
- ultrasound contrast agents (p. 78)

The use of an ultrasound contrast agent is appropriate if two or more myocardial segments cannot be seen clearly on the rest images.

Imaging of the LV must show each of the myocardial segments in at least one and, where possible, two views. The standard stress echo windows and views are

- left parasternal window
  - parasternal long-axis view
  - parasternal short-axis view
- apical window
  - apical four-chamber view
  - apical two-chamber view

The apical three-chamber (long-axis) view can be used as an alternative to the parasternal long-axis view where necessary. With conventional 2D echo, each view has to be obtained in turn. However, the real-time 3D (RT3D) multislice imaging and the real-time 3D full-volume (RT3DFV) data acquisition offer an opportunity to image *all* of the LV myocardial segments at once, which can make image acquisition faster and also allows more flexible 'slicing' of the LV to permit better alignment between views obtained at different levels of stress.

Take your time in acquiring the baseline images – these are the benchmark for comparison with the stress images, so it is important that they are as good as they can be. Make a mental note of the position and angulation of the probe that you used for each view – when you repeat the images during the stress part of the study, you'll be under pressure to find the same views in a much shorter time. The baseline echo should also include an assessment of

- chamber dimensions (including the aortic root)
- overall left and right ventricular function
- valvular structure and function

Acquire images digitally so that images acquired from the same view (but at different stages of the study) can later be displayed side by side for direct comparison, making identification of any

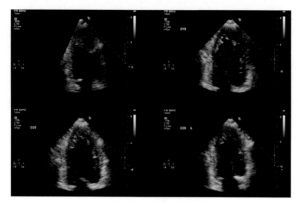

View	Apical two-chamber
Modality	2D

Figure 9.1   Stress echo 'quad screen' view.

regional wall motion abnormalities easier. This comparison is typically done in a 'quad screen' view, with images acquired at baseline, low-level stress, peak stress and recovery displayed side by side (**Figure 9.1**).

As you acquire the images, assess the wall motion of each myocardial segment and score it appropriately. Describe the wall motion of each segment using one of the following terms:

- X = unable to interpret (suboptimal image quality)
- 1 = normal or hyperkinetic
- 2 = hypokinetic
- 3 = akinetic
- 4 = dyskinetic
- 5 = aneurysmal (diastolic deformation)

Wall motion is assessed according to the degree of excursion of the endocardium and, in particular, by the degree of wall thickening – normal segments have an excursion of >5 mm and thicken by >50% during systole. Assess each segment at baseline, low-level stress (where appropriate), peak stress and in recovery. The clearest way to summarize the scores is in the form of a chart, as shown for a 16-segment model in **Figure 9.2**.

Terminate the stress echo study if

- maximum target heart rate (220 – age) is attained
- maximal exercise workload or pharmacological dose is attained
- the patient experiences severe chest pain or intolerable symptoms
- there are new (or worsening) regional wall motion abnormalities in ≥2 adjacent myocardial segments, or with ventricular dilatation
- there is a global reduction of LV systolic function
- there is a clear ECG evidence of ischaemia (new ST segment depression >2 mm)
- systolic blood pressure falls by >20 mmHg below baseline or from a previous level
- blood pressure increases to >220/120 mmHg
- there are sustained arrhythmias

When each myocardial region has been scored, the **wall motion score index** (WMSI) can be calculated at baseline and for each level of stress. This is calculated by adding together the total wall

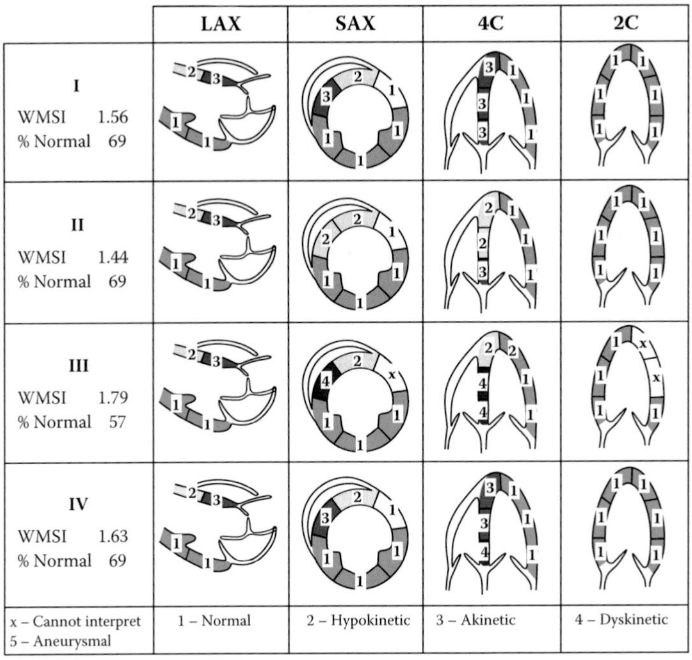

	LAX	SAX	4C	2C
I WMSI 1.56 % Normal 69				
II WMSI 1.44 % Normal 69				
III WMSI 1.79 % Normal 57				
IV WMSI 1.63 % Normal 69				
x – Cannot interpret 5 – Aneurysmal	1 – Normal	2 – Hypokinetic	3 – Akinetic	4 – Dyskinetic

Figure 9.2   Stress echo wall motion scores. *Abbreviation:* WMSI: Wall motion score index.

motion score (i.e., the individual scores for all the segments that can be scored), and then dividing this by the number of scored segments. If all the segments are normokinetic, the WMSI will be 1.0. If any regional wall motion abnormalities are present, the WMSI will be greater than 1.0. An additional quantitative measure is the percentage of scored segments that are normokinetic.

If the study has confirmed myocardial ischaemia, note the heart rate at which ischaemia was first evident (this is only possible with dobutamine or bicycle stress echo, where repeated imaging occurs at different levels of stress). **Ischaemic threshold** is the heart rate at which ischaemia first occurred and is calculated as a percentage, using the following equation:

$$\text{Ischaemic threshold} = \frac{\text{Heart rate when ischaemia first occurred}}{220 - \text{Patient's age (in years)}} \times 100$$

Ischaemic threshold is particularly useful in assessing cardiovascular risk in patients due to undergo non-cardiac surgery. An ischaemic threshold <60% or ischaemia in ≥3–5 segments is an indicator of high risk.

ADDITIONAL INFORMATION

A normal stress echo study is defined as showing normal wall motion at rest and with stress. Those patients with a normal exercise stress echo have an annual risk of cardiac death or non-fatal myocardial infarction of <1% and are therefore regarded as being in a 'low-risk' group. The annual risk for those with a normal pharmacological stress echo is a little higher which is thought to reflect the fact that many of these patients are unable to exercise because of comorbidities. Several factors indicate high risk, including extensive regional wall motion abnormalities (four to five segments) at rest or induced with stress, or the presence of a low ischaemic threshold (<60%–70%).

STRESS PROTOCOLS

Exercise stress

Exercise stress can be undertaken using either a treadmill or semi-supine on a bicycle: Treadmill exercise limits the echo assessment to baseline and peak stress (i.e., immediately post-exercise), whereas semi-supine bicycle exercise means that images can be acquired during the test at different levels of exertion. Bicycle exercise offers greater sensitivity for ischaemia detection than treadmill exercise. 'Peak' stress images must all be acquired within 60 seconds of completing exercise, before the effects of exercise start to wear off and the patient enters the recovery phase.

For treadmill exercise, a symptom-limited Bruce (or modified Bruce) protocol is recommended, with the level of exercise increasing at 3 minute intervals. For bicycle exercise, the World Health Organization 25 Watt programme is recommended, with workload increased in increments of 25 W every 2–3 minutes. Exercise usually continues (all else being equal) until the patient attains their maximum age-predicted target heart rate (220 − Patient's age in years), although the test's sensitivity is usually satisfactory once at least 85% of the target heart rate has been attained.

Dobutamine stress

Dobutamine stress protocols begin with an IV infusion of dobutamine at 5 µg/kg/min, increasing the infusion rate at 3-minute intervals to 10, 20, 30 and 40 µg/kg/min with the aim of reaching the patient's maximum age-predicted target heart rate. If patients are failing to approach their target heart rate with the dobutamine infusion alone, IV atropine can also be administered in divided doses of 0.25 mg every minute (up to a maximum of 1 mg) to increase heart rate. Acquisition of images at low/intermediate levels of dobutamine stress as well as at peak stress allows for the assessment of myocardial viability.

Vasodilator stress

Vasodilator stress usually causes a relatively small increase in heart rate together with a mild fall in blood pressure. It is less sensitive than exercise or dobutamine stress for detecting mild/moderate coronary disease, and so vasodilator stress should be used only when exercise or dobutamine stress are contraindicated.

Dipyridamole stress is performed with an IV infusion of 0.56 mg/kg dipyridamole given over 4 minutes, followed by no infusion for 4 minutes. If no end points have been reached by this time, a further infusion of 0.28 mg/kg is given over 2 minutes. Baseline images are acquired prior to the infusion and the stress images are acquired after the first 4-minute infusion and, if given, the second infusion. Adverse effects of dipyridamole can be treated using 240 mg IV aminophylline.

Adenosine stress is performed with an IV infusion of 140 µg/kg/min adenosine given over 4–6 min (to a maximum of 60 mg). Baseline images are acquired prior to the infusion and stress images are acquired 3 minutes into the infusion.

Regadenoson stress is administered at a dose of 400 µg as an IV bolus (given over 5–10 seconds). Baseline images are acquired prior to the bolus and stress images are acquired 1–2 minutes after the bolus is given.

Vasodilator stress permits the evaluation of myocardial perfusion in addition to the regional wall motion assessment, improving the overall sensitivity of the test. Myocardial perfusion stress echo (MPSE) involves the administration of a myocardial contrast agent (Chapter 10) so that it perfuses the myocardium, and then delivering a brief 'power flash' of ultrasound with a high mechanical index to destroy the bubbles within the heart. This instantaneously clears the bubbles from the myocardium, which turns black. Within the next 5 seconds, the myocardial contrast reappears as new bubbles reperfuse the myocardium, and perfusion defects can be identified as areas in which the contrast fails to replenish as soon as might be expected.

STRESS ECHO AND VALVULAR DISEASE

Aortic stenosis

Assessing the severity of aortic stenosis in patients with impaired LV function can be difficult. One measure of aortic stenosis severity is aortic valve area, calculated by the continuity equation (p. 143). In the presence of impaired LV function, a reduced aortic valve area may be the result of aortic stenosis, but it can also result from the reduced cardiac output failing to open the aortic valve cusps to their full extent during systole. Aortic valve gradient (velocity) does not help, as gradients underestimate the severity of aortic stenosis in the presence of impaired LV function.

It can therefore be difficult to assess whether a patient with 'low flow, low gradient aortic stenosis' has a significantly stenosed valve ('true' aortic stenosis) or whether the findings are primarily the result of reduced valve opening secondary to low cardiac output ('functional' aortic stenosis). 'Low flow, low gradient aortic stenosis' has been defined as an aortic valve orifice area of <1.0 cm^2 and a mean valve gradient of <35 mmHg in a patient with a LV ejection fraction of $<40\%$.

Dobutamine stress echo can be useful in this situation. To distinguish between 'true' and 'functional' aortic stenosis, dobutamine is initially infused at 5 μg/kg/min with increases, if necessary, 2.5–5 μg/kg/min at 5-minute intervals to a maximal dose of 20 μg/kg/min. If there is true (fixed) aortic stenosis, the aortic valve area will remain essentially unchanged (usually remaining at <1.0 cm^2), but the mean valve gradient will increase (usually to a value of $\geq35–40$ mmHg). If the 'stenosis' is functional, the valve area will increase relatively more (usually to ≥1.2 cm^2), and the mean gradient relatively less (<40 mmHg at peak stress), with the dobutamine infusion.

It is important to look for any regional wall motion abnormalities during such a study, which would indicate coexistent myocardial ischaemia, and also to assess the overall LV response to dobutamine. For the stress echo to be useful, there needs to be LV 'contractile reserve', indicated by an increase in stroke volume of 20% or more with dobutamine stress. In the absence of any contractile reserve, it is not possible to draw any conclusions about the severity of the aortic stenosis. Patients with contractile reserve have a better perioperative mortality than those without.

Mitral stenosis

In patients with mitral stenosis, stress echo can be helpful in those whose symptoms appear disproportionate to resting haemodynamic measurements and also those who are asymptomatic but who appear to have severe stenosis. Doppler studies of the mitral and tricuspid valves can be performed during stress, and those who have exertional breathlessness with a mean mitral valve gradient of >15 mmHg and a pulmonary artery systolic pressure of >60 mmHg are likely to benefit from intervention.

AFTER THE STRESS ECHO STUDY

Following the stress echo study, continue to monitor the patient carefully until they are asymptomatic and any ECG, echo or haemodynamic changes have returned to baseline. Patients should rest in the echo department for 30 minutes before going home, and they should be driven home by a companion. Where possible, discuss the results of the study with the patient before they leave. If the results are not immediately available, advise the patient how and when they will hear the results of the study.

Begin your study report with the patient's demographic details and a summary of the indication for the study. Comment on the image quality and whether a contrast agent was used. Describe the stress protocol and the adequacy of the patient's response to it, noting in particular any symptoms (e.g., chest pain) and/or ECG changes, together with changes in heart rate and blood pressure. If an exercise protocol was used, include the exercise duration and peak heart rate attained; for a pharmacological protocol, include information on the drug(s) and doses administered. Review all the images and record the wall motion scores at each level of stress, summarizing them in your stress echo report in an easily understood visual format (as in **Figure 9.2**). Finally, conclude your report with a summary of your interpretation of the findings with regard to ischaemia, infarction and viability. If you have undertaken any valvular assessments as part of the study, include these details in your report too.

Further reading

Lancellotti P et al. The clinical use of stress echocardiography in non-ischaemic heart disease: recommendations from the European Association of Cardiovascular Imaging and the American Society of Echocardiography. *European Heart Journal – Cardiovascular Imaging* (2016). PMID 27880640.

Pellikka PA et al. Guidelines for performance, interpretation, and application of stress echocardiography in ischemic heart disease: from the American Society of Echocardiography. *Journal of the American Society of Echocardiography* (2020). PMID 31740370.

Steeds RP et al. Stress echocardiography in coronary artery disease: a practical guideline from the British Society of Echocardiography. *Echo Research and Practice* (2019). PMID 30921767.

CHAPTER 10

Contrast echo

There are two very different types of echo contrast studies, using:

- agitated saline bubble contrast
- transpulmonary contrast agents

AGITATED SALINE BUBBLE CONTRAST

An agitated saline bubble contrast study is simple to perform and is used primarily to detect an intracardiac shunt, most commonly a patent foramen ovale (PFO, p. 266) or atrial septal defect (ASD). Normally the presence of an intracardiac shunt will allow blood to flow from the left atrium to the right atrium (high pressure to low pressure), but if there is a momentary increase in right atrial pressure, the blood flow will transiently reverse from right to left.

A Valsalva manoeuvre, in which the patient is asked to hold their breath and 'bear down' for 10 seconds, is one such method of increasing the right atrial pressure. It is important to note that it is at the *release* of the Valsalva manoeuvre that right atrial pressure transiently exceeds left atrial pressure (because of the sudden increase in venous return at the end of the manoeuvre) and right-to left shunting can occur if a shunt is present.

A right-to-left shunt can also result from a pulmonary arteriovenous malformation (PAVM). These extracardiac shunts are much rarer than intracardiac ones, and they cause a permanent right-to-left shunt (as opposed to a transient one).

To detect a shunt, a suspension of tiny air bubbles is injected intravenously while an echo is performed. Normally the bubbles fill the right heart where they are clearly visible on echo (**Figure 10.1**), but they are then filtered out as they pass through the lungs – no bubbles will therefore be seen in the left heart. If bubbles *are* seen within the left heart, this indicates that the agitated saline bubble contrast (and hence blood) is managing to cross into the left heart via a right-to-left shunt, bypassing the lungs.

By studying the timing and quantity of bubbles appearing in the left heart, it's possible to distinguish between an intracardiac shunt (PFO/ASD) and an extracardiac shunt (i.e., a PAVM).

To demonstrate a right-to-left shunt, you can use 'agitated' saline:

- draw up 8.5 mL of normal saline and 0.5 mL of air into a 10 mL Luer lock syringe
- using a three-way tap, connect this to another (empty) 10 mL Luer lock syringe, and then attach this to an intravenous cannula sited in the patient's antecubital vein
- withdraw 1 mL of the patient's blood into the syringe containing the saline–air mixture

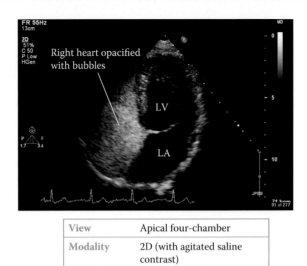

Figure 10.1   Agitated saline bubble contrast study. *Abbreviations:* LA: Left atrium, LV: Left ventricle.

- with the three-way tap turned off to the patient, repeatedly squirt the saline–blood–air mixture back and forth between the two syringes for a few seconds until a suspension of tiny air bubbles is created in the mixture.
- obtain a good apical four-chamber view with your echo probe
- with the patient performing a Valsalva manoeuvre, ensure you are recording the echo images and rapidly inject the 10 mL mixture. As you do so, ask the patient to release the Valsalva manoeuvre
- watch carefully for air bubbles appearing in the left atrium as the patient releases the Valsalva – note the approximate quantity of bubbles that cross and their timing (count the number of cardiac cycles between the agitated saline injection/Valsalva release and the appearance of bubbles in the left heart)

As a general rule of thumb, the appearance of bubbles in the left heart within three cardiac cycles is likely to indicate an intracardiac shunt, whereas a later appearance of bubbles is more likely to indicate an extracardiac shunt.

An agitated saline contrast study can be performed during transthoracic (TTE) or transoesophageal (TOE) echo. Although the image quality is better with TOE, patients usually perform a better Valsalva manoeuvre during TTE.

An additional use of agitated saline bubble contrast is to assist with echo guidance during pericardiocentesis. If there is doubt about whether the pericardiocentesis needle is in the pericardial cavity, a small amount of agitated saline can be injected through the pericardiocentesis needle. If the needle is in the right place, the bubbles will appear within the pericardial effusion. If the pericardiocentesis needle has inadvertently punctured the heart, the bubbles will be seen within one of the cardiac chambers instead.

TRANSPULMONARY CONTRAST AGENTS

One of the limitations of TTE is image quality, which can be suboptimal in patients with poor echo windows. Good image quality is particularly important to obtain clear endocardial border definition for accurate left ventricular (LV) function assessment, for instance, during stress echocardiography, and also to help identify LV masses and morphological abnormalities. The use of transpulmonary contrast agents – sometimes referred to as ultrasound enhancing agents (UEAs) – is one way in which image quality can be enhanced.

As we have already seen, agitated saline bubble contrast does not normally pass through the lungs and so it is of little value in LV opacification. Transpulmonary contrast agents are different – they are specifically designed to pass though the lungs and reach the left heart. In order to achieve this, the bubbles within these echo contrast agents must be very small, usually measuring around 1–10 µm in diameter. The exact composition of the bubbles varies between manufacturers, but they typically consist of a shell (e.g., lipid, phospholipid, albumin) enclosing a cavity filled with gas (e.g., perfluoropropane, sulfur hexafluoride). Echo contrast agents include SonoVue® (known in North America as Lumason®), Optison® and Luminity® (known in North America as Definity®). The licensing and availability of these agents may vary from country to country.

Echo contrast microbubbles are not just passive reflectors of ultrasound. Instead, when they are struck by an incident ultrasound beam, the microbubbles resonate, emitting an ultrasound signal of their own at higher harmonics than the incident beam. The use of appropriate settings on the echo machine (e.g., harmonic imaging, intermittent imaging) optimizes the detection of the 'resonant' signal generated by the microbubbles while at the same time suppressing the usual ultrasound signal returned from the surrounding tissues.

Echo contrast agent microbubbles are relatively 'fragile' and tend to be disrupted by the intensity of conventional ultrasound – the use of a low mechanical index (low-MI imaging) reduces this, although in some situations a higher MI can be used to deliberately disrupt the microbubbles (for example, to assess myocardial perfusion by disrupting the microbubbles in the myocardium with a brief high-MI pulse, and then observing how quickly the microbubbles are replenished – see the box **Myocardial Contrast Echo**).

Clinical applications

Echo contrast agents provide opacification of the cardiac chambers and enhance the delineation of the LV endocardial border, making them useful in cases where image quality is suboptimal and two or more contiguous LV segments cannot be seen with conventional imaging. This improves the accuracy of LV volume and ejection fraction measurements and is especially valuable in the assessment of regional wall motion during stress echo studies (Chapter 9).

Improved imaging of the LV endocardium can also help in the identification of morphological abnormalities, including isolated ventricular non-compaction, apical hypertrophic cardiomyopathy, intracardiac masses such as tumours and thrombus, and LV aneurysm.

The enhanced LV imaging obtained with echo contrast agents can be particularly useful when performing portable studies in the intensive care unit, where the inability to position the patient optimally means that image quality is frequently suboptimal. Echo contrast agents can also improve spectral Doppler signals, aiding in the assessment of valvular disease and LV diastolic function. Enhancement of a weak tricuspid regurgitation spectral Doppler signal can be particularly helpful in aiding the assessment of pulmonary artery systolic pressure (p. 202).

For full details about the safe and appropriate use of echo contrast agents, refer to the relevant product datasheet.

MYOCARDIAL CONTRAST ECHO

An unlicensed use of echo contrast agents is in myocardial contrast echo (MCE) to assess the myocardial perfusion. The principle behind the MCE is that the presence of microbubbles within the capillaries of the myocardium increases the intensity of the myocardial signal on echo. After an administration of echo contrast, the microbubbles enter the myocardial capillaries, and these microbubbles can then be destroyed using a series of high-energy ultrasound pulses. The sonographer then observes the replenishment of microbubbles as more blood (carrying intact microbubbles) flows into the capillaries of the myocardium. The intensity of the myocardial signal and the speed at which the microbubbles are replenished can be assessed, both of which are indicators of tissue blood flow. Normally the microbubbles are fully replenished within five cardiac cycles (or just two to three cycles during stress). A delay in replenishment and a reduced signal intensity indicates reduced myocardial blood flow, as seen in the presence of coronary artery disease.

Further reading

Montrief T et al. Point-of-care echocardiography for the evaluation of right-to-left cardiopulmonary shunts: a narrative review. *Canadian Journal of Anaesthesia* (2020). PMID 32944839.

Muskula PR et al. Safety with echocardiographic contrast agents. *Circulation: Cardiovascular Imaging* (2017). PMID 28377467.

Porter TR et al. Clinical applications of ultrasonic enhancing agents in echocardiography: 2018 American Society of Echocardiography guidelines update. *Journal of the American Society of Echocardiography* (2018). PMID 29502588.

Senior R et al. Clinical practice of contrast echocardiography: recommendation by the European Association of Cardiovascular Imaging (EACVI) 2017. *European Heart Journal – Cardiovascular Imaging* (2017). PMID 28950366.

CHAPTER 11

Tissue Doppler imaging

In Chapter 5, we saw how tissue Doppler imaging (TDI) has an important role to play, alongside speckle tracking, in the evaluation of myocardial mechanics. TDI is most commonly associated with the assessment of **LV diastolic function**, and this is discussed in detail in Chapter 18. However, it also has applications in assessing

- LV systolic function
- right ventricular (RV) function
- coronary artery disease
- cardiomyopathies
- valvular heart disease
- LV dyssynchrony
- constrictive pericarditis and restrictive cardiomyopathy (p. 242)

TDI has greater sensitivity than the 'conventional' echo parameters for the detection of subclinical myocardial abnormalities and is therefore of interest in the early detection of myocardial disorders.

PERFORMING TDI

Pulsed-wave TDI

Pulsed-wave TDI permits the measurement of myocardial velocity in a specific region with excellent temporal resolution. To perform pulsed-wave TDI, the sonographer places the sample volume in the region of interest. In the assessment of left ventricular (LV) longitudinal contraction, the sample volume is placed in the myocardium within 1 cm of the insertion of the mitral valve leaflets, either medially (septally) or laterally, in the apical four-chamber view (**Figure 11.1**). In each location, a pulsed-wave TDI recording is made using a low gain setting, an aliasing velocity 15–20 cm/s and a sweep speed of 100 mm/s.

The resultant pulsed-wave TDI recording (**Figure 11.2**) shows a mitral annular velocity towards the transducer which corresponds to the annular myocardium moving towards the apex as the LV contracts longitudinally during systole (S'). This is followed by an early myocardial velocity (e') which corresponds to early diastolic relaxation, the myocardium moving away from the transducer, and finally by a further movement away from the transducer, corresponding to atrial contraction (a').

For LV assessments, measurements can be quoted for both medial and lateral velocities, and also mean values can be calculated by averaging the medial and lateral values.

DOI: 10.1201/9781003304654-11

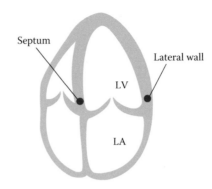

Figure 11.1   Positioning of sample volume for pulsed-wave tissue Doppler imaging (TDI) of the mitral annulus. *Abbreviations:* LA: Left atrium, LV: Left ventricle.

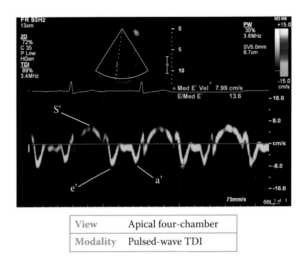

View	Apical four-chamber
Modality	Pulsed-wave TDI

Figure 11.2   Pulsed-wave trace of medial mitral annulus (septal wall) obtained with tissue Doppler imaging (TDI).

For RV assessments, pulsed-wave TDI can be undertaken at the lateral tricuspid annulus (ensure that the lateral tricuspid annulus and basal RV free wall segment are aligned with the Doppler cursor). This allows measurement of the peak systolic velocity at the tricuspid valve annulus (RV S′), which is a reflection of RV systolic function.

Colour TDI

As with 'standard' colour Doppler, colour TDI is based upon the principle of pulsed-wave Doppler. Rather than using pulsed-wave TDI to measure myocardial velocity at a single sample volume, in colour TDI, the myocardial velocity is assessed at multiple points within a preselected area. The information is displayed on screen with colour-coding of myocardial velocity according to its direction and the *mean* velocity within each sample volume. Movement away from the transducer is shown as blue, and towards the transducer is shown as red (**Figure 11.3**).

As noted earlier, it's important to recall that pulsed-wave TDI measures **peak** velocity, whereas colour TDI measures **mean** velocity. Thus, the velocity values generated from colour Doppler are generally around 25% lower than for pulsed-wave Doppler, and so pulsed-wave and colour TDI are not interchangeable.

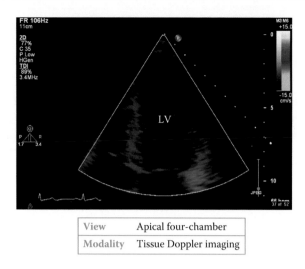

View	Apical four-chamber
Modality	Tissue Doppler imaging

Figure 11.3   Colour tissue Doppler imaging. *Abbreviation:* LV: Left ventricle.

CLINICAL APPLICATIONS OF TDI

Reference intervals for TDI measurements in normal individuals have been published. **Table 11.1** shows the data published by Chahal et al. (2010) obtained from 453 healthy subjects aged 35–75 years.

Both S′ and e′ values decrease with aging (and a′ values increase). The British Society of Echocardiography provides age-specific reference intervals for normal mean mitral annular S′ values as follows:

- *Age 20–40 years:* mean S′ > 6.4 cm/s
- *Age 40–60 years:* mean S′ > 5.7 cm/s
- *Age >60 years:* mean S′ > 4.9 cm/s

The use of these TDI-derived values in the assessment of LV diastolic function is discussed in detail in Chapter 18.

LV systolic function

Measurement of lateral mitral annular velocity (S′) provides an assessment of longitudinal LV contraction during systole and has been shown to correlate well with LV ejection fraction. If S′ is >6 cm/s, this usually indicates a normal ejection fraction.

In addition to providing information on global LV systolic function, TDI can be used to assess regional systolic function by measuring myocardial velocities within each LV segment. A fall in S′ is a sensitive indictor of myocardial ischaemia or infarction.

Myocardial deformation

As discussed in Chapter 5, myocardial velocity measurements obtained using TDI can be used to assess myocardial deformation. If the velocities at two points in the myocardium are known, then the difference between these velocities gives a measure of strain rate (i.e., the rate at which these two

Table 11.1   Reference intervals for S′ and e′ obtained using tissue Doppler imaging

	Medial	Lateral	Mean
S′ (cm/s)	6.0–10.9	6.7–14.6	6.8–12.2
e′ (cm/s)	5.8–11.9	7.9–17.6	7.3–14.1

Source: Chahal et al., 2010.

regions are moving closer together or farther apart). If you want to measure strain itself using TDI, then you need to integrate strain rate over time to obtain a value for strain.

A colour overlay can be used to display myocardial strain on the 2D greyscale image to assist in the identification of areas of abnormal contractility.

Although widely available, TDI has several limitations in the assessment of myocardial deformation, not least its angle dependency. TDI can only assess deformation that occurs parallel to the ultrasound beam, and therefore directed towards (or away from) the ultrasound probe. Speckle tracking offers significant advantages over TDI for the evaluation of myocardial deformation, and it is discussed in Chapter 12.

RV systolic function

Measurement of the peak systolic velocity at the tricuspid valve annulus gives a measure of RV systolic function, with a normal value of 14 ± 2 cm/s. A value <11.5 cm/s provides a relatively high sensitivity and specificity for indicating impaired RV systolic function.

LIMITATIONS OF TDI

TDI provides valuable information on cardiac function. However, it also has certain limitations. Like all Doppler techniques, TDI is heavily angle dependent in that it can only measure motion parallel to the direction of the ultrasound beam. Furthermore, TDI is unable to distinguish between active motion (i.e., myocardial contraction/relaxation) and passive motion (where a region of myocardium is 'pulled' by an adjacent segment).

Further reading

Chahal NS et al. Normative reference values for the tissue Doppler imaging parameters of left ventricular function: a population-based study. *European Journal of Echocardiography* (2010). PMID 19910319.

Kadappu KK et al. Tissue Doppler imaging in echocardiography: value and limitations. *Heart, Lung and Circulation* (2015). PMID 25465516.

Nagueh SF et al. Recommendations for the evaluation of left ventricular diastolic function by echocardiography: an update from the American Society of Echocardiography and the European Association of Cardiovascular Imaging. *European Heart Journal – Cardiovascular Imaging* (2016). PMID 27037982.

Pellerin D et al. Tissue Doppler, strain, and strain rate echocardiography for the assessment of left and right systolic ventricular function. *Heart* (2003). PMID 14594870.

Waggoner AD et al. Tissue Doppler imaging: a useful echocardiographic method for the cardiac sonographer to assess systolic and diastolic ventricular function. *Journal of the American Society of Echocardiography* (2001). PMID 11734780.

CHAPTER 12

Speckle tracking

In Chapter 5, we saw how myocardial mechanics can be expressed in terms of strain and strain rate. Speckle tracking provides a means for measuring these parameters, and it offers significant advantages over the alternative technique of tissue Doppler imaging (TDI). Unlike TDI, speckle tracking does not require the prospective acquisition of any extra images during a standard echo examination but instead simply relies upon the retrospective processing of good quality greyscale images. Speckle tracking is not dependent upon alignment with the ultrasound beam, which makes it relatively straightforward to assess strain in the longitudinal, radial and circumferential planes (**Figure 5.1**, p. 32).

BASIC PRINCIPLES

The interaction of ultrasound with myocardial tissue generates speckles within the myocardium, which can be clearly appreciated on a greyscale echo image (particularly if the gain setting of the echo machine is increased). The pattern of these speckles is relatively stable and also unique to each region of the myocardium, which means that they can act as a 'myocardial footprint' allowing the movement of the myocardium to be tracked from one frame to the next.

This tracking of the speckles is performed by sophisticated software. It's not feasible to track the position of a single speckle throughout the cardiac cycle, because of small changes in their relative location and intensity as the myocardium deforms. However, it is possible for the software to track the location of a grouping of speckles.

To achieve this, the software identifies the speckles within a defined region of interest in the initial frame of a greyscale cine loop – this region of interest is called a kernel. In the next frame of the loop, the software will search for the kernel – the same pattern of speckles – within a search area around the location of the original kernel (**Figure 12.1**). A 'best match' algorithm is used to identify the new location of the kernel, and then this process is repeated from one to the next. In order to ensure that the kernel does not move too far between frames (which would make tracking it much harder), it's important to use a high frame rate during the acquisition of the cine loop, typically 40–90 frames per second at a normal heart rate.

Multiple kernels can be tracked simultaneously, allowing for evaluation of the whole myocardium within a single view. Typically, there will be 3 kernels in the radial direction and 30–50 kernels in the longitudinal direction, with kernels grouped into myocardial segments according to the standard 17-segment model (Chapter 17), and the data for each segment averaged accordingly.

By following the motion of the kernel throughout the cardiac cycle, its displacement can be calculated and also the time taken for the displacement to occur, giving each kernel's velocity at any

DOI: 10.1201/9781003304654-12

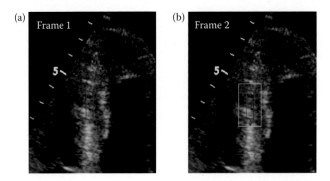

Figure 12.1   Tracking the kernel location between frames. (a) In Frame 1, the kernel (red box) identifies the speckle pattern of interest. (b) In the second frame of the cine loop, the software then looks for the best match within the search area (white box). (Image © Dr Grant Heatlie, University Hospital of North Staffordshire.)

moment during the cardiac cycle. This can be measured in any plane (longitudinal, radial and circumferential) as speckle tracking is not limited to measuring motion only perpendicular to the ultrasound beam, unlike TDI.

Two kernels can be considered as a bar of myocardium with a kernel at each end, and so by assessing the relative motion of the two kernels, it becomes possible to measure strain – the change in the distance between the two kernels (the length of the 'bar'), relative to the original distance, being the strain. Factoring in the time taken for this change to occur provides the strain rate.

The speckle tracking software can plot curves of segmental displacement, velocity, strain and strain rate in the longitudinal, radial and circumferential planes (**Figure 12.2**). Normal longitudinal

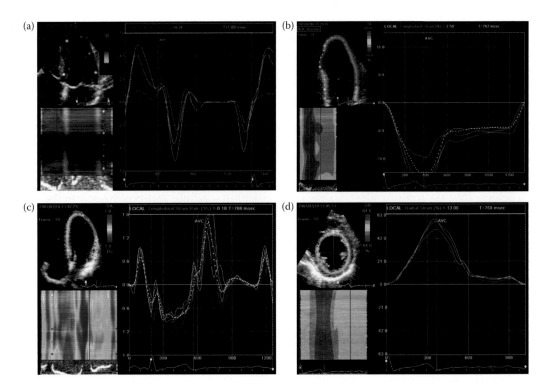

Figure 12.2   The normal curves for (a) longitudinal velocity, (b) longitudinal strain, (c) longitudinal strain rate and (d) radial strain. Note that the longitudinal velocity and longitudinal strain rate curves are almost mirror images, and also that longitudinal strain and radial strain are also almost mirror images of each other. (Image © Dr Grant Heatlie, University Hospital of North Staffordshire.)

strain is negative during systole, when the heart shortens in the longitudinal plane, but is positive in the radial plane, as the myocardium thickens radially during systole. Longitudinal and radial strain curves therefore look like mirror images. The software can overlay the calculated data in colour-coded format on the 2D greyscale images, making it easier to visualize segmental abnormalities.

ROTATIONAL MECHANICS

In addition to its motion in the longitudinal, radial and circumferential planes, the left ventricle also rotates about its long axis during systole due to helical fibres in its wall. Looking at the left ventricle from the apex, the apex rotates clockwise and the base anticlockwise, giving the ventricle as a whole a 'twisting' motion. This twist (and the associated twisting and untwisting rates) can be measured using speckle tracking, but it is not commonly used in the clinical setting.

SEGMENTAL AND GLOBAL VALUES

Strain and strain rate can be measured segmentally and globally. Although it's possible to calculate the global longitudinal, radial and circumferential strains, most publications refer to global *longitudinal* strain (GLS).

Segmental values describe the average values within a particular segment of the myocardium, and global values can be calculated by averaging segmental values. If some segments are badly tracked, generating questionable data, it's possible to exclude these from the calculation of a global average (but no more than one segment per view should be excluded).

When reporting your speckle tracking results, it's important to describe the methods you have used in your analysis. You should also clarify whether any global calculations were made in a single imaging plane or were obtained from the entire ventricle.

Because of the difference in software between vendors, there are no universally applicable reference intervals for strain and strain rate results. In one meta-analysis involving 2597 subjects, normal GLS values varied from −15.9% to −22.1% (Yingchoncharoen et al., 2013). It's therefore important to be familiar with the reference intervals applicable for the software you are using.

CLINICAL APPLICATIONS OF SPECKLE TRACKING

Over the last decade, speckle tracking has entered mainstream practice and its value in the assessment of myocardial diseases is well-recognized. Segmental abnormalities in particular can help to identify the aetiology of cardiomyopathies, such as cardiac amyloidosis.

In patients with cardiac amyloidosis, there is a reduction in GLS but with relative sparing of the apex, as shown by colour-coded bull's-eye maps of segmental strain which show a characteristic 'cherry on top' pattern (**Figure 29.6**, p. 232). Similarly, patients with hypertrophic cardiomyopathy typically have the greatest reduction in strain values in the location with most hypertrophy and myocardial fibrosis.

Global measures of strain can be useful in the early recognition of myocardial abnormalities before they become clinically apparent. As such, there has been much interest in the role of GLS in identifying subclinical cardiotoxicity in oncology patients. The British Society of Echocardiography has included GLS in their cardio-oncology guidelines, in which probable subclinical cardiotoxicity is defined by a decline in LVEF by >10% (absolute percentage points) to an LVEF ≥50% with an accompanying fall in GLS >15%. Possible subclinical cardiotoxicity is defined by a decline in LVEF by <10% (absolute percentage points) to an LVEF <50%, or by a relative reduction in GLS >15% from the baseline value.

There are also roles for speckle tracking in the echo assessment of hypertension, aortic stenosis and ischaemic heart disease. Speckle tracking is not limited to the assessment of the left ventricle, with growing interest in its potential for assessing the right ventricular and left atrial myocardial dynamics too.

Further reading

Collier P et al. A test in context: myocardial strain measured by speckle-tracking echocardiography. *Journal of the American College of Cardiology* (2017). PMID 28231932.

Dobson R et al. British Society for Echocardiography and British Cardio-Oncology Society guideline for transthoracic echocardiographic assessment of adult cancer patients receiving anthracyclines and/or trastuzumab. *Echo Research and Practice* (2021). PMID 34106116.

Johnson C et al. Practical tips and tricks in measuring strain, strain rate and twist for the left and right ventricles. *Echo Research and Practice* (2019). PMID 31289687.

Moharram MA et al. Myocardial tissue characterisation using echocardiographic deformation imaging. *Cardiovascular Ultrasound* (2019). PMID 31730467.

Shah AM et al. Myocardial deformation imaging: current status and future directions. *Circulation* (2012). PMID 22249531.

Voigt JU et al. Definitions for a common standard for 2D speckle tracking echocardiography: consensus document of the EACVI/ASE/Industry task force to standardize deformation imaging. *European Heart Journal – Cardiovascular Imaging* (2015). PMID 25525063.

Yingchoncharoen T et al. Normal ranges of left ventricular strain: a meta-analysis. *Journal of the American Society of Echocardiography* (2013). PMID 23218891.

CHAPTER 13

3D echo

The heart is a 3D structure and a full understanding of its anatomy and physiology can only be gained by considering its structure and function in all three dimensions. Using 2D echo, this is usually achieved by the sonographer mentally reconstructing a 3D image from the information obtained in multiple 2D imaging planes.

The ability to generate a 3D visualization of the heart using the echo machine and/or post-processing software is known as 3D echo. The facility to do this 'live' during image acquisition is called real-time 3D (RT3D) echo, which is sometimes referred to as 4D echo as it incorporates the three dimensions of space plus the additional dimension of time.

The last two decades have seen significant advances in 3D echo, underpinned by the development of ever more sophisticated transducers (improving both usability and image quality) together with advances in both hardware and software that permit high-quality real-time imaging with greater automation and ease-of-use.

3D TECHNOLOGY

Contemporary 3D echo systems use fully sampled matrix array transducers to perform volume scanning, in contrast to the sector scanning performed by a 2D transducer. A 2D transducer typically contains 128 elements arranged in a linear fashion. The ultrasound beam is steered across one plane (y-axis, azimuth plane) creating a tomographic slice of the heart. In contrast, matrix array transducers contain nearly 3,000 elements arranged in the form of a rectangular grid and capable of parallel processing. The ultrasound beam can be steered in two different planes – the y-axis (similar to 2D imaging) and the z-axis (elevation plane) – to produce a pyramidal volume dataset (**Figure 13.1**).

Each element in the 3D transducer has to be controlled independently, and this poses a major technical challenge because the large number of wiring connections required would ordinarily necessitate a large and unwieldy cable to connect the transducer to the echo machine. Manufacturers have been able to get around this problem by incorporating sophisticated microelectronics inside the 3D transducer, which allow some processing (beamforming) to take place within the transducer itself. The amount of data that has to be transmitted between the transducer and the echo machine is reduced as a result, and so a smaller cable can be used. Because of the microelectronics within the transducer, 3D transducers are generally larger and heavier than the 2D transducers. However, refinements in transducer technology have enabled the most recent generation of matrix array transducers (e.g., Philips xMATRIX X5-1 or GE 4Vc-D) to be significantly smaller in size and weight, and 3D technology is available for both transthoracic and transoesophageal transducers.

DOI: 10.1201/9781003304654-13

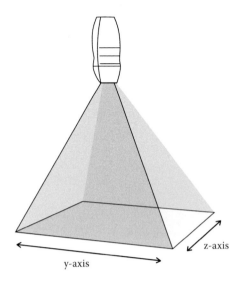

Figure 13.1   The ultrasound beam from a 3D matrix array transducer is steered in two different planes to create a pyramidal volume dataset.

Similar to 2D imaging, there is an inverse relationship between frame rate (temporal resolution), sector width and spatial resolution (scan lines) in 3D echo. An increase in one of these factors will cause a decrease in the other two. In 3D echo, frame rate is more properly referred to as volume rate, as it's the number of 3D *volumes* acquired each second that is measured, not the number of frames per se.

Manufacturers have developed several techniques such as parallel processing and multi-beat imaging to try to balance the competing trade-offs of sector width and spatial and temporal resolution. In practice, image optimization is usually achieved by selecting the appropriate acquisition mode and by using a small-volume dataset. In this way, diagnostic quality image can be obtained with a suitable sector width and an appropriate balance between spatial and temporal resolution.

ACQUISITION MODES

There are two methods of data acquisition in 3D echo:

- real-time (live) 3D imaging
- multi-beat imaging

Each mode has advantages and disadvantages, and it's important to select the appropriate mode according to the clinical information you need to acquire.

Real-time (live) 3D imaging

Real-time (live) 3D imaging acquires several pyramidal volume datasets each second (the 'volume rate') and displays the images as a real-time display. As the information is updated in real time, the image orientation and plane can be changed by rotating the transducer. Analysis can be done with minimal post-processing and the image display can be rotated (independent of the transducer position) to view the heart from different orientations.

Whilst this method is useful to assess the real-time motion of a cardiac structure, it is limited by spatial and temporal resolution. Real-time imaging is available in the following modes:

- *Live 3D*: Any 2D image can be converted to a 3D image by single-button activation in this mode. To allow sufficient spatial and temporal resolution, the software automatically defaults to a narrow sector width of approximately 300 × 600 pyramidal volume (**Figure 13.2**). The sector

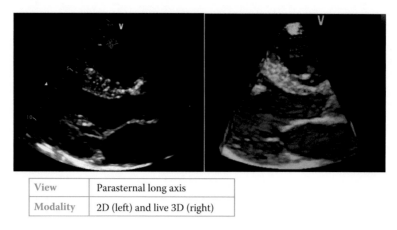

View	Parasternal long axis
Modality	2D (left) and live 3D (right)

Figure 13.2   Live 3D image (right-hand panel) of a parasternal long-axis view obtained from a single beat. (Image © Dr Thomas Mathew, Trent Cardiac Centre.)

width can be increased to visualize a larger structure, but the scan density (spatial resolution) and frame rate (temporal resolution) will go down.

- *3D zoom*: This is an extension of live 3D that allows a focused real-time view of a structure of interest. By adjusting the lateral and elevation width using a crop box placed on a pre-acquired image, the system automatically crops the adjacent structures to provide a real-time display of the structure of interest (**Figure 13.3**). This can be a useful way of assessing structures such as the mitral valve, left atrial appendage or interatrial septum.

- *Live 3D colour*: Colour flow can be superimposed on a live 3D image to assess blood flow in real time.

- *Multiplane imaging*: One unique feature of the matrix array transducer is to display 2D images in multiple planes. For example, acquisition of a four-chamber view from the apical window will simultaneously display two-chamber and three-chamber views (**Figure 13.4**). The first image is often the reference image and the others can be changed depending on the operator-chosen angle. Although strictly not a 3D image, this feature is useful in situations where the assessment of multiple imaging planes from the same cardiac cycle is useful (e.g., stress echo).

Multi-beat imaging

Multi-beat imaging, in contrast to real-time/live 3D imaging, acquires several wedge-shaped volumes over a number of cardiac cycles and stitches them together to create a full-volume display. Once acquired, the images cannot be altered by manipulation of the probe as in real-time 3D imaging.

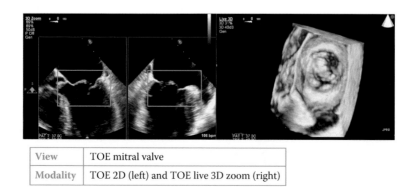

View	TOE mitral valve
Modality	TOE 2D (left) and TOE live 3D zoom (right)

Figure 13.3   Live 3D zoom view. The left-hand panel shows the crop box placed on the structure of interest (mitral valve) on a pre-acquired image. The right-hand panel shows the live 3D zoom view of the mitral valve as viewed from the left atrium. (Image © Dr Thomas Mathew, Trent Cardiac Centre.)

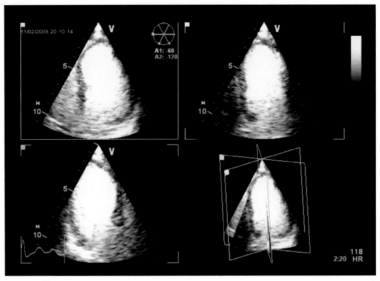

View	Apical long axis
Modality	Multiplane (four-, two- and three-chamber)

Figure 13.4 Multiplane imaging. Simultaneous display of four-, two- and three-chamber (apical long-axis) views from a single acquisition from the apex. Contrast has been administered to improve endocardial definition. (Image © Dr Thomas Mathew, Trent Cardiac Centre.)

Multi-beat imaging allows the acquisition of a pyramidal 3D dataset with much greater temporal and spatial resolution than can be achieved with real-time 3D imaging. In addition, it can be used to assess a larger structure such as the left or right ventricle (or indeed the entire heart). However, the fact that the 3D dataset is stitched together from images acquired over several cardiac cycles means that this method is susceptible to artifacts caused by ECG gating and probe movement (see Stitching Artifact, p. 95). Multi-beat imaging can be used with and without colour flow mapping.

SELECTING AN ACQUISITION MODE

Selection of an appropriate acquisition mode depends upon the clinical context. In general, live 3D imaging is used to assess a small structure (e.g., cardiac valves, left atrial appendage, interatrial septum, locating the origin of a regurgitant jet using colour flow) or when real-time information is required (e.g., while guiding an interventional procedure). Multi-beat imaging is used when a wider sector or high temporal or spatial resolution is required and is also the method of choice for chamber or valve quantification.

THE 3D EXAMINATION

There is no formal protocol for a 3D examination. In clinical practice, it is often used as a focused study to complement 2D imaging. Firstly, a good quality 2D image of the region of interest is identified. Then, small-volume 3D datasets are acquired using live 3D or 3D zoom, making sure the structure is fully included within the volume. At the end, a full-volume multi-beat acquisition is obtained for advanced offline analysis. Although a 3D dataset can be acquired from any conventional echo window, there are recommended views for assessing specific cardiac structures (**Table 13.1**).

Table 13.1   Recommended views for assessing cardiac structures in 3D echo

Structure	Recommended view
Left ventricle	Apical four-chamber view
Right ventricle	Apical four-chamber view
Mitral valve	Parasternal long-axis and apical four-chamber views
Aortic valve	Parasternal long-axis view
Pulmonary valve	Right ventricular outflow view
Tricuspid valve	Apical four-chamber view
Interatrial septum	Apical four-chamber view

POST-PROCESSING

Once the 3D images are acquired, the dataset has to be processed for analysis. This again depends upon the mode of acquisition. Live 3D imaging can be analysed with minimal post-processing, whereas multi-beat imaging requires detailed post-processing. Some aspects of the post-processing are done by the ultrasound machine, but the rest is carried out by the operator.

As soon as the image is acquired, the intracardiac structures are reconstructed within the computer memory by a process called **volume rendering**. An example of a volume-rendered image acquired by multi-beat imaging is shown in **Figure 13.5a**. As opposed to a live 3D image (**Figure 13.2**), the region of interest is not easily seen. This is analogous to a surgeon looking at the heart from outside and not being able to visualize the intracardiac structures without removing the walls.

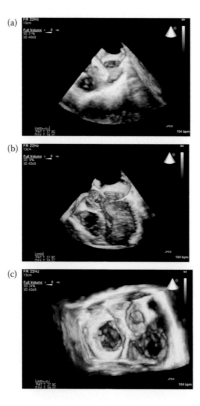

Figure 13.5   (a) Volume-rendered full-volume image acquired over four cardiac cycles. Structures within the volume dataset are not easy to visualize without post-processing. (b) The dataset has been cropped to view a five-chamber view. (c) The dataset has been cropped and rotated to show mitral, tricuspid and aortic valves. (Image © Dr Thomas Mathew, Trent Cardiac Centre.)

By electronically segmenting and sectioning the dataset, either automatically using pre-sets or manually using a crop box/crop plane, the region of interest can be identified. This process is called **cropping** and is unique to 3D echo. The processed image can then be displayed in any anatomical plane (**Figure 13.5b**) or rotated around the centre point to view from different angles (**Figure 13.5c**). It is also possible to generate 2D slices from the 3D dataset.

IMAGE DISPLAY

Once a dataset is acquired and processed, the images can be displayed in three different formats:

- volume rendering
- surface rendering
- 2D tomographic slices

Volume rendering

Volume rendering is the commonest method of display. This technique uses multiple algorithms (specific to each manufacturer) to display a 3D image on a 2D screen (**Figure 13.6**). This can be used for images obtained both from live 3D and from multi-beat imaging. The images can be cropped to view a specific structure of interest and can also be rotated to be viewed from different orientations. Volume-rendered images are commonly used to study the complex spatial relationship of cardiac anatomy and are most useful for evaluating valve pathology and congenital heart disease.

Surface rendering

Surface rendering is a technique that allows a structure or an organ to be visualized in a solid appearance. To use this technique, the acquired image is opened in a specific software package and the surface of the structure tracked either manually or by using a semi-automatic border detection algorithm. There are several online and offline software packages that provide this facility, and they are specific to each manufacturer.

Surface rendering is commonly used to assess ventricular volumes and function. For the analysis of the left ventricle, the user identifies certain landmarks (such as the medial and lateral mitral annulus and the apex). The software then automatically tracks the endocardium using these landmarks to create a 'cast' of the ventricle, producing a time–volume curve from which global and regional function can be assessed (**Figure 13.7**).

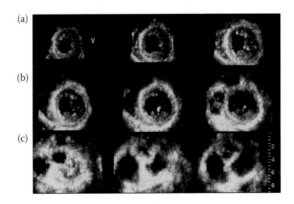

Figure 13.6 Volume-rendered displays. (a) 2D tomographic slice of a prosthetic mitral valve. (b) Live 3D image from a similar angle. (c) Live 3D zoom view (cropped and rotated to show the surgical view). (Image © Dr Thomas Mathew, Trent Cardiac Centre.)

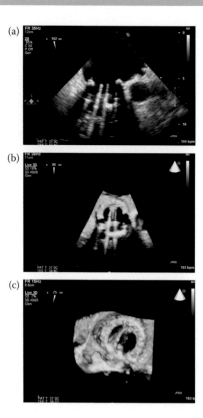

Figure 13.7 Surface-rendered display. Semiautomatic tracking of the endocardium using dedicated software to create a cast of the left ventricle. Systolic and diastolic volumes are calculated by the software. (Image © Dr Thomas Mathew, Trent Cardiac Centre.)

2D tomographic slices

The 3D full-volume dataset can be sliced or cropped to obtain multiple 2D views. This can be achieved using either pre-set buttons or an operator-selected arbitrary plane. Images can be displayed in any conventional imaging plane (four-chamber, two-chamber or short-axis) or a unique cutting plane which is not usually possible by transducer manipulation using 2D imaging.

The advantage of this mode is the simultaneous display of 2D images in multiple planes from the same dataset, permitting better evaluation of structure and function. A typical example is the display of multiple short-axis views of the left ventricle (**Figure 13.8**) obtained from parallel tomographic slices during the same cardiac cycle, making the assessment of regional and global function more accurate.

3D ECHO ARTIFACTS

Three-dimensional echo is subject to the usual artifacts of 2D imaging, such as side lobe and attenuation artifacts (p. 19), but two types of artifacts are specific to this technique and are commonly encountered in practice:

- stitching artifact
- dropout artifact

Stitching artifact

To produce a smooth full-volume display, the sub-volumes acquired from each cardiac cycle should be at the same time and space. Improper ECG gating, or motion related to respiration or transducer movement, will result in artifacts when the volumes are stitched together (**Figure 13.9**).

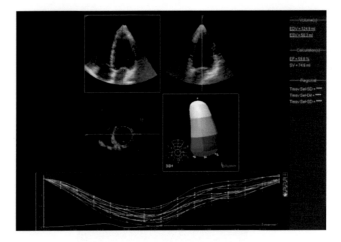

Figure 13.8 Multiple short-axis views obtained by transecting a full-volume dataset of the left ventricle. (Image © Dr Thomas Mathew, Trent Cardiac Centre.)

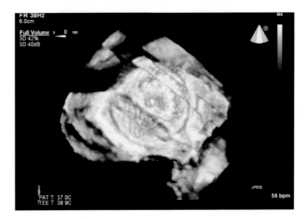

Figure 13.9 Stitching artifacts caused by respiratory motion in a ventilated patient. (Image © Dr Thomas Mathew, Trent Cardiac Centre.)

This occurs with multi-beat image acquisition and is common in patients with an irregular heart rhythm or on mechanical ventilators. In patients with regular heart rhythm, this can be minimized by appropriate ECG triggering and a combination of breath holding and a steady transducer position. In patients with irregular heart rhythm, it remains a challenge, and in these situations maximum information should be obtained using real-time imaging.

Dropout artifact

Dropout artifacts are due to low gain settings and appear as 'false holes' on thin structures due to the poor echo signal intensity. Avoidance of dropout artifacts requires appropriate gain settings, especially time-gain compensation (which cannot be recovered during post-processing). Interpretation of a dropout artifact requires extensive experience and additional information from 2D imaging.

CLINICAL APPLICATIONS OF 3D ECHO

There are three main uses of 3D echo in current clinical practice:

- assessment of ventricular size and function
- assessment of morphology and function
- guiding interventional procedures

Assessment of ventricular size and function

Although 2D echo is routinely used to assess ventricular function (Chapter 16), it relies heavily on geometric assumptions and manual tracing of the endocardial border. In addition, foreshortening of the apex is common with 2D imaging which leads to underestimation of volumes. These factors limit the reproducibility of this technique.

Using 3D echo, the volume of the left ventricle is calculated from the entire endocardial surface without the need for assumptions about its shape. The true length of the ventricle can be adjusted to avoid foreshortening, and tracking of the endocardium is done by semi-automatic border detection algorithms. Several studies have shown an improved accuracy of left ventricular volume quantification by 3D echo compared to 2D echo, and 3D echo has a close approximation with other modalities such as cardiovascular magnetic resonance imaging (p. 102). Currently, the 3D transthoracic and transoesophageal assessment of left ventricular volume and ejection fraction is recommended over the use of 2D echo.

Assessment of right ventricular (RV) volume and function is also possible and has been validated in a selected group of patients. But the inability to obtain a full volume of the RV from one sector angle and difficulty in tracking the thin RV endocardium limit its use in all patients.

> **REFERENCE INTERVALS FOR 3D ECHO**
>
> It is important to be aware that the 3D echo reference intervals for left ventricular (LV) volumes and function are not the same as those derived from 2D echo. Generally speaking, LV volumes assessed by 3D echo are larger than those assessed by 2D echo, and the 3D echo reference intervals are closer to those seen with cardiovascular magnetic resonance imaging. When interpreting measurements obtained using 3D echo, be sure to use an appropriate dataset for your reference intervals.

Assessment of morphology and function

The ability to visualize an image in 3D and the facility to crop and view a structure from any anatomical plane make 3D echo an invaluable tool in the assessment of morphology and function. This is mostly useful in the assessment of valvular and congenital heart disease. It has already made a major impact in the diagnosis and treatment of mitral valve disease and is routinely recommended for its assessment. Similarly, 3D echo has provided additional insights into the understanding of various congenital heart diseases such as Ebstein's anomaly and atrio-ventricular septal defects (Chapter 33).

Guiding interventional procedures

Perioperative imaging of the mitral valve is routinely carried out during mitral valve surgery. In addition, 3D echo is a popular imaging modality for percutaneous structural heart disease interventions. The ability to reproduce a real-time anatomic view using live 3D imaging provides effective and accurate guidance to the operator. Currently, percutaneous closure of atrial and ventricular septal defects in children are done almost entirely under transoesophageal 3D echo guidance and many other procedures such as transcatheter aortic valve implantation, mitral clip, device occlusion of the left atrial appendage, paravalvular leak closure and catheter ablation use transoesophageal 3D echo guidance in addition to fluoroscopy.

LIMITATIONS AND FUTURE DIRECTIONS

Although 3D echo is a major advance in the field of echo, the uptake of this technique into routine practice has been limited by a number of factors. Until recently, separate transducers were required for 2D and 3D imaging. This is because the early generation 3D transducers did not provide sufficient quality for 2D and Doppler imaging. The latest generation of transthoracic and transoesophageal transducers have overcome this problem, enabling a single transducer to be used for the full echo examination.

Because of the trade-offs between sector size and spatial and temporal resolution, live 3D imaging has tended to use narrow sector widths. However, gradual improvements in processing power are steadily reducing the limitations of these trade-offs, allowing larger volume real-time 3D imaging with ever-improving image quality.

Direct measurement on a 3D image is not possible. All measurements and analysis are currently done using special software packages and are specific to the manufacturer. This is time-consuming and expensive. The availability of generic software packages capable of online and offline analyses will make the technique more user-friendly and will enable images to be stored and retrieved using any picture archiving and communications system.

Although the use of 3D echo by an experienced operator improves diagnostic accuracy and confidence, clinical evidence supporting its superiority over 2D echo remains somewhat limited. More studies confirming its value in clinical decision-making will enable this technique to realize its full potential in clinical practice.

Further reading

Lang RM et al. EAE/ASE recommendations for image acquisition and display using three-dimensional echocardiography. *European Heart Journal: Cardiovascular Imaging* (2012). PMID 22275509.

Lang RM et al. 3-Dimensional echocardiography: latest developments and future directions. *Journal of the American College of Cardiology: Cardiovascular Imaging* (2018). PMID 30522687.

Simpson J et al. Three-dimensional echocardiography in congenital heart disease: an expert consensus document from the European Association of Cardiovascular Imaging and the American Society of Echocardiography. *European Heart Journal: Cardiovascular Imaging* (2016). PMID 27655864.

Vegas A. Three-dimensional transesophageal echocardiography: principles and clinical applications. *Annals of Cardiac Anaesthesia* (2016). PMID 27762247.

CHAPTER 14

Intravascular ultrasound and epicardial echo

INTRAVASCULAR ULTRASOUND

Intravascular ultrasound (IVUS) provides direct imaging of the coronary arteries, using a miniature ultrasound probe that can be passed down the coronary arteries via a catheter. IVUS probes use very high-frequency ultrasound (typically 20–50 MHz) to image the wall of the artery, revealing not just the diameter of the lumen but also the characteristics of any atherosclerotic plaques (**Figure 14.1**).

Coronary angiography (p. 104) commonly underestimates the severity of coronary atherosclerosis, particularly when the atheroma is diffusely distributed. IVUS plays an important role in clarifying the extent of coronary atheroma and can help identify obstructive disease that might be overlooked by angiography alone. IVUS has also provided an insight into the phenomenon of coronary artery remodelling, in which the arterial diameter can increase as plaque accumulates, preserving the diameter of the lumen (so the vessel looks unobstructed on angiography) even though significant atheroma is present (as revealed by IVUS).

IVUS can also be helpful in guiding coronary artery stenting in percutaneous coronary intervention procedures, helping the operator determine the optimal length and diameter of stent for the lesion being treated. Performing an IVUS study immediately after stent deployment allows an assessment of how well-deployed the stent is, i.e., whether it is fully expanded and well-apposed to the walls of the artery.

EPICARDIAL ECHO

The use of TOE during surgical procedures has grown over recent years, not only in the assessment of structural heart disease during cardiac surgery but also in monitoring cardiac performance more generally. However, not all patients can undergo such an intraoperative TOE examination, and in these cases, epicardial echo provides a useful alternative (**Table 14.1**).

Epicardial echo involves placing an echo probe directly on the surface of the heart while the heart is exposed during a sternotomy. The probe must of course be kept sterile, and so it is placed within a sterile sheath together with some acoustic gel. As there are no intervening structures during epicardial echo, an echo probe with a higher frequency than a normal transthoracic probe can be used and this will enhance image quality. Seven standard views are recommended by the American Society of Echocardiography and the Society of Cardiovascular Anesthesiologists (**Table 14.2**).

DOI: 10.1201/9781003304654-14

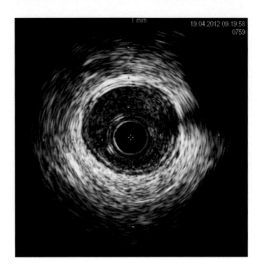

Figure 14.1   Intravascular ultrasound.

Table 14.1   Indications for epicardial echo

Epicardial echo can be used as an alternative to intraoperative TOE in patients where:

- There are oesophageal abnormalities that contraindicate the passage of a TOE probe
- Attempts to pass a TOE probe have been unsuccessful
- Areas need to be inspected that cannot be clearly visualized with intraoperative TOE

Abbreviation: TOE: Transoesophageal echo.

Table 14.2   Epicardial echo views and transthoracic echo (TTE) equivalents

Epicardial echo view	Equivalent TTE view
Aortic valve short axis	Parasternal aortic valve short axis
Aortic valve long axis	Suprasternal aortic valve long axis
Left ventricular basal short axis	Modified parasternal mitral valve basal short axis
Left ventricular mid short axis	Parasternal mid-left ventricle short axis
Left ventricular long axis	Parasternal long axis
Two-chamber	Modified parasternal long axis
Right ventricular outflow tract	Parasternal short axis

Further reading

Mintz GS et al. American College of Cardiology clinical expert consensus document on standards for acquisition, measurement and reporting of intravascular ultrasound studies (IVUS). A report of the American College of Cardiology Task Force on Clinical Expert Consensus Documents. *Journal of the American College of Cardiology* (2001). PMID 11300468.

Neumann FJ et al. 2018 ESC/EACTS guidelines on myocardial revascularization. *European Heart Journal* (2019). PMID 30165437.

Räber L et al. Clinical use of intracoronary imaging. Part 1: guidance and optimization of coronary interventions. An expert consensus document of the European Association of Percutaneous Cardiovascular Interventions. *European Heart Journal* (2018). PMID 29790954.

Reeves ST et al. Guidelines for performing a comprehensive epicardial echocardiography examination: recommendations of the American Society of Echocardiography and the Society of Cardiovascular Anesthesiologists. *Journal of the American Society of Echocardiography* (2007). PMID 17400124.

CHAPTER 15

Alternative cardiac imaging techniques

Echo is not the only technique for diagnostic imaging of the heart. Several cardiac imaging techniques are available, some of which provide similar information to echo (e.g., assessment of left ventricular [LV] function with cardiovascular magnetic resonance imaging [MRI]) and some of which can provide additional information about the heart that echo alone cannot obtain (e.g., visualization of coronary artery stenoses with coronary angiography). Knowledge of these alternative imaging techniques can help you decide when another test might replace or supplement an echo study.

NUCLEAR CARDIOLOGY

Nuclear cardiology uses radioactive isotopes, administered intravenously, to image the heart and to provide information about myocardial perfusion (myocardial perfusion imaging) and ventricular function (radionuclide ventriculography).

Uses of nuclear cardiology

Myocardial perfusion imaging uses a radiopharmaceutical (e.g., thallium-201 or technetium-99m-labelled radiopharmaceutical) to assess myocardial blood flow, providing valuable information about coronary artery disease with a high degree of sensitivity and specificity (**Figure 15.1**).

After the radiopharmaceutical has been administered intravenously, its distribution in the myocardium can be assessed using single-photon emission computed tomography (SPECT) imaging. Imaging is performed at rest and again after stress (exercise or pharmacological), and comparison of the rest and stress images allows identification of areas of normal perfusion, reversible ischaemia (normal perfusion at rest but reduced perfusion after stress) and fixed ischaemia (reduced perfusion at rest and after stress). The use of ECG gating also allows myocardial function to be assessed with the calculation of a LV ejection fraction.

Radionuclide ventriculography gives an accurate assessment of ventricular function. It is most commonly performed using red blood cells labelled with technetium-99m which are administered intravenously. The count rate of the radioactivity can be measured using a gamma camera over many cardiac cycles and, with the use of ECG gating, the average count rate at different stages of the cardiac cycle can be calculated. From this, an accurate measure of ejection fraction can be derived.

Disadvantages of nuclear cardiology

The principal drawback of nuclear cardiology is the patient's exposure to ionizing radiation. The typical effective radiation dose of a ^{99m}Tc dynamic cardiac scan is 6 mSv, equivalent to 2.7 years' exposure to natural background radiation. For a ^{201}Tl myocardial perfusion scan, the typical dose

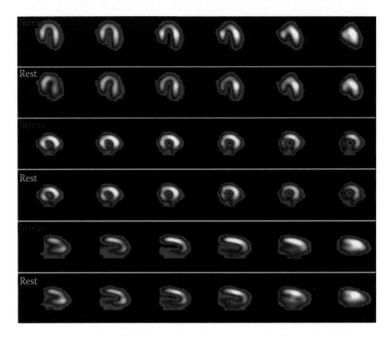

Figure 15.1   Myocardial perfusion imaging (showing inferior wall defect).

is 18 mSv, equivalent to 8 years' background radiation (for comparison, the typical dose of a single chest X-ray is 0.014 mSv, equivalent to about 2 days' background radiation).

CARDIOVASCULAR MAGNETIC RESONANCE IMAGING

MRI is a highly versatile technique for cardiovascular imaging and provides both anatomical and functional information. Cardiovascular MRI is performed with a scanner containing a large super-conducting magnet; radio waves are transmitted into the heart, aligning hydrogen nuclei, and as the nuclei subsequently 'relax', they emit radio waves of their own which can be detected by the scanner. The detected signal can then be used to reconstruct an image of the heart (**Figure 15.2**).

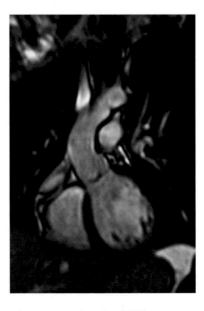

Figure 15.2   Cardiovascular magnetic resonance imaging (MRI) scan.

Uses of cardiovascular MRI

One of the great advantages of cardiovascular MRI over many other cardiac imaging techniques is the wide range of information that it can provide: In addition to anatomical information (usually with excellent image quality), cardiovascular MRI can also measure blood flow velocities, making it suitable for the assessment of valvular abnormalities and shunts. Its uses include the assessment of

- cardiac chamber dimensions and function
- valvular heart disease
- cardiomyopathies
- cardiac masses
- congenital heart disease
- pericardial disease
- aortic abnormalities

Cardiovascular MRI does not have the spatial resolution to image the coronary arteries very well, but it can nevertheless aid in the assessment of coronary artery disease. A cardiovascular MRI scan can be combined with pharmacological stress, as for stress echo, to identify myocardial ischaemia, necrosis and viability. The use of a gadolinium-based contrast agent can provide valuable information on myocardial perfusion and viability.

Disadvantages of cardiovascular MRI

Although cardiovascular MRI does not involve exposure to ionizing radiation, it does expose the patient to a powerful magnetic field and is therefore contraindicated in patients with certain types of metallic implants (e.g., some pacemakers and implantable defibrillators). Some patients with claustrophobia are unable to tolerate the enclosed conditions found in many MRI scanners. For certain cardiovascular MRI studies, patients require an intravenous injection of a gadolinium-based contrast agent, and in patients with renal impairment, this may pose a risk of nephrogenic systemic fibrosis.

CARDIAC COMPUTED TOMOGRAPHY

The development of multislice computed tomography (MSCT) has led to the increasing use of CT scanning to image the heart. MSCT scanners contain a gantry carrying an X-ray source and a number of detectors that rotate around the patient. Multiple image 'slices' are obtained as the patient is moved through the gantry during the scan, and an ECG is also recorded. The slices are then processed by the appropriate software, and the ECG data can be used to 'gate' the images so that the heart can be examined at different points in the cardiac cycle. Processing of the imaging data allows the heart to be viewed in any plane and from any angle, either as a 3D volume-rendered image or as cross-sectional slices (**Figure 15.3**).

Cardiac CT scanners typically have 64 or more slices, and many offer 256 or 320 slices. Cardiac CT scanning is very fast, as it typically takes no more than 15 seconds to acquire the images. However, some patient preparation is required, as cardiac studies require the injection of an intravascular contrast agent and many patients also require a beta-blocker to slow their heart rate. Examining and reporting the images usually takes 10–30 minutes, depending on the complexity of the case.

Uses of cardiac CT

The main use of MSCT is in the assessment of the coronary arteries. A calcium score can be obtained, which reflects the amount of calcification present in the coronary arteries; this information can then be used to estimate the patient's risk of future cardiovascular events. The coronary arteries themselves can be imaged with the use of contrast (CT angiography [CTA]), and plaque

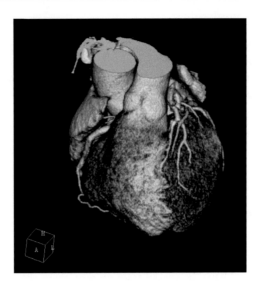

Figure 15.3   Cardiac computed tomography (CT) (volume-rendered image).

disease can be identified. The functional significance of coronary plaques can be evaluated with the CT perfusion imaging and also by the CT evaluation of fractional flow reserve (FFR_{CT}). High-risk coronary lesions can be identified using plaque characterization, and advanced techniques to measure wall shear stress and perivascular inflammation have been developed.

MSCT can also be used to image the cardiac chambers, allowing measurements to be made, and movie images show ventricular function. Cardiac masses can be examined, as can congenital abnormalities. Unfortunately, cardiac CT does not provide information on blood flow, but it does allow valvular morphology to be assessed.

Disadvantages of cardiac CT

Cardiac CT involves exposure to ionizing radiation, and patients do need to have a relatively slow (and regular) pulse and must be able to hold their breath during the scan. For the assessment of the heart valves and chambers, echo and/or MRI is generally the preferred modality, but for coronary artery visualization, cardiac CT offers a valuable non-invasive modality (and an alternative to cardiac catheterization).

CARDIAC CATHETERIZATION

Cardiac catheterization allows imaging of the coronary arteries and cardiac chambers (using a contrast agent) and also the measurement of intracardiac pressures and oxygen saturations. It is an invasive technique, requiring a catheter to be passed to the heart via a peripheral vessel.

In the case of a left heart study, the catheter is passed under local anaesthetic into the radial or femoral artery and then guided to the heart under fluoroscopic screening. Once the catheter is in position, a contrast agent is injected to visualize the left and right coronary arteries in turn (coronary angiography, **Figure 15.4**). Larger volumes of contrast can be used to visualize the LV and aorta. Intracardiac pressure measurements can be taken, and blood can be sampled from the tip of the catheter to assess the oxygen saturation. For a right heart study, the catheter is passed via the femoral vein and again allows intracardiac pressure and oxygen saturation measurements. Cardiac output can also be calculated.

Uses of cardiac catheterization

Cardiac catheterization is most commonly used to assess the coronary arteries in cases of suspected coronary artery disease. Although echo can provide information about myocardial ischaemia

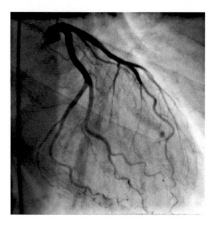

Figure 15.4 Coronary angiogram (showing left coronary artery).

(e.g., regional LV wall motion abnormalities), it cannot visualize the coronary arteries themselves. Cardiac catheterization also has a role to play in supplementing the echo assessment of valvular, LV and congenital cardiac abnormalities.

Disadvantages of cardiac catheterization

Cardiac catheterization is an invasive procedure, carrying a risk of trauma to the vessels where catheters are inserted; it also carries the risk of arrhythmias, myocardial infarction, stroke and death. There is also exposure to radiation and an intravascular contrast agent.

IMAGING FOR SUSPECTED STABLE ANGINA

The National Institute for Health and Clinical Excellence (NICE) has produced guidance on the appropriate selection of cardiac imaging tests for intermittent stable chest pain in people with suspected stable angina. For those with no prior diagnosis of coronary artery disease, if clinical assessment indicates typical or atypical angina, then 64-slice (or more) CT coronary angiography should be offered. This is also the case if the clinical assessment indicates non-anginal chest pain, but a 12-lead resting ECG has been done that indicates ST-T changes or Q waves. However, where patients already have a background history of confirmed coronary artery disease, then non-invasive functional imaging should be offered instead when there is uncertainty about whether their chest pain is caused by myocardial ischaemia. See the full NICE guidance at www.nice.org.uk/guidance/CG95 for further details.

Further reading

Kelion A et al. *Nuclear Cardiology.* 2nd ed. (Oxford University Press, 2017).

Mitchell A et al. *Cardiac Catheterization and Coronary Intervention.* 2nd ed. (Oxford University Press, 2020).

Pfeiffer MP et al. Cardiac MRI: a general overview with emphasis on current use and indications. *Medical Clinics of North America* (2015). PMID 26042886.

Serruys PW et al. Coronary computed tomographic angiography for complete assessment of coronary artery disease: JACC state-of-the-art review. *Journal of the American College of Cardiology* (2021). PMID 34384554.

Stirrup J et al. *Cardiovascular Computed Tomography.* 2nd ed. (Oxford University Press, 2019).

PART III: CLINICAL CASES

CHAPTER 16

The left ventricle and its systolic function

In many echo departments, assessment of left ventricular (LV) function is the single commonest echo request. One reason for this is that symptoms and signs that can indicate heart failure are common and echo is a non-invasive, straightforward and relatively inexpensive technique for confirming whether LV dysfunction is present. This chapter will cover the assessment of LV dimensions and overall LV systolic function. The assessment of regional systolic function, in the context of coronary artery disease, is discussed in Chapter 17, and LV diastolic function is covered in Chapter 18.

The key challenge in using echo to assess the LV lies in summarizing the size and function of a complex 3D structure using just a handful of parameters. Trying to represent the LV within a limited number of measurements is fraught with pitfalls, not least when using volumetric measures that rely on assumptions about the geometrical shape of the LV, which are not necessarily correct, particularly if the shape of the LV is distorted or abnormalities are limited just to one or two areas of the ventricular wall. The key is to use common sense – if there is a clear discrepancy between your 'eyeball' assessment of the LV and the figures coming out of your calculations, highlight this in your report.

A comprehensive echo evaluation of the LV includes the assessment of:

- LV dimensions
  - LV shape
  - wall thickness
  - cavity size
- LV mass
- LV systolic function
  - global function
  - regional function (see Chapter 17)
- LV diastolic function (see Chapter 18)
- LV outflow tract (LVOT) morphology (see Chapter 29)
- LV masses or thrombus (see Chapter 32)

If you haven't already done so, you may also find it helpful to read the chapters on myocardial mechanics (Chapter 5), tissue Doppler imaging (Chapter 11) and speckle tracking (Chapter 12).

LV DIMENSIONS

In measuring LV dimensions, it is important not to 'miss the wood for the trees' – as LV measurements only provide a selective snapshot of the LV in the regions where the measurements are taken, you must ensure that your report also includes a description of any abnormalities that

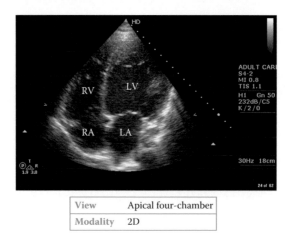

View	Apical four-chamber
Modality	2D

Figure 16.1 Dilated left ventricle. *Abbreviations*: LA: Left atrium, LV: Left ventricle, RA: Right atrium, RV: Right ventricle.

are not reflected in the figures alone. Take time to 'eyeball' the LV as a whole in several views (at least part of the LV is visible in almost every standard view of the heart), and if the overall shape is abnormal, be sure to describe this (**Figure 16.1**). A good example of this is the presence of an LV aneurysm, in which case describe its location and identify whether it is a true aneurysm or a pseudoaneurysm (Chapter 17), or the presence of a localized area of hypertrophy in hypertrophic cardiomyopathy.

Linear LV measurements

Linear LV measurements should be made using 2D echo in the parasternal long-axis view, immediately below the mitral valve leaflet tips and perpendicular to the LV long axis (**Figure 16.2**). The routine use of M-mode echo to make LV measurements is discouraged by the British Society of Echocardiography, although it can be used if the LV long axis is perpendicular to the ultrasound

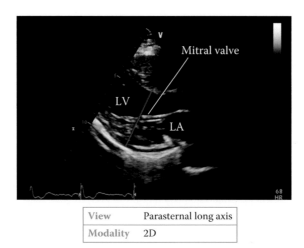

View	Parasternal long axis
Modality	2D

Figure 16.2 Measurement of LV internal diameter in diastole (red line) using 2D echo. *Abbreviations*: LA: Left atrium, LV: Left ventricle.

END-DIASTOLE AND END-SYSTOLE

A review of the echo literature reveals several definitions of end-diastole and end-systole. The routine use of the ECG to identify these time points is discouraged, except where it is unavoidable, as it can be affected by the choice of ECG lead and the presence of conduction defects. The British Society of Echocardiography advocates the following definitions:

End-diastole is defined as the frame before mitral valve closure. If this is not feasible (for instance, if the mitral valve is not visible in the view in question), then surrogates include the frame with the largest LV cavity size, the start of the QRS complex on the ECG or the ECG R wave.

End-systole is defined as the frame where the aortic valve initially closes. When using pulsed-wave (PW) Doppler, a 'closure click' is seen at this point. A surrogate definition, where necessary, is the frame before mitral valve opening.

beam. Be sure to identify end-diastole and end-systole (see the box **End-Diastole and End-Systole**) and the endocardial/epicardial borders correctly.

At the level of the mitral valve leaflet tips, measure the following LV dimensions perpendicular to the LV long axis at end-diastole:

- IVSd (interventricular septal thickness in diastole)
- LVIDd (LV internal diameter in diastole)
- LVPWd (LV posterior wall thickness in diastole)

Then, at end-systole measure

- LVIDs (LV internal diameter in systole)

The echo machine will display the measurements as you make them and will sometimes also display a number of calculated parameters (e.g., ejection fraction, fractional shortening) based on these measurements (**Figure 16.2**).

Table 16.1 shows the linear LV measurement reference intervals for males and females.

Table 16.1   Linear left ventricular measurement reference intervals for males and females

	Normal	Mild	Moderate	Severe
Males				
LVIDd (mm)	37–56	57–61	61–65	>65
LVIDs (mm)	22–41	41–45	46–50	>50
IVSd (mm)	6–12	–	–	–
LVPWd (mm)	6–12	–	–	–
Females				
LVIDd (mm)	35–51	52–55	56–59	>59
LVIDs (mm)	20–37	38–42	43–46	>46
IVSd (mm)	5–11	–	–	–
LVPWd (mm)	6–12	–	–	–

Abbreviations: IVSd: Interventricular septal thickness in diastole, LVIDd: Left ventricular internal diameter in diastole, LVIDs: Left ventricular internal diameter in systole, LVPWd: Left ventricular posterior wall thickness in diastole.

Source: Reference intervals reproduced with permission of the British Society of Echocardiography.

COMMON PITFALLS

Pitfalls in the assessment of LV dimensions include

- failure to take measurements at the correct time points (end-systole or end-diastole)
- failure to take measurements perpendicular to the long axis of the LV
- failure to identify the endocardium correctly – be particularly careful to avoid mistaking chordae tendineae for the endocardium of the LV posterior wall

Volumetric LV measurements

Volumetric measurements are based upon the principle that LV volumes can be calculated from 2D measurements of the LV as long as certain assumptions about the shape of the LV apply. The more distorted the LV is (e.g., as a result of an aneurysm), the less reliable such volumetric measurements become.

Biplane Simpson's method

The biplane Simpson's method is the best (and most commonly used) way of calculating LV volumes. It is also known as biplane disc summation, as it works on the principle that the LV cavity can be considered a stack of elliptical discs of differing sizes from base to apex. If the volume of each disc is known (from its area and thickness), then the overall LV volume is equal to the volume of all the discs added together.

Echo machines automate much of the process and require the operator simply to measure the length of the LV (long axis) and to trace the outline of the LV endocardium in two planes: The apical four- and two-chamber views. Doing this requires the following:

1. In the apical four-chamber view, obtain the best view you can of the LV, paying particular attention to endocardial border definition and avoidance of foreshortening. The use of an echo contrast agent (Chapter 10) may help delineate the endocardium if the image quality is suboptimal.

2. Freeze a loop and find the end-diastolic image. Now trace the endocardial contour from the mitral valve annulus all the way down to the apex and then back up to the annulus on the opposite side. Ignore any papillary muscle that may be visible. The machine will normally join up the start and finish points with a straight line across the mitral valve, to enclose the entire LV cavity within the traced area. The machine will then automatically split the traced area into a stack of discs (usually 20).

3. Measure the length of the LV long axis from the apex to the midpoint of the mitral valve. The machine will now use these measurements to calculate LV end-diastolic volume (LVEDV, **Figure 16.3**).

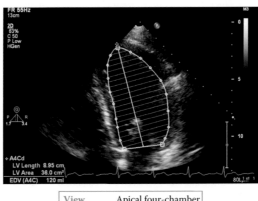

View	Apical four-chamber
Modality	2D

Figure 16.3   Measurement of LV volume using the modified Simpson's rule method. *Abbreviations:* EDV: End-diastolic volume, LV: Left ventricular.

4. Although a measurement taken in just one plane will give you a value for LVEDV and LVESV, this does make the assumption that each of the discs is circular. Repeating the measurements in the apical two-chamber view takes better account of the elliptical cross section of the LV and any regional wall motion abnormalities.

5. Scroll to the end-systolic frame and repeat Steps 2–4 to obtain the LV end-systolic volume (LVESV).

Area–length method

The area–length method can be useful for estimating LV volumes when the endocardium cannot be seen clearly enough to allow accurate tracing. However, it does make major assumptions (and simplifications) about the shape of the LV:

1. In the parasternal short-axis view, at mid-LV (papillary muscle) level, freeze a loop and find the end-diastolic frame. Perform planimetry by tracing the endocardial border to calculate the cross-sectional area (CSA) of the LV cavity at this level in cm^2. Ignore the presence of the papillary muscles as you trace the endocardium.

2. In the apical four-chamber view, in the end-diastolic frame, measure the length of the LV long axis from the apex to the midpoint of the mitral valve in cm.

3. The LVEDV, in mL, is given by the following formula:

$$LVEDV = \frac{5 \times Area \times Length}{6}$$

4. Scroll to the end-systolic frame and repeat Steps 1–3 to obtain the LVESV.

Both LVEDV and LVESV should be indexed for the patient's body surface area (BSA), measured in m^2. The Mosteller formula is commonly used to calculate BSA:

$$BSA(m^2) = \sqrt{\frac{Height\ (cm) \times Weight\ (kg)}{3600}}$$

Table 16.2 shows the volumetric LV measurement reference intervals for males and females.

Table 16.2 Volumetric left ventricular measurement reference intervals for males and females

	Normal	Mildly dilated	Moderately dilated	Severely dilated
Males				
LVEDVi (mL/m²)	30–79	80–91	92–103	>103
LVESVi (mL/m²)	9–31	32–36	37–42	>42
LVEDV (mL)	53–156	–	–	–
LVESV (mL)	15–62	–	–	–
Females				
LVEDVi (mL/m²)	29–70	71–81	82–91	>91
LVESVi (mL/m²)	8–27	28–32	33–37	>37
LVEDV (mL)	46–121	–	–	–
LVESV (mL)	13–47	–	–	–

Abbreviations: LVEDV: Left ventricular end-diastolic volume, LVESV: Left ventricular end-systolic volume, LVEDVi: Left ventricular end-diastolic volume (indexed), LVESVi: Left ventricular endsystolic volume (indexed).

Source: Reference intervals reproduced with permission of the British Society of Echocardiography.

> **LV VOLUMES AND 3D ECHO**
>
> Three-dimensional echo gets around many of the problems inherent in assessing LV volumes using 2D echo. Because 3D echo can visualize the whole LV, volume calculations do not require any assumptions to be made about LV geometry. The assessment of LV volumes (and mass) using 3D echo is well-validated and shown to be more accurate (and reproducible) than 2D techniques (Chapter 13).

LV MASS

LV hypertrophy (LVH) is defined as an increase in overall LV myocardial mass which can result from either pressure overload or volume overload on the LV. Although it is common to think of LVH as equating to an increase in LV wall thickness, it is possible to have an increased myocardial mass (and therefore LVH) even with little or no wall thickening, for example, when the LV dilates in cases of chronic aortic regurgitation.

The echo assessment of LVH includes

- geometry of the LVH (concentric, eccentric, asymmetric)
- measurement of LV dimensions
- calculation of LV mass
- assessment of LV function (systolic and diastolic)
- a search for underlying causes, such as aortic stenosis or coarctation of the aorta

The geometry of LVH can be described qualitatively, and also quantitatively in terms of relative wall thickness (RWT):

$$RWT = \frac{IVSd + LVPWd}{LVIDd}$$

where,
  IVSd is the interventricular septal thickness in diastole;
  LVPWd is the LV posterior wall thickness in diastole;
  LVIDd is the LV internal diameter in diastole.

An RWT >0.42 defines **concentric** LVH (typically seen in response to increased *afterload*), whereas an RWT ≤0.42 indicates **eccentric** LVH (typically seen in response to increased *preload*), and there is evidence that concentric LVH carries a worse prognosis than eccentric LVH. There is also a scenario where LV mass is normal, but RWT is increased, and this is termed **concentric remodelling**.

LV mass using linear measurements

As described earlier under the 'Linear LV Measurements' section, use 2D (or M-mode) echo to obtain the following measurements (in cm) at end-diastole:

- IVSd
- LVIDd
- LVPWd

LV mass, in grams, can then be calculated using the following formula:

$$LV\ mass = \{[0.8 \times 1.04 \times ((LVIDd + LVPWd + IVSd)^3 - (LVIDd)^3)]\} + 0.6$$

Although this method has been widely used historically, it has a tendency to overestimate LV mass. It is particularly vulnerable to measurement errors, as the cubing of the linear measurements means that even small errors can become relatively large.

LV mass using volumetric measurements

Volumetric calculations of LV mass are based on measuring the LV cavity volume, as outlined above, and subtracting this from the total volume of the LV (enclosed within the epicardium). This subtraction leaves the 'shell' volume, i.e., the volume occupied by the ventricular myocardium. The LV mass then equals this 'shell' volume multiplied by the myocardial density (1.05 g/mL). There are several ways of going about this.

The **area–length formula** is based on the method used to calculate LVEDV, outlined under the 'Volumetric LV Measurements' section:

1. In the parasternal short-axis view, mid-LV (papillary muscle) level, freeze a loop and find the end-diastolic frame. Perform planimetry by tracing the endocardial border to calculate the endocardial CSA (A_2) of the LV at this level in cm². Ignore the presence of the papillary muscles as you trace the endocardium.
2. In the same view, perform planimetry by tracing the *epicardial* border to calculate the epicardial CSA (A_1) of the LV in cm².
3. Calculate the mean wall thickness (t) in cm using the following formula:

$$t = \sqrt{\frac{A_1}{\pi}} - \sqrt{\frac{A_2}{\pi}}$$

4. In the apical four-chamber view, in the end-diastolic frame, measure the length (L) of the LV long axis from the apex to the midpoint of the mitral valve in cm.
5. LV mass, in grams, is given by the following formula:

$$LV\ mass = 1.05 \times \left\{ [(5/6) \times A_1 \times (L + t)] - [(5/6) \times A_2 \times L] \right\}$$

The **truncated ellipsoid formula** is based on similar measurements but is more complex. Here the length of the LV long axis (L), as measured from the apical four-chamber view, is split into two by the short-axis plane in which the planimetry of the LV CSAs was performed. The distance from the apex to the short-axis plane is denoted by 'a', and from this plane to the mitral annulus plane by 'd', both measured in cm. There is also a further variable 'b', which is the short-axis radius given by the following formula:

$$b = \sqrt{\frac{A_2}{\pi}}$$

LV mass, in grams, is given by the following formula:

$$LV\ mass = 1.05 \times \pi \left\{ (b+t)^2 \left[\left\{ \frac{2}{3}(a+t) + d - \frac{d^3}{3(a+t)^2} \right\} - b^2 \left\{ \frac{2}{3}a + d - \frac{d^3}{3a^2} \right\} \right] \right\}$$

Table 16.3 shows the LV mass reference intervals for males and females.

Table 16.3   Left ventricular mass reference intervals for males and females

	Normal	Mild	Moderate	Severe
Males				
LVMi (g/m²)	40–110	111–127	128–145	>145
LV mass (g)	72–219	–	–	–
Females				
LVMi (g/m²)	33–99	100–115	116–131	>131
LV mass (g)	51–173	–	–	–

Abbreviations: LV: Left ventricle, LVMi: Left ventricular mass (indexed).
Source: Reference intervals reproduced with permission of the British Society of Echocardiography.

COMMON PITFALLS

Pitfalls in the assessment of LV mass include the following:

- Linear measurements:
  - small measurement errors can become greatly magnified because of the cubing of LV dimensions in the linear LV mass formula
  - do not use linear measurements in cases with distorted LV geometry (e.g., isolated areas of hypertrophy)
- Volumetric measurements:
  - failure to trace the endocardium or epicardium accurately

---

LEFT VENTRICULAR SYSTOLIC FUNCTION

The assessment of LV systolic function forms a cornerstone of any echo study and is an essential part of the management of patients with suspected systolic heart failure, which is a common condition with considerable morbidity and mortality.

Heart failure

Heart failure affects 1%–2% of the adult population and is particularly common in the elderly, affecting ≥10% of those aged over 70 years. Heart failure is regarded as a clinical syndrome in which patients have the symptoms and signs of heart failure (**Table 16.4**) together with objective evidence of a structural or functional cardiac abnormality at rest.

Heart failure symptoms and signs can be an indicator of impaired LV systolic function, but can also occur despite normal systolic function (e.g., in diastolic dysfunction, see Chapter 18). Patients with

Table 16.4   Clinical features of heart failure

Symptoms	Signs
May be asymptomatic	Tachycardia, gallop rhythm
Breathlessness	Tachypnoea
Fatigue	Elevated jugular venous pressure
Ankle swelling	Cardiomegaly
	Pulmonary congestion/Oedema
	Peripheral oedema
	Ascites
	Hepatomegaly

the symptoms and/or signs of heart failure are categorized according to their LV ejection fraction (LVEF) as follows:

- *LVEF ≤40%*: HFrEF (Heart failure with reduced ejection fraction)
- *LVEF 41–49%*: HFmrEF (Heart failure with mildly reduced ejection fraction)
- *LVEF ≥50%*: HFpEF (Heart failure with preserved ejection fraction)

There are many causes of systolic heart failure, including

- coronary artery disease
- hypertension
- valvular disease
- viral myocarditis
- cardiomyopathy (Chapter 29)
- cardiotoxic drugs, e.g., anthracyclines, trastuzumab
- arrhythmias
- alcohol

The diagnostic algorithm for someone with symptoms and/or signs suspicious of heart failure begins with a blood test to check the patient's N-terminal pro-B-type natriuretic peptide (NT-pro-BNP) level. In the United Kingdom, the National Institute for Health and Care Excellence (2018) recommends referral for a specialist assessment and echo as follows:

- *NT-pro-BNP >2000 ng/L*: Urgent assessment and echo (within 2 weeks)
- *NT-pro-BNP 400–2000 ng/L*: Assessment and echo (within 6 weeks)

Heart failure is less likely with an NT-pro-BNP <400 ng/L and the diagnosis should be reconsidered, with discussion with a heart failure specialist if appropriate.

LV ejection fraction

Measurement of LVEF is the cornerstone of the echo assessment of suspected heart failure. LVEF is the most widely quoted measure of LV systolic performance, and expresses (as a percentage) the proportion of blood pumped out of the LV with each heartbeat.

LVEF is calculated from the LVEDV and LVESV obtained, as described earlier, using 2D echo in the four- and two-chamber views:

$$LVEF = \frac{LVEDV - LVESV}{LVEDV} \times 100\%$$

The reference intervals for LVEF are the same for males and females, as shown in **Table 16.5**. A normal ejection fraction (EF) is ≥55%. The British Society of Echocardiography guidelines no longer make a distinction between 'mild' and 'moderate' impairment of LV systolic function – patients with an LVEF of 36%–49% are described simply as having 'impaired LVEF'.

It is also possible to estimate EF using linear rather than volumetric measurements (Teicholz method). However, this takes no account of variations in regional wall motion and is highly prone to inaccuracies, so it should be avoided.

Table 16.5   Left ventricular ejection fraction (LVEF) reference intervals

Normal	Normal LVEF	Borderline low LVEF	Impaired LVEF	Severely impaired LVEF
LVEF (%)	≥55	50–54	36–49	≤35

Source: Reference intervals reproduced with permission of the British Society of Echocardiography.

Other echo parameters of LV systolic function

Apart from LVEF, there are several other echo parameters for the quantification of LV systolic function, and these are discussed next. As the assessment of LV function is based on many of the linear and/or volumetric measurements already discussed in this chapter, the same pitfalls apply. The calculations assume that the LV has a regular geometrical shape and that the function of each segment of the LV is the same. It is therefore important to be aware of the limitations of each of the following methods and to use them judiciously. The key point is to use common sense – if there is a clear discrepancy between how LV function appears to you and the figures coming out of your calculations, highlight this in your report.

Fractional shortening

Fractional shortening (FS) is a measure of the percentage change in LV dimensions between diastole and systole. A normal FS lies in the range of 25%–43%. FS is calculated from the LVIDd and LVIDs:

$$FS = \frac{LVIDd - LVIDs}{LVIDd} \times 100\%$$

Stroke distance

Stroke distance (SD) is the average distance travelled by the blood leaving the LV with each heartbeat. In the apical five-chamber view, use PW Doppler to measure the velocity time integral (VTI) of outflow in the LVOT to give VTI_{LVOT} (in cm). Place the sample volume at the level of the aortic valve annulus, just proximal to the cusps. SD equals the VTI_{LVOT}. A normal SD is in the range of 18–22 cm.

Stroke volume

Stroke volume (SV) is the quantity of blood ejected into the aorta by the LV with each heartbeat. It can be measured as follows:

1. In the parasternal long-axis view, measure the diameter of the LVOT in cm at the level of the aortic valve annulus, just proximal to the cusps (**Figure 16.4**), and use this to calculate the CSA of the LVOT in cm²:

$$CSA_{LVOT} = 0.785 \times (LVOT\,Diameter)^2$$

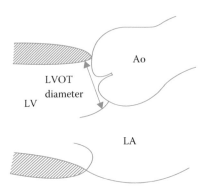

Figure 16.4 Measurement of LVOT diameter. *Abbreviations:* Ao: Aorta, LA: Left atrium, LV: Left ventricle, LVOT: Left ventricular outflow tract.

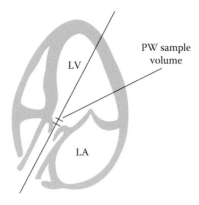

Figure 16.5 Positioning of sample volume for pulsed-wave (PW) Doppler of left ventricular outflow tract velocity time integral (VTI). *Abbreviations:* LA: Left atrium, LV: Left ventricle.

2. In the apical five-chamber view, use PW Doppler to measure the VTI of outflow in the LVOT. Place the sample volume at the level of the aortic valve annulus, at the same point where the LVOT diameter was measured (**Figure 16.5**) and obtain a PW trace of flow in the LVOT to measure VTI_{LVOT} (in cm) (**Figure 16.6**).

3. The LV SV, in mL/beat, can then be calculated from the following formula:

$$SV = CSA_{LVOT} \times VTI_{LVOT}$$

A normal SV lies in the range of 60–100 mL/beat. The calculation of SV depends on a good alignment of the Doppler interrogation angle with the direction of flow and upon the assumption that flow in the LVOT is laminar and the LVOT cross section is circular. It is essential to measure the LVOT diameter as accurately as possible. In principle, SV can be measured anywhere in the heart where a CSA and VTI can be measured, but in practical terms, measurement at the LVOT is relatively straightforward.

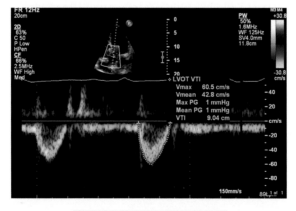

View	Apical five-chamber
Modality	PW Doppler

Figure 16.6 Pulsed-wave (PW) Doppler of left ventricular outflow tract (LVOT). *Abbreviations:* PG: Pressure gradient, V_{max}: Peak velocity, V_{mean}: Mean velocity, VTI: Velocity time integral.

Stroke volume index

Stroke volume index (SVI) is SV adjusted for BSA, measured in mL/beat/m^2:

$$SVI = \frac{SV}{BSA}$$

Cardiac output

Cardiac output (CO) can be calculated from the SV and the heart rate (HR, in beats/min). A normal CO is 4–8 L/min:

$$CO = \frac{SV \times HR}{1000}$$

Cardiac index

Cardiac index (CI) is CO adjusted for BSA, measured in L/min/m^2:

$$CI = \frac{CO}{BSA}$$

Rate of ventricular pressure rise (dP/dt)

With normal LV systolic function, the rate of rise in ventricular pressure (dP/dt) during systole is rapid. If systolic function is impaired, dP/dt starts to fall. The measurement of dP/dt requires the presence of mitral regurgitation:

1. In the apical four-chamber view, use CW Doppler to obtain a spectral trace of mitral regurgitation, ensuring careful alignment of the ultrasound beam with the regurgitant jet. Set the sweep speed as high as possible to 'spread out' the trace and make it easier to mark the relevant time points.

2. Using the trace, mark the points where the regurgitant jet velocity reaches 1 m/s and also 3 m/s. Measure the time interval (dt) between these two points in seconds (**Figure 16.7**).

3. At 1 m/s, the pressure gradient driving the regurgitant jet is 4 mmHg (Bernoulli equation), and at 3 m/s the gradient is 36 mmHg, giving a change in pressure gradients (dP) between the two velocities of 32 mmHg.

4. dP/dt is therefore calculated, in mmHg/s, by dividing the measured time interval (dt) into 32. The longer the duration of dt, and the smaller the value for dP/dt, the worse the LV systolic function. A normal LV will have a dP/dt >1200 mmHg/s (and a dt <0.027 second), whereas a severely impaired LV usually has a dP/dt <800 mmHg/s (and a dt >0.04 second).

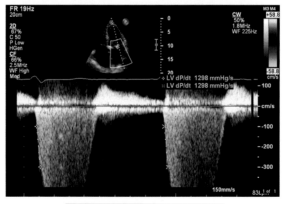

View	Apical four-chamber
Modality	CW Doppler

Figure 16.7 Measurement of the rate of rise in ventricular pressure (dP/dt). *Abbreviations:* CW: Continuous wave, LV: Left ventricle.

Do not use dP/dt if there is *acute* mitral regurgitation, or if there is significant aortic stenosis or hypertension.

Mitral valve E-point septal separation

Mitral valve E-point septal separation (EPSS, the distance between the E point or maximal anterior movement of the anterior mitral leaflet and the septum) is measured in the parasternal long-axis view using M-mode. EPSS is a reflection of mitral valve inflow and correlates with LV SV (as long as there is no significant mitral regurgitation). Normally, the mitral valve EPSS is between 0 and 5.3 mm, and a value >7 mm is indicative of impaired LV systolic function.

Further reading

Harkness A et al. Normal reference intervals for cardiac dimensions and function for use in echocardiographic practice: a guideline from the British Society of Echocardiography. *Echo Research and Practice* (2020). PMID 32105051.

Iyengar SS et al. Concentric vs. eccentric left ventricular hypertrophy: does it matter? It is all "blood pressure centered". *American Journal of Hypertension* (2021). PMID 33950166.

Lang RM et al. Recommendations for cardiac chamber quantification by echocardiography in adults: an update from the American Society of Echocardiography and the European Association of Cardiovascular Imaging. *Journal of the American Society of Echocardiography* (2015). PMID 25559473.

McDonagh TA et al. 2021 ESC guidelines for the diagnosis and treatment of acute and chronic heart failure. *European Heart Journal* (2021). PMID 34447992.

National Institute for Health and Care Excellence. (2018). https://www.nice.org.uk/guidance/ng106

CHAPTER 17

Coronary artery disease and regional left ventricular function

Chapter 16 looked at the global assessment of left ventricular (LV) dimensions and function. However, abnormalities of LV function can affect one or more specific areas of the LV wall and then the LV is said to show a regional wall motion abnormality (RWMA). RWMA is the result of coronary artery disease affecting the function of the myocardium, because the blood supply to a particular area of myocardium has become either reduced (ischaemia) or blocked altogether, causing death (necrosis) of the myocytes. The identification of RWMA by echo can therefore reveal a great deal about the status of the coronary circulation.

THE CORONARY ARTERIES

Normal coronary artery anatomy

As discussed in Chapter 2, the coronary circulation normally arises as two separate vessels from the sinuses of Valsalva – the left coronary artery (LCA) from the left sinus and the right coronary artery (RCA) from the right sinus (**Figure 2.5**, p. 5). The initial portion of the LCA is the left main stem which soon divides into the left anterior descending (LAD) and circumflex (Cx) arteries. The LAD runs down the anterior interventricular groove and the Cx runs in the left atrioventricular groove. The RCA runs in the right atrioventricular groove, and in most people gives rise to the posterior descending artery which runs down the posterior interventricular groove.

All the arteries supply branches to the myocardium in their respective territories, and as there is some anatomical variation from one person to the next, there can be a little variability in which vessel is responsible for supplying blood to each territory. Nonetheless, each vessel's territory is fairly well-defined and so wall motion abnormalities in a particular region give an indication of the coronary vessel(s) likely to be involved.

Regional left ventricular function

The LV is conventionally split into 16 or 17 different regions or 'segments'. In the 16-segment model, the LV is sliced longitudinally into three (basal, mid-cavity and apical). Both basal and mid-cavity slices contain six segments and the apical slice contains four segments. The American Heart Association's 17-segment model contains all these segments plus one more – an apical 'cap' (**Figure 17.1**). The 16-segment model remains popular for echo purposes, but if you are going to compare echo findings with other modalities (e.g., nuclear cardiology), then it is better to use the 17-segment model. Whichever model you choose, ensure that your nomenclature is consistent.

In the 17-segment model, the six segments in each of the basal and mid-cavity slices are termed anterior, anteroseptal, inferoseptal, inferior, inferolateral and anterolateral. The boundaries of the septum are defined by the attachment of the right ventricle (RV), and each of the six circumferential

DOI: 10.1201/9781003304654-17

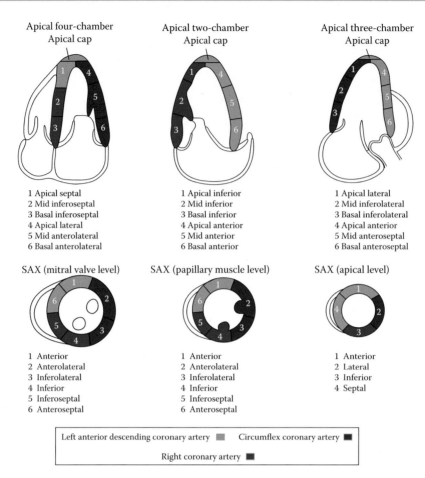

Figure 17.1   The 17-segment model of LV segmentation. *Abbreviation:* SAX: Short axis.

segments occupies 60° in the short-axis view. As the LV narrows towards the apex, there are just four apical segments – anterior, septal, inferior and lateral. The apical cap is at the very tip of the ventricle, where there is no LV cavity.

Each segment is assigned to one of the coronary arteries (LAD, Cx or RCA), as indicated by the colour-coding in **Figure 17.1**, although there can be some overlap depending on each individual's coronary anatomy. Normal wall motion during systole is indicated by an endocardial excursion >5 mm and by wall thickening >50%. Inspect each segment in turn, where possible in two separate views, and score it according to its motion:

- X = unable to interpret (suboptimal image quality)
- 1 = normal or hyperkinetic
- 2 = hypokinetic
- 3 = akinetic
- 4 = dyskinetic
- 5 = aneurysmal (diastolic deformation)

MYOCARDIAL ISCHAEMIA AND INFARCTION

Myocardial ischaemia results from the development of an atherosclerotic plaque in one or more coronary arteries, limiting the flow of blood to the myocardium downstream. This normally does not cause symptoms until the lumen is obstructed by ≥70%, at which point the patient develops exertional chest discomfort and/or breathlessness. The chest discomfort is typically central in location and heavy or tight in character, and may radiate into the neck and jaw and down one or both arms. The symptoms are rapidly relieved with rest and/or nitrates.

An acute coronary syndrome occurs when an atherosclerotic plaque ruptures, exposing the lipid-rich core to the bloodstream. This leads to the rapid formation of a thrombus which acutely obstructs flow down the coronary artery. If this leads to necrosis of a portion of myocardium, cardiac markers (e.g., troponins) will be released into the circulation, and the detection of these markers is one of the key diagnostic features of a myocardial infarction. Unstable symptoms without a rise in cardiac markers is termed unstable angina.

Echo assessment of myocardial ischaemia and infarction

The areas of myocardial ischaemia and infarction typically lead to hypokinetic, akinetic, dyskinetic or aneurysmal myocardial segments. By assessing wall motion in each of the LV segments, a comprehensive picture of LV regional wall motion can be compiled and likely abnormalities in the supplying coronary arteries identified. The assessment of regional LV function includes an assessment of LV dimensions, morphology and global LV systolic and diastolic function (see Chapters 16 and 18).

Myocardial ischaemia is frequently assessed by stress echo (see Chapter 9), in which any changes in wall motion are evaluated in response to exercise or pharmacological stress. In the classical ischaemic response, the myocardium is normokinetic at rest, but its wall motion worsens on stress.

Stress echo can also have an important role following **myocardial infarction**, identifying areas where the myocardium is still viable. The areas of myocardial necrosis are typically akinetic or hypokinetic at rest and remain unchanged with stress. However, sometimes improvement in wall motion is seen with stress, indicating that the myocardium is still viable but is stunned or hibernating. Stunned myocardium is likely to improve spontaneously with time, whereas hibernating myocardium will usually only improve with coronary revascularization.

Echo can help in the differential diagnosis of acute chest pain, which includes not just acute coronary syndromes but also conditions such as aortic dissection (p. 249) and pulmonary embolism. Echo is also important in the diagnosis of many of the complications of myocardial infarction, discussed later in this chapter.

Management of myocardial ischaemia and infarction

Myocardial ischaemia

Stable angina is managed with drugs to relieve symptoms and to reduce the risk of coronary thrombosis. Symptomatic relief can be obtained with glyceryl trinitrate used as required and with one or more regular anti-ischaemic agents (beta-blockers, calcium channel blockers, nitrates, nicorandil, ivabradine or ranolazine). Cardioprotective drugs include aspirin, statins and angiotensin-converting enzyme (ACE) inhibitors.

Unstable angina is also managed with cardioprotective and anti-ischaemic drugs, but with the addition of antithrombin therapy such as fondaparinux and antiplatelet agents such as ticagrelor, prasugrel or clopidogrel.

Coronary revascularization has an important role in patients with troublesome symptoms or a high risk of coronary events. Revascularization can be achieved with percutaneous coronary intervention (PCI) or coronary artery bypass grafting (CABG).

Myocardial infarction

Myocardial infarctions are subgrouped and managed according to the accompanying ECG changes. The presence of ST segment elevation defines an ST elevation myocardial infarction (STEMI) in which urgent restoration of coronary blood flow with primary PCI is required. Other ECG changes

(ST segment depression, T wave inversion) are seen in a non-STEMI (NSTEMI), in which the mainstay of therapy is aggressive treatment with antiplatelet and antithrombotic drugs and reduction in myocardial oxygen demand, followed by coronary angiography and coronary revascularization (as guided by symptoms and risk stratification).

COMPLICATIONS OF MYOCARDIAL INFARCTION

Cardiogenic shock

The development of hypotension after myocardial infarction is most commonly an indicator of extensive damage to the myocardium and consequent 'pump failure'. This is associated with a high mortality (around 50%) even with aggressive treatment. Urgent echo is required to assess the LV function and to rule out other causes of hypotension post-myocardial infarction such as papillary muscle rupture, ventricular septal defect (VSD) and cardiac rupture.

Echo is also important for assessing the RV in cases of suspected RV infarction (which can occur with an inferior myocardial infarction or on its own). RV infarction causes hypotension and a raised jugular venous pressure but in the absence of pulmonary oedema.

Echo assessment

Assess the dimensions and the global and regional function of both the LV and RV. Look for evidence of papillary muscle rupture or cardiac rupture and assess the interventricular septum to rule out VSD (see below).

Papillary muscle rupture

Acute severe mitral regurgitation can occur following myocardial infarction as a result of papillary muscle dysfunction or rupture. Papillary muscle dysfunction most commonly occurs in inferior myocardial infarction; where rupture occurs, it is often due to rupture of the posteromedial papillary muscle (which has a single blood supply, usually from the RCA or Cx artery) rather than the anterolateral papillary muscle (which has a dual blood supply). Patients may present with acute pulmonary oedema, cardiogenic shock and a new systolic murmur. Urgent surgical intervention is required.

Echo assessment

Use 2D imaging to assess the structure of the mitral valve leaflets, annulus, papillary muscles and chordae. In cases of papillary muscle rupture, look for evidence of a flail mitral leaflet with an attached piece of papillary muscle, and its chordal attachments, prolapsing into the left atrium (LA) during systole.

Use Doppler assessment to examine the nature and extent of mitral regurgitation, as outlined in Chapter 21. Assess the LV dimensions and function and LA dimensions (in acute severe mitral regurgitation, the LA will not have had time to dilate).

Be alert to alternative diagnoses – haemodynamic decompensation with a new systolic murmur can also occur in post-infarction VSD (described below).

Post-infarction ventricular septal defect

Rupture of the interventricular septum, due to a focal area of myocardial necrosis, causes an acquired VSD. There is usually a sudden deterioration in the patient's condition and a new harsh systolic murmur. It is associated with a high mortality and requires urgent surgical intervention.

Echo assessment

Assess the interventricular septum using 2D and colour Doppler to identify the location and size of the VSD – some post-infarction VSDs are small and can be challenging to find. Do not forget that post-infarction VSDs can be multiple, so check to see if there is more than one jet on colour

Doppler. Anterior infarcts are usually associated with apical VSDs, whereas inferior infarcts tend to cause VSDs in the basal inferoseptum (and have a worse prognosis).

Post-infarction VSDs can be 'simple', with a direct channel between the ventricles, or 'complex', tracking through the myocardium, sometimes for several centimetres (particularly in the case of inferior infarcts). Doppler imaging will show a left-to-right shunt, with a high-velocity jet. Assess the LV and RV dimensions and function. Surgeons are particularly interested in the size and function of the RV which helps predict prognosis.

Left ventricular aneurysm

Aneurysmal dilatation of the LV can occur in areas where the infarcted myocardium has become weakened and thinned. Patients may have clinical features of impaired LV function and persistent ST segment elevation on the ECG.

Echo assessment

Identify the region of the LV affected with reference to the usual segmental nomenclature. Look for the characteristic dyskinetic wall motion within the aneurysmal segment. In contrast with pseudoaneurysms (see below), 'true' aneurysms have a wide 'neck', which is at least half the diameter of the aneurysm itself (**Figure 17.2**) and are lined by myocardium rather than pericardium.

Look for evidence of mural thrombus, which can form as a consequence of impaired wall motion. Undertake a full assessment of LV systolic and diastolic function.

Mural thrombus

Mural thrombus can occur where stasis of blood occurs, for example within an LV aneurysm or on an akinetic segment (**Figure 32.3**, p. 259). Embolic risk is generally low, but is greater with mobile or protuberant thrombus than it is with laminated thrombus. Mural thrombus is most commonly seen at the LV apex following an anterior infarct. It can also be seen in the RV following an RV infarct. The assessment of intracardiac thrombus is described on page 258.

Ventricular rupture and cardiac tamponade

Rupture of the ventricular free wall is uncommon (occurring in 2.7% of myocardial infarctions), but is usually a devastating complication, causing rapid haemorrhage into the pericardium and fatal cardiac tamponade in around 75% of cases. However, sometimes the ventricular rupture can be contained by adhesions or thrombosis, causing a more stable (but nonetheless still extremely dangerous) situation which can, if time permits, be repaired surgically.

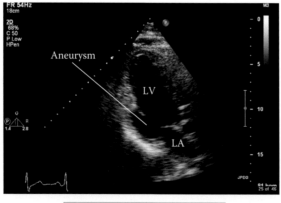

View	Apical three-chamber
Modality	2D

Figure 17.2   Left ventricular (LV) inferolateral wall aneurysm. *Abbreviation:* LA: Left atrium.

A chronic ventricular rupture is known as a pseudoaneurysm. The distinction between a 'true' aneurysm and a pseudoaneurysm is that the wall of a true aneurysm is composed of myocardium, but with a pseudoaneurysm, the myocardium has been breached and the pseudoaneurysm is lined by pericardium.

Echo assessment

Look for evidence of a pericardial effusion with associated thrombus in the pericardial space, particularly a localized effusion adjacent to an area of akinetic myocardium, and check for evidence of flow between the ventricle and the pericardium on colour Doppler. Assess the location and dimensions of the rupture (most cases involve the anterior wall) and the pericardial effusion and look for features of cardiac tamponade. The presence of a pericardial effusion after myocardial infarction does not, in itself, confirm a ventricular rupture, but should nonetheless raise a suspicion that a rupture may have occurred.

A pseudoaneurysm is well-demarcated from the surrounding myocardium and has a narrow 'neck', which is less than half the diameter of the aneurysm itself. Pseudoaneurysm most commonly affects the inferolateral (posterior) wall. Thrombus may be present within the aneurysm.

DRESSLER'S SYNDROME

A pericardial effusion may be seen following a myocardial infarction and is assessed as outlined in Chapter 30. Pericardial effusion occurring 1–8 weeks after the myocardial infarction is likely to be due to Dressler's syndrome, a form of pericarditis also known as post-myocardial infarction syndrome. Patients may present with pleuritic chest pain, fever and a pericardial friction rub. Dressler's syndrome is thought to be an autoimmune response, caused by the release of myocardial antigens, and is also seen in some patients after cardiac surgery (post-pericardiotomy syndrome).

Further reading

Collet JP et al. 2020 ESC Guidelines for the management of acute coronary syndromes in patients presenting without persistent ST-segment elevation. *European Heart Journal* (2020). PMID 32860058.

Damluji AA et al. Mechanical complications of acute myocardial infarction: a scientific statement from the American Heart Association. *Circulation* (2021). PMID 34126755.

Ibanez B et al. 2017 ESC guidelines for the management of acute myocardial infarction in patients presenting with ST-segment elevation. *European Heart Journal* (2017). PMID 28886621.

Knutti J et al. 2019 ESC Guidelines for the diagnosis and management of chronic coronary syndromes. *European Heart Journal* (2019). PMID 31504439.

National Institute for Health and Care Excellence. (2020). https://www.nice.org.uk/guidance/ng185

CHAPTER 18

Left ventricular diastolic function

The echo evaluation of left ventricular (LV) diastolic function is essential in patients presenting with symptoms or signs of heart failure. However, the original echo guidelines for diastolic function were complex and were applied inconsistently in clinical practice. As a result, the European Association of Cardiovascular Imaging and the American Society of Echocardiography jointly published a simplified guideline in 2016, and that guideline forms the foundation for this chapter.

Diastolic dysfunction is thought to reflect impaired relaxation of the LV, with or without reduced restoring forces, together with increased stiffness of the LV chamber. There are several conditions where the LV becomes less compliant:

- ageing
- hypertension
- LVH
- myocardial ischaemia
- aortic stenosis
- infiltrative cardiomyopathies

Impairment of LV relaxation increases the LV end-diastolic pressure, and this consequently impacts on the pulmonary circulation, leading to pulmonary congestion and breathlessness.

ECHO ASSESSMENT IN PATIENTS WITH A NORMAL LEFT VENTRICULAR EJECTION FRACTION

For patients with a normal left ventricular ejection fraction (LVEF), which in this context means an LVEF ≥50%, four echo parameters form the foundation of a diastolic function assessment:

- septal e′ velocity <7 cm/s or lateral e′ velocity <10 cm/s
- average E/e′ ratio >14
- tricuspid regurgitation (TR) velocity >2.8 m/s
- left atrial (LA) volume index >34 mL/m^2

The measurement of these four parameters is discussed in more detail below. The aim is to measure all four if possible (but as many of them as you can if not) in order to determine whether or not diastolic dysfunction is present. LV diastolic function is **normal** if more than half of the measured parameters do not meet the cut-off values specified above. Conversely, diastolic **dysfunction** is diagnosed if more than half the parameters meet these cut-off values. The study is **inconclusive** if precisely half the parameters do not meet the cut-off values (**Figure 18.1**).

DOI: 10.1201/9781003304654-18

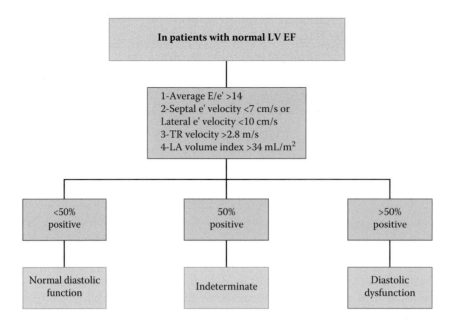

Figure 18.1   Algorithm for diagnosis of LV diastolic dysfunction in subjects with normal LVEF. *Abbreviations:* LA: Left atrial, LVEF: Left ventricular ejection fraction, TR: Tricuspid regurgitation. (From Nagueh SF et al., 2016. With permission of Oxford University Press and the European Society of Cardiology.)

Don't forget that any assessment of the LV diastolic function also needs to include a full assessment of the LV dimensions, mass and systolic function, as outlined in Chapter 16. Remember to look for features indicative of the underlying aetiology of diastolic dysfunction (e.g., aortic stenosis, ischaemic heart disease). The patient's heart rate (and rhythm) and blood pressure should also be recorded as part of a diastolic function study.

Septal e′ velocity and lateral e′ velocity

The method for measuring the mitral annular septal e′ velocity and lateral e′ velocity using tissue Doppler imaging was described in Chapter 11. Measure both velocities where possible. The abnormal cut-off value for septal e′ velocity is <7 cm/s and for lateral e′ velocity is <10 cm/s. Only one of these results (septal or lateral) needs to be below the cut-off value for one of the four diastolic dysfunction criteria to have been met.

Average E/e′ ratio

To calculate the average E/e′ ratio, begin by measuring the mitral E velocity. Perform pulsed-wave (PW) Doppler in the apical four-chamber view with a 1–3 mm sample volume placed between the tips of the mitral valve leaflets (**Figure 18.2**). Obtain a PW Doppler trace and measure the peak E velocity (**Figure 18.3**).

Next, calculate the average of the septal and the lateral mitral annular e′ velocities that you measured earlier. The average E/e′ ratio is calculated by dividing the peak mitral E wave velocity by the *average* e′ velocity. Although it's possible to quote separate E/e′ ratios for both the septal and the lateral mitral annulus, for simplicity, it's better to average the septal and lateral e′ values and use this average e′ to calculate the average E/e′ ratio.

The abnormal cut-off value for average E/e′ is >14.

Sometimes it's not possible to measure one of the mitral annular velocities, in which case an average e′ can't be calculated. In this case, you can calculate the septal E/e′ or the lateral E/e′ instead, depending upon which one you were able to measure. However, the abnormal cut-off values are slightly different if you do this: The cut-off value is >15 for a septal E/e′ and >13 for a lateral E/e′.

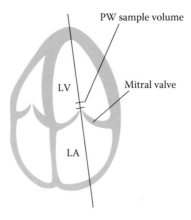

Figure 18.2 Positioning of sample volume for pulsed-wave (PW) Doppler of mitral valve inflow. *Abbreviations:* LA: Left atrium, LV: Left ventricle.

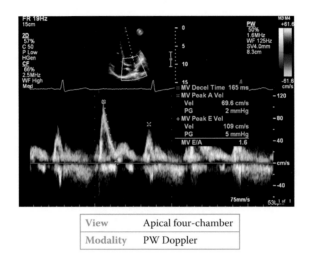

View	Apical four-chamber
Modality	PW Doppler

Figure 18.3 Pulsed-wave (PW) Doppler of mitral valve (MV) inflow. *Abbreviations:* PG: Pressure gradient, Vel: Velocity.

Tricuspid regurgitation velocity

Peak TR velocity is measured by visualizing the tricuspid valve in both the apical four-chamber view and the parasternal right ventricular inflow view, using continuous wave Doppler carefully aligned with the TR jet. The abnormal cut-off value for peak TR velocity is >2.8 m/s.

Left atrial volume index

See Chapter 19 for details on how to measure the left atrial volume index (LAVi). The abnormal cut-off value for LAVi is >34 mL/m².

GRADING LEFT VENTRICULAR DIASTOLIC DYSFUNCTION

The approach we've discussed so far is intended to decide whether or not LV diastolic dysfunction is present in patients with a normal LVEF. However, patients who have a reduced LVEF, or those who have a normal LVEF but also have myocardial disease, are likely to have some degree of diastolic dysfunction. In this situation, our aim is not to *detect* diastolic dysfunction, but instead to *grade* the diastolic function.

This approach begins with the assessment of mitral inflow by measuring

- E/A ratio
- peak E velocity

Measure the peak mitral inflow E and A velocities using PW Doppler in the apical four-chamber view (**Figure 8.3**). The E/A ratio is simply the ratio between the peak E and peak A wave velocities:

$$\text{E/A ratio} = \frac{\text{Peak E wave velocity}}{\text{Peak A wave velocity}}$$

Once you have measured these parameters, the algorithm shown in **Figure 18.4** will allow you to make a start on estimating LV filling pressures (i.e., mean left atrial pressure, LAP) and grading

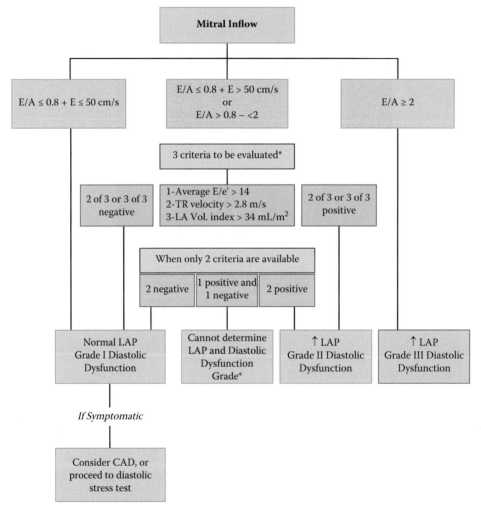

(*: LAP indeterminate if only 1 of 3 parameters available. Pulmonary vein S/D ratio <1 applicable to conclude elevated LAP in patients with depressed LV EF)

Figure 18.4   Algorithm for estimation of LV filling pressures and grading LV diastolic function in patients with depressed LVEFs and patients with myocardial disease and normal LVEF. *Abbreviations:* CAD: Coronary artery disease, LA: Left atrial, LAP: Left atrial pressure, LVEF: Left ventricular ejection fraction, TR: tricuspid regurgitation. (From Nagueh SF et al., 2016. With permission of Oxford University Press and the European Society of Cardiology.)

LV diastolic function. Mean LAP correlates better with mean pulmonary capillary wedge pressure than does LV end-diastolic pressure and is a better correlate with symptoms of pulmonary congestion.

The grading of LV diastolic dysfunction and estimation of mean LAP begins with the mitral inflow parameters. If the E/A ratio is ≤0.8 and the peak E velocity is ≤50 cm/s, the mean LAP is normal and Grade 1 diastolic dysfunction is diagnosed. At the opposite end of the scale, if the E/A ratio is ≥2, then the LAP is elevated and Grade III diastolic dysfunction is diagnosed.

Things are more complex if the E/A ratio is ≤0.8 and the peak E velocity is >50 cm/s, or if the E/A ratio is >0.8 and <2. In this scenario, more parameters must be measured in order to discriminate between the degrees of diastolic dysfunction. These parameters are as follows:

- average E/e' ratio >14
- TR velocity >2.8 m/s
- LAVi >34 mL/m²

The average E/e' ratio, TR velocity and LAVi are all measured as described earlier in this chapter. If all three parameters have been measured, and two of three or three of three are negative, then the LAP is normal and Grade I diastolic dysfunction is diagnosed. However, if two of three or three of three are positive, then the LAP is elevated and Grade II diastolic dysfunction is diagnosed.

Sometimes only two parameters can be measured. In this case, if both are negative, then the LAP is normal and Grade I diastolic dysfunction is diagnosed. Conversely, if both are positive, then the LAP is elevated and Grade II diastolic dysfunction is diagnosed. If one is positive and one is negative (or if only one parameter can be measured), then the LAP and diastolic dysfunction grade cannot be determined.

In patients with reduced LVEF, if one of the three parameters is not available, then it is possible to use pulmonary vein S/D ratio as an alternative parameter. To measure pulmonary venous flow, perform PW Doppler in the apical four-chamber view with a 2–3 mm sample volume placed 0.5 cm inside one of the pulmonary veins (the right upper pulmonary vein is usually easiest to locate, **Figure 18.5**).

Pulmonary vein flow normally consists of three components: The S wave represents forward flow into the left atrium during ventricular systole, and the smaller D wave represents forward flow

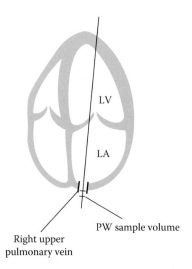

Figure 18.5   Positioning of a sample volume for pulsed-wave Doppler of pulmonary venous flow. *Abbreviations:* LA: Left atrium, LV: Left ventricle.

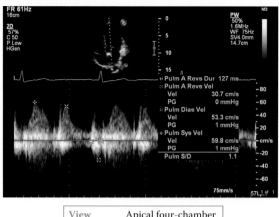

View	Apical four-chamber
Modality	PW Doppler

Figure 18.6   Pulsed-wave (PW) Doppler of pulmonary venous flow. *Abbreviations:* Dur: duration, PG: Pressure gradient, Revs: Reversal, S/D: S (systolic) wave/D (diastolic) wave, Vel: Velocity.

during ventricular diastole. If the patient is in sinus rhythm, the S and D waves are followed by an 'a' wave, representing flow reversal in the pulmonary vein during atrial systole.

Obtain a PW Doppler trace (**Figure 18.6**) and measure:

- peak systolic (S wave) velocity
- peak diastolic (D wave) velocity

Pulmonary vein S/D ratio is simply the ratio between the peak S and peak D wave velocities:

$$\text{S/D ratio} = \frac{\text{Peak S wave velocity}}{\text{Peak D wave velocity}}$$

A pulmonary vein S/D ratio <1 is consistent with increased LAP.

CONDITIONS THAT AFFECT MITRAL INFLOW

Unfortunately, there are some clinical conditions which affect mitral inflow and/or mitral annular dynamics, which means that the algorithm shown in **Figure 18.4** cannot be reliably used to evaluate LV filling pressures. These conditions include

- atrial fibrillation
- mitral stenosis
- moderate or severe mitral regurgitation
- moderate or severe mitral annular calcification
- mitral valve repair or replacement
- constrictive pericarditis
- left bundle branch block
- ventricular pacing
- LV assist devices
- heart transplantation

Depending upon the condition, it is sometimes possible to use alternative echo parameters to evaluate LV filling pressures, such as the peak acceleration rate of the mitral E velocity, the isovolumic relaxation time or the deceleration time of the pulmonary venous diastolic velocity. A detailed discussion of all these alternatives is beyond the scope of this book, but can be found in the ASE/EACVI guidelines (Nagueh SF et al., 2016).

Reporting of results

There are many ways of reporting on diastolic function in an echo report. Whatever descriptive approach you use, it is important to include all of the key parameters that you have used in your evaluation, together with a description of relevant pathology (e.g., LV hypertrophy) and relevant clinical features (e.g., heart rate and rhythm). Your conclusion should include the presence or absence of diastolic dysfunction and (where appropriate) an evaluation of the LV filling pressures:

- normal diastolic function
- Grade I diastolic dysfunction (normal LAP)
- Grade II diastolic dysfunction (moderately elevated LAP)
- Grade III diastolic dysfunction (markedly elevated LAP)
- indeterminate

Further reading

Henein MY et al. Diastolic function assessment by echocardiography: a practical manual for clinical use and future applications. *Echocardiography* (2020). PMID 32426907.

Nagueh SF et al. Recommendations for the evaluation of left ventricular diastolic function by echocardiography: an update from the American Society of Echocardiography and the European Association of Cardiovascular Imaging. *European Heart Journal – Cardiovascular Imaging*, 7 (15), 1335, 2016. PMID 27422899.

Sunil Kumar S et al. Impact of updated 2016 ASE/EACVI vis-à-vis 2009 ASE recommendation on the prevalence of diastolic dysfunction and LV filling pressures in patients with preserved ejection fraction. *Journal of Cardiovascular Imaging* (2021). PMID 33511798.

CHAPTER 19

The left atrium

The left atrium (LA) can be thought of as having three key haemodynamic functions. During left ventricular systole and its subsequent isovolumic relaxation phase, the LA acts as a **reservoir** for oxygenated blood returning to the heart from the lungs. During early diastole, the LA then acts as a passive **conduit** for this blood to enter the left ventricle. In late diastole, atrial contraction actively **boosts** left ventricular filling (unless the patient is in atrial fibrillation).

ECHO ASSESSMENT OF THE LEFT ATRIUM

The left atrium (LA) can be seen in several views:

- Left parasternal window
  - parasternal long-axis view
  - parasternal short-axis view (at aortic valve level)
- Apical window
  - apical four-chamber view
  - apical two-chamber view
  - apical three-chamber (long-axis) view
- Subcostal window
  - subcostal long-axis view

An echo evaluation of the LA includes the assessment of

- LA morphology
- LA volume
- LA function

LEFT ATRIAL MORPHOLOGY

Inspect the overall size and shape of the LA and check for the presence of any masses (e.g., tumour, thrombus). Also be alert for the presence of spontaneous echo contrast, particularly in the presence of atrial fibrillation and/or mitral stenosis. Although best seen on transoesophageal echo, spontaneous echo contrast may also be evident during transthoracic imaging. LA masses and spontaneous echo contrast are discussed further in Chapter 32.

The left atrial appendage is not easily seen on transthoracic echo but may be visible in the apical two-chamber view. The pulmonary veins can sometimes also be hard to spot but are generally best seen in the apical four-chamber view (especially the right upper pulmonary vein, **Figure 18.5**, p. 131).

COR TRIATRIATUM

Cor triatriatum is a rare congenital abnormality in which the LA is partitioned into two chambers by a membrane, best seen in the apical four-chamber view. The membrane contains one or more perforations allowing blood to flow between the two chambers, but nonetheless there is a degree of obstruction to LV inflow which can be assessed using PW Doppler. Cor triatriatum dexter is the name given to this condition when it occurs in the right atrium.

LEFT ATRIAL VOLUME

The causes of LA dilatation (**Figure 19.1**) include

- mitral valve disease
- dilated cardiomyopathy
- restrictive cardiomyopathy
- LV diastolic dysfunction
- atrial fibrillation or flutter
- high-output states (e.g., anaemia)
- 'athlete's heart'

The British Society of Echocardiography recommends that LA size should be assessed by measuring LA volume, indexed for body surface area.

The LA volume is measured using the biplane Simpson's method:

1. In the apical four-chamber view, obtain the best view you can of the LA, paying particular attention to avoidance of foreshortening.
2. Freeze a loop and find the end-systolic image, immediately prior to mitral valve opening. Now trace the endocardial border around the LA to obtain an area measurement in cm². Ignore any pulmonary veins that may be visible.

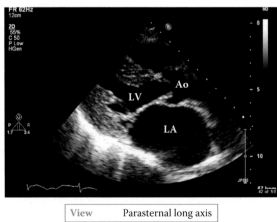

View	Parasternal long axis
Modality	2D

Figure 19.1   Dilated left atrium (LA), with left ventricular (LV) hypertrophy. *Abbreviation:* Ao: Aorta.

Table 19.1   Left atrial (LA) volume indexed: Reference ranges

	Normal	Borderline	Dilated
LA volume index (mL/m²)	<34	34–38	>38

Source: Reference intervals reproduced with permission of the British Society of Echocardiography.

3. Measure the length of the LA long axis in cm from the midpoint of the mitral annulus to the superior border (back wall) of the LA.

4. Repeat the measurements in the apical two-chamber view.

5. If the echo machine does not calculate LA volume for you, it can be calculated as follows:

$$\text{LA volume} = \frac{0.85 \times \text{LA Area (4 – Chamber view)} \times \text{LA Area (2 – Chamber view)}}{\text{LA Length}}$$

This formula gives the LA volume in mL, and this can be indexed for body surface area to give the left atrial volume index (LAVi) in mL/m². Reference ranges for LAVi are given in **Table 19.1**, with the values being the same for males and females.

It should be noted that the area–length method for calculating LA volume is *not* interchangeable with the biplane Simpson's method (volumes calculated using the area–length method is larger). Similarly, LA volumes measured using 3D echo are significantly larger than those calculated from 2D echo measurements. The reference ranges in **Table 19.1**, therefore, only apply to LA volumes calculated using the biplane Simpson's method.

The *routine* use of linear LA measurements is no longer encouraged. However, there are scenarios in which a linear LA measurement can be useful, such as in risk assessment in patients with hypertrophic cardiomyopathy (LA diameter is one of the parameters used in predicting risk of sudden cardiac death in this condition). If a linear LA diameter is required, then it can be measured at end-systole in the parasternal long-axis view, using either 2D or M-mode imaging.

LEFT ATRIAL FUNCTION

The assessment of LA function can be challenging and time-consuming, and it is not commonly performed in everyday clinical practice. The problem with parameters such as peak A wave velocity on mitral inflow (**Figure 18.3**, p. 129) is their dependence upon loading conditions which makes their interpretation difficult.

The most widely used technique for assessing the LA function is a volumetric method based upon the LA volume measured at different times. Three volumes need to be measured:

- **LAVmax**, which is the maximal LA volume measured at the end of systole (immediately prior to mitral valve opening)

- **LAVmin**, which is the minimal LA volume measured at the end of diastole (at the time of mitral valve closure)

- **LAVpre-a**, which is the LA volume measured immediately prior to atrial contraction (at the onset of the P wave on the ECG)

Using these measured volumes, the following parameters can be calculated:

1. **LA reservoir volume**, reflecting the expansion volume or 'reservoir' function of the LA:

$$\text{LA reservoir volume} = \text{LAV}_{max} - \text{LAV}_{min}$$

From this, it's possible to calculate the **LA expansion index**:

$$LA\ expansion\ index = \frac{LAV_{max} - LAV_{min}}{LAV_{min}} \times 100$$

And also the **LA diastolic emptying index**:

$$LA\ diastolic\ emptying\ index = \frac{LAV_{max} - LAV_{min}}{LAV_{max}} \times 100$$

2. **LA active pumping volume**, reflecting the stroke volume or 'boost' function of the LA:

$$LA\ active\ pumping\ volume = LAV_{pre-a} - LAV_{min}$$

From this, it's possible to calculate the **LA active emptying index**:

$$LA\ active\ emptying\ index = \frac{LAV_{pre-a} - LAV_{min}}{LAV_{pre-a}} \times 100$$

And also the **LA active emptying per cent of total emptying**:

$$LA\ active\ emptying\ per\ cent\ of\ total\ emptying = \frac{LAV_{pre-a} - LAV_{min}}{LAV_{max} - LAV_{min}} \times 100$$

3. **LA conduit volume**, which reflects the 'conduit' function of the LA, i.e., the proportion of blood which flows 'passively' through the LA and into the left ventricle. This parameter requires the calculation of LA stroke volume (SV_{LA}, which equals the LA active pumping volume above) and of left ventricular stroke volume (SV_{LV}, p. 116):

$$LA\ conduit\ volume = SV_{LV} - SV_{LA}$$

From this, it's possible to calculate the **LA passive emptying index**:

$$LA\ passive\ emptying\ index = \frac{LAV_{max} - LAV_{pre-a}}{LAV_{max}} \times 100$$

And also the **LA passive emptying per cent of total emptying**:

$$LA\ passive\ emptying\ of\ total\ emptying = \frac{LAV_{max} - LAV_{pre-a}}{LAV_{max} - LAV_{min}} \times 100$$

Further reading

Badano LP et al. Left atrial volumes and function by three-dimensional echocardiography: reference values, accuracy, reproducibility, and comparison with two-dimensional echocardiographic measurements. *Circulation: Cardiovascular Imaging* (2016). PMID 27412658.

Harkness A et al. Normal reference intervals for cardiac dimensions and function for use in echocardiographic practice: a guideline from the British Society of Echocardiography. *Echo Research and Practice* (2020). PMID 32105051.

Rosca M et al. Left atrial function: pathophysiology, echocardiographic assessment, and clinical applications. *Heart* (2011). PMID 22058287.

CHAPTER 20

The aortic valve

ECHO VIEWS OF THE AORTIC VALVE

The aortic valve is usually assessed in the

- Left parasternal window
  - parasternal long-axis view
  - parasternal short-axis view (aortic valve level)
- Apical window
  - apical five-chamber view

The **parasternal long-axis view** (**Figure 7.2**, p. 44) bisects the aortic valve, showing the right coronary cusp anterior to the non-coronary cusp. Two-dimensional imaging shows the structure of the aortic valve and allows an assessment of cusp mobility. An M-mode study of the valve, at the level of the cusp tips, shows the cusps opening at the start of systole (**Figure 20.1**). The aortic root as a whole moves anteriorly during systole, being pushed forward by the expanding left atrium (LA) as it fills during diastole. Conditions that enhance LA filling, such as mitral regurgitation, exaggerate this anterior motion of the aortic root. The aortic valve cusps close at the end of systole to make a single thin closure line. This M-mode pattern of normal aortic valve cusp motion is described as 'box-shaped'. While in this view, use colour Doppler to assess the valvular flow.

The **parasternal short-axis view** (**aortic valve level**) shows the valve 'face on' and all three cusps can be seen together with the surrounding cardiac structures (**Figure 7.5**, p. 47). Colour Doppler shows the location and extent of any valvular regurgitation.

The **apical five-chamber view** allows further 2D inspection of the valve (**Figure 7.9**, p. 51) and a colour Doppler assessment of any regurgitant flow.

In this view, a good alignment of continuous wave (CW) Doppler with the valve can usually be obtained, allowing an assessment of forward (and any regurgitant) flow. The normal aortic valve has a peak forward flow velocity of <1.7 m/s and a valve area of > 2.0 cm^2.

Additional information can also be obtained from the

- Right parasternal window
- Apical three-chamber (long-axis) view
- Subcostal window
  - subcostal short-axis view
- Suprasternal window
  - aorta view

DOI: 10.1201/9781003304654-20

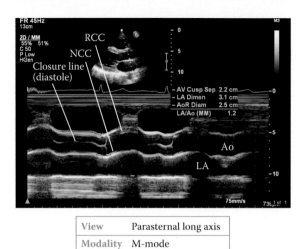

View	Parasternal long axis
Modality	M-mode

Figure 20.1 M-mode of normal aortic valve. *Abbreviations:* Ao: aorta, LA: Left atrium, NCC: Non-coronary cusp, RCC: Right coronary cusp.

The **right parasternal window** provides an additional view from which the aortic valve can be interrogated using CW Doppler (e.g., using a stand-alone pencil probe). The **apical three-chamber (long-axis) view** is similar in many ways to the parasternal long-axis view but offers the advantage of a suitable angle for CW Doppler assessment (**Figure 7.11**, p. 52). The **subcostal short-axis view** is seldom used but can visualize the aortic valve in short axis when good views cannot be obtained from the standard locations. The **suprasternal window (aorta view)** allows Doppler assessment of flow in the descending thoracic aorta, which is useful in aortic regurgitation.

AORTIC STENOSIS

Aortic stenosis is the obstruction of blood flow from the left ventricle (LV) due to a narrowing of the aortic valve, or an obstruction just below or above the level of the valve.

Causes of aortic stenosis

Calcific degeneration of the aortic valve is one of the commonest causes of aortic stenosis. This is characterized by progressive fibrosis and calcification of the aortic valve, beginning at the base of the cusps. The early stage of this process is often referred to as 'aortic sclerosis', but this term is somewhat misleading – it implies a benign process, but in fact aortic sclerosis is often a prelude to the development of significant stenosis later on.

Bicuspid aortic valve (p. 270) is also a common cause of aortic stenosis in the West and is thought to be responsible for around half of cases of severe aortic stenosis in adults. The stenotic process is similar to that seen in calcific degeneration but occurs at a younger age. Fibrosis typically starts in a patient's teens, with gradual calcification in their 30s onwards. Patients who require surgery for stenosis of a bicuspid aortic valve do so on average 5 years earlier than those with calcific degeneration of a tricuspid aortic valve.

Rheumatic aortic stenosis is less common than rheumatic mitral stenosis, and the two often coexist in the same patient. There is fusion of the commissures of the aortic valve cusps and the cusps themselves become fibrotic and eventually calcified.

Sub- and supravalvular obstruction cause a form of aortic stenosis in which the valve itself is unaffected but the obstruction lies below or above the valve. Subvalvular aortic stenosis can result from a *fixed* obstruction in the LV outflow tract (LVOT), usually a fibromuscular ridge or membrane, and may be associated with other congenital heart defects in up to half of cases. It can also result from a *dynamic* obstruction in the LVOT, causing obstruction predominantly in mid–late

Table 20.1 Clinical features of aortic stenosis

Symptoms	Signs
Often asymptomatic	Slow-rising pulse
Angina	Low systolic blood pressure and narrow pulse pressure
Exertional dizziness and syncope	Sustained apex beat (as a result of left ventricular hypertrophy)
Breathlessness	Soft aortic component to second heart sound (A$_2$)
	Ejection click
	Ejection systolic murmur
	Signs of heart failure in advanced cases

systole, as in hypertrophic obstructive cardiomyopathy (p. 227). In supravalvular aortic stenosis, which is uncommon, there is a fixed obstruction in the ascending aorta, just above the sinuses of Valsalva, due to a diffuse narrowing or a discrete membrane.

Clinical features of aortic stenosis

The clinical features of aortic stenosis are summarized in **Table 20.1**. Many cases of aortic stenosis are detected incidentally, either because of a systolic murmur heard during a routine examination or as an incidental finding during an echocardiogram for other indications. The appearance of symptoms has significant implications on the patient's outlook: Those with angina as a result of aortic stenosis have an average life expectancy of 5 years, those with exertional syncope 3 years and those with heart failure just 1 year.

Echo assessment of aortic stenosis

2D and M-mode

Use 2D and M-mode echo to assess the structure of the valve (**Figure 20.2**):

- Is it a tricuspid aortic valve, or is it bicuspid (or pseudobicuspid), unicuspid or quadricuspid? If there is cusp fusion, describe which cusps are involved.
- Is there any thickening of the cusps? How severe?
- Is there any calcification of the cusps? How severe (mild – isolated spots, moderate – larger spots, severe – extensive)? Is this diffuse or focal? If focal, which area of each cusp is affected? Is there calcification in the LVOT or aorta?

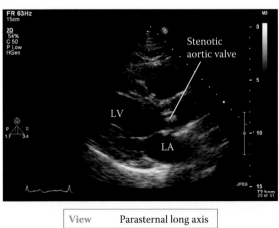

View	Parasternal long axis
Modality	2D

Figure 20.2 Moderate aortic stenosis. *Abbreviations:* LA: Left atrium, LV: Left ventricle.

- Is cusp mobility normal or restricted? Grade any cusp restriction as mild (restricted in basal third only), moderate (affecting basal and middle third) or severe (affecting entire cusp).
- Is there any systolic doming of the cusps?
- Is there an asymmetric closure line (suggesting a bicuspid valve)?
- Is there any evidence of sub- or supravalvular stenosis?

Planimetry of the aortic valve orifice area in the parasternal short-axis view (aortic valve level) can be challenging, particularly with heavily calcified cusps, and is not routinely recommended. It can sometimes be useful, however, if Doppler estimation of aortic valve effective orifice area (see below) cannot be performed reliably.

SUB- OR SUPRAVALVAR AORTIC STENOSIS

Always be alert to this possibility if the transaortic pressure gradient is unexpectedly high in the presence of an aortic valve that does not look stenosed. If you suspect sub- or supravalvular stenosis, use pulsed-wave (PW) Doppler to assess blood flow at different levels above and below the valve to detect where the main flow acceleration occurs. Use 2D echo to look carefully for a discrete membrane causing obstruction above or below the valve.

Colour Doppler

Colour Doppler imaging will show an increase in flow velocity and/or turbulent flow at valve level and downstream of the stenosis. If turbulence is seen proximal to the aortic valve, look carefully for any evidence of LVOT obstruction.

CW and PW Doppler

Use CW Doppler to obtain a trace of forward flow through the aortic valve (**Figure 20.3**). Obtain traces from multiple windows (apical, suprasternal, right parasternal, subcostal), and make recordings with both an imaging probe and a stand-alone 'pencil' probe. Optimize your gain and sweep speed, setting the sweep speed at 50–100 mm/s. Average your measurements from three beats in sinus rhythm (5–10 consecutive beats in atrial fibrillation), ignoring any tracings obtained from ectopic beats (and the beat following an ectopic).

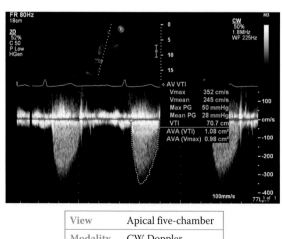

View	Apical five-chamber
Modality	CW Doppler

Figure 20.3 Doppler assessment of valve gradient in moderate aortic stenosis. *Abbreviations:* AVA: Aortic valve area, PG: Pressure gradient, V_{max}: Peak velocity, V_{mean}: Mean velocity, VTI: Velocity time integral.

In severe aortic stenosis, the CW Doppler trace is rounded in shape with the peak velocity occurring in mid-systole. In mild aortic stenosis, the trace has a more triangular shape with an earlier peak. You should trace around the dense outer edge of the spectral Doppler envelope.

The CW Doppler trace will give **peak velocity** (V_{max}), which is one of the key parameters used in assessing aortic stenosis severity. You can use V_{max} to calculate the peak transaortic pressure gradient (ΔP_{max}) via the simplified Bernoulli equation:

$$\Delta P_{max} = 4 \times V^2_{max}$$

If peak velocity in the LVOT is >1.0 m/s, use the full Bernoulli equation for greater accuracy:

$$\Delta P_{max} = 4 \times \left(V^2_2 - V^2_1 \right)$$

where V_2 is the peak transaortic velocity, assessed by CW Doppler, and V_1 is the peak LVOT velocity, assessed by PW Doppler. Since peak velocity and peak gradient are related, there is little to gain from quoting both figures in your report, and so peak velocity is the parameter usually given.

PEAK-TO-PEAK AND INSTANTANEOUS GRADIENTS

Transaortic gradient can also be assessed during cardiac catheterization, by measuring the fall in systolic pressure on withdrawing a catheter across the aortic valve. The gradient measured in this way is a **peak-to-peak** gradient – it is the difference between the peak pressure in the LV and the peak pressure in the aorta (which do not occur simultaneously – see **Figure 2.6**, p. 8). In contrast, the gradient measured by echo Doppler is an **instantaneous** gradient – it measures the maximum instantaneous pressure difference between the two chambers. Instantaneous gradients are greater than peak-to-peak gradients, and so peak transaortic gradients measured by echo will be higher than gradients measured by cardiac catheterization.

The **mean gradient** (ΔP_{mean}) can be obtained by tracing the Doppler envelope, from which the echo machine can calculate a mean value by averaging the instantaneous gradients throughout the trace. Alternatively, ΔP_{mean} can be estimated from the ΔP_{max} using the following equation:

$$\Delta P_{mean} = \frac{\Delta P_{max}}{1.45} + 2 \text{ mmHg}$$

Conditions that increase stroke volume (e.g., aortic regurgitation, pregnancy) increase transaortic flow during systole and can therefore lead to an *overestimation* of transaortic pressure gradients. Conversely, transaortic pressure gradients are *underestimated* in the presence of impaired LV function. These problems can, to some extent, be compensated for by using the continuity equation to calculate the **aortic valve area**, also known as effective orifice area (EOA_{AV}). To do this:

1. Measure the diameter of the LVOT in the parasternal long-axis view, from inner-edge to inner-edge. It is now recommended that the measurement be made at the insertion point of the aortic valve cusps (which is more reproducible than the 'historic' approach of measuring the LVOT 1 cm below the valve). Use your LVOT diameter measurement to calculate the cross-sectional area (CSA) of the LVOT:

$$CSA_{LVOT} = 0.785 \times (\text{LVOT diameter})^2$$

2. Now measure the velocity time integral (VTI) of flow in the LVOT (using PW Doppler) and across the aortic valve (using CW Doppler) to give VTI_{LVOT} and VTI_{AV}, respectively.

3. Use the continuity equation to calculate aortic valve EOA as follows:

$$EOA_{AV} = \frac{CSA_{LVOT} \times VTI_{LVOT}}{VTI_{AV}}$$

If you measure the LVOT diameter in centimetres, this will give you a valve area in cm². Some versions of the continuity equation use the ratio of peak velocities in the LVOT and across the aortic valve instead of using VTIs – although the results are often very similar, they are not identical and it is better to use VTI for the calculation. It is also important to note that direct measurement of aortic valve area by planimetry is not routinely recommended due to its inherent inaccuracy.

You will find more information on the assessment of aortic stenosis in the setting of impaired LV function in Chapter 9.

COMMON PITFALLS

Pitfalls in the echo assessment of aortic stenosis include:

- a poor Doppler signal outline, which may lead the sonographer to 'miss' the true peak of the Doppler velocity signal
- failure to align the Doppler beam with the flow through the aortic valve, which leads to an underestimation of transaortic peak velocity (the extent of error increases rapidly with misalignment of more than 20°)
- accidentally mistaking a mitral regurgitation trace for an aortic stenosis trace (particularly when using a pencil probe), and thus making measurements from the wrong valve
- overestimation of the severity of stenosis because of coexistent aortic regurgitation
- underestimation of the severity of aortic stenosis because of coexistent mitral stenosis or impairment of LV function
- inappropriate use of the continuity equation (it cannot be used if there are serial stenoses, i.e., sub/supravalvular stenoses, or if the LVOT is not circular, as in hypertrophic obstructive cardiomyopathy or subvalvular stenosis)

Associated features

If aortic stenosis is present:

- assess any coexistent aortic regurgitation.
- assess any coexistent disease affecting the other valves (as patients undergoing aortic valve surgery may also require any other valvular abnormalities to be corrected at the same time).
- *assess LV dimensions and function*: Obstruction to LV outflow by the aortic valve raises LV pressure, leading to LV hypertrophy (indexed LV mass is a prognostic marker in aortic stenosis). Subsequently dilatation occurs with impairment of function.
- assess aortic root morphology and dimensions (aortic root dilatation is a common finding in aortic stenosis).
- if the aortic valve is bicuspid, check for the presence of coarctation of the aorta (bicuspid aortic valve and coarctation of the aorta are sometimes associated).

Severity of aortic stenosis

Severity of aortic stenosis can be quantified by

- peak velocity (V_{max})
- mean gradient (P_{mean})
- valve area
- indexed valve area
- velocity ratio

In the presence of a calcified aortic valve with restricted motion, a peak velocity ≥ 4.0 m/s or a mean gradient of ≥ 40 mmHg is indicative of severe aortic stenosis (**Table 20.2**). Be aware, truly severe aortic stenosis in the *absence* of calcification/restriction is unusual, except in rare cases of congenital aortic stenosis.

Indexing of aortic valve area is not routinely required, but can be helpful in cases where the patient has a small body habitus (BSA <1.7 m²). Calculation of **velocity ratio** is also not routinely needed, but can be considered when the LVOT area cannot be reliably measured. Velocity ratio, also known as the dimensionless index, is simply

$$\text{Velocity ratio} = \frac{\text{VTI}_{\text{LVOT}}}{\text{VTI}_{\text{AV}}}$$

A velocity ratio <0.25 is consistent with severe aortic stenosis.

Once severe aortic stenosis is confirmed with confidence, the focus of your echo study (and report) should turn to prognostic factors that will help with clinical decision-making, such as LV ejection fraction, LV mass, pulmonary hypertension, whether there has been a rapid progression in aortic valve peak velocity (>0.3 m/s per year), whether there is 'very severe' stenosis (**Table 20.2**) and (optionally) whether the global longitudinal strain is more positive than −14%.

If the peak velocity is <4.0 m/s and the mean gradient is <40 mmHg, then this indicates non-severe aortic stenosis. Calculate the aortic valve area, where possible. If the aortic valve area is ≥ 1.0 cm², this confirms non-severe aortic stenosis.

However, sometimes these parameters can give conflicting results – for instance, the valve area may indicate severe aortic stenosis (<1.0 cm²), but the velocity and gradient do not (peak velocity <4.0 m/s, mean gradient <40 mmHg).

If the patient's LV systolic function is satisfactory (LVEF $\geq 50\%$), then first of all confirm that the discrepant results are not simply the result of a small body habitus by indexing the valve area. An indexed valve area of ≥ 0.60 cm²/m² would indicate that this is the case, and that their aortic stenosis is non-severe.

However, if the indexed valve area still suggests severe aortic stenosis (<0.60 cm²/m²), and you have reviewed the quality of your measurements to rule out measurement error, then consider 3D planimetry (if available) of the LVOT to obtain a more accurate measurement of LVOT CSA and thereby a more accurate calculation of valve area.

If this doesn't help, then calculate the stroke volume index (SVi) by measuring LV stroke volume (p. 116) and indexing it for body surface area; an SVi <35 mL/m² indicates low flow. If low flow is confirmed, this may explain why the velocity/gradient is low despite a small valve area.

Table 20.2   Indicators of aortic stenosis severity

	Mild	Moderate	Severe	Very severe
Peak velocity (m/s)	2.5–2.9	3.0–3.9	4.0–4.9	≥ 5.0
Mean gradient (mmHg)	<20	20–39	40–59	≥ 60
Valve area (cm²)	>1.5	1.0–1.5	<1.0	≤ 0.6
Valve area/BSA (cm²/m²)	>0.85	0.60–0.85	<0.60	
Velocity ratio	>0.5	0.25–0.5	<0.25	

Abbreviation: BSA: Body surface area.
Source: Reference intervals reproduced with permission of the British Society of Echocardiography.

If so, then circumstantial evidence can make severe aortic stenosis more likely – for instance, a mean gradient >35 mmHg, or a valve area <0.8 cm², or the presence of an increased LV mass. However, this is always a challenging scenario to unpick, and it is recommended that such a case be reviewed at a multidisciplinary team meeting. Measurement of valvular–arterial impedance (Zva) is no longer routinely recommended in these cases.

If there are discrepant results and LV systolic function is impaired (LVEF ≤40%), then there are two possibilities:

- in 'true-severe' aortic stenosis (in which the valve area is truly <1.0 cm²), the velocities/gradients are low simply as a consequence of the poor cardiac output
- in "pseudo-severe' aortic stenosis (in which the valve area is actually ≥1.0 cm²), the valve area is actually being underestimated as a result of reduced valve opening because of the poor cardiac output

In such a scenario, double check all your measurements and look carefully at the aortic valve (to judge whether its appearance is consistent with severe aortic stenosis). A dobutamine stress echo can be very helpful in distinguishing between 'true' and 'functional' aortic stenosis, and is described in more detail on page 74.

Rarely the conflicting parameters can be the other way around – i.e., the velocities/gradients indicate severe aortic stenosis (peak velocity ≥4.0 m/s, mean gradient ≥40 mmHg) but the valve area does not (≥1.0 cm²). This is known as 'high gradient, high valve area' aortic stenosis and tends to result from measurement error. These patients have elevated aortic valve calcium levels on CT scanning and should be regarded as having severe aortic stenosis unless proven otherwise.

Management of aortic stenosis

Echo surveillance

Advise patients with aortic stenosis to report symptoms immediately. Patients with severe aortic stenosis should be considered for surgery or, if surgery is not undertaken, undergo echo and cardiology review every 6 months. Those with moderate stenosis should be reassessed with an echo and a cardiology review every 12–18 months (peak velocity 3.5–3.9 m/s) or every 18–24 months (peak velocity 3.0–3.4 m/s). Those with mild stenosis need an echo every 3–5 years, and a cardiology review if symptomatic.

Drug therapy

There is no specific drug therapy to reverse aortic stenosis.

Surgery

Surgical replacement of the valve is the definitive treatment for aortic stenosis. Biological replacement valves are generally preferred for older patients or those who wish to avoid the need for long-term anticoagulation, while mechanical replacement valves are preferred for younger patients. Alternatively, transcatheter aortic valve replacement (TAVR) offers a percutaneous approach in appropriate cases.

Surgery is indicated for severe symptomatic aortic stenosis. Consider asymptomatic patients for surgery if they have LV systolic dysfunction, or if they develop symptoms (or a fall in blood pressure or complex ventricular arrhythmias) on exercise testing. Replacement of a moderate or severely stenosed aortic valve is usually advisable if patients are due to undergo heart surgery for another reason, such as bypass grafting or mitral valve surgery.

AORTIC REGURGITATION

Aortic regurgitation is the flow of blood from the aorta back through the aortic valve during diastole. It can result from a problem with the aortic valve itself or from a problem with the aortic root affecting an otherwise normal valve.

Causes of aortic regurgitation

Valvular causes include

- calcific degeneration of the aortic valve
- bicuspid aortic valve, causing incomplete closure of the valve
- infective endocarditis
- rheumatic aortic valve disease
- connective tissue diseases (e.g., rheumatoid arthritis, systemic lupus erythematosus)

Aortic root causes result from dilatation and/or distortion of the aortic root. These include

- hypertension
- Marfan syndrome
- Ehlers–Danlos syndrome
- osteogenesis imperfecta
- aortic dissection
- sinus of Valsalva aneurysm
- cystic medial necrosis
- syphilitic aortitis
- Behçet disease

Some conditions, such as ankylosing spondylitis, can affect both the aortic valve and the aortic root.

Clinical features of aortic regurgitation

The clinical features of aortic regurgitation are summarized in **Table 20.3**. Chronic aortic regurgitation places a volume overload on the LV, which, with time, dilates and becomes increasingly impaired, at which point the patient may develop symptoms and signs of heart failure. The disease process can therefore be insidious, although once heart failure does develop, patients often decline rapidly. Infective endocarditis and aortic dissection can cause acute aortic regurgitation, in which the patient can have clinically severe regurgitation but the usual markers of severity (such as LV dilatation) have not had time to develop.

Echo assessment of aortic regurgitation

2D and M-mode

Use 2D and M-mode echo to assess the structure of both the aortic valve and the aortic root:

- Is it a normal tricuspid aortic valve, or is it bicuspid (or pseudobicuspid), unicuspid or quadricuspid? Are the valve cusps thickened or calcified?
- Is there commissural fusion (indicative of rheumatic aortic valve disease)?

Table 20.3   Clinical features of aortic regurgitation

Symptoms	Signs
May be asymptomatic	Collapsing pulse
Symptoms of heart failure – breathlessness, orthopnoea, paroxysmal nocturnal dyspnoea	Low diastolic blood pressure and wide pulse pressure
Symptoms may also indicate the aetiology (e.g., fever in infective endocarditis)	Displaced apex beat (as a result of left ventricular dilatation)
	Early diastolic murmur
	Signs of heart failure in advanced cases

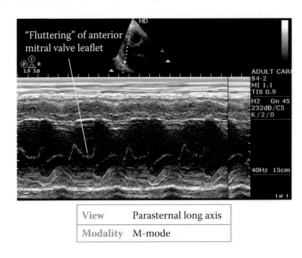

View	Parasternal long axis
Modality	M-mode

Figure 20.4   Aortic regurgitation causing 'fluttering' of anterior mitral valve leaflet.

- Are there any features of aortic stenosis (which may coexist with regurgitation)?
- Is there any prolapse? Which cusps are affected?
- Are there any features of infective endocarditis (vegetations, aortic root abscess)?
- Is there dilatation of the aortic root and/or any indication of dissection?

Severe aortic regurgitation is more likely to be seen in association with a structurally abnormal valve exhibiting flailing, restriction, perforation or a wide coaptation defect.

Use M-mode to interrogate the *mitral* valve. The diastolic jet of aortic regurgitation may hit the anterior mitral valve leaflet, causing fluttering of the leaflet, which can be seen on M-mode echo (**Figure 20.4**). This pushes the anterior leaflet backwards during diastole, causing 'reverse doming' and premature closure of the mitral valve and thereby partly obstructing the normal flow of blood through the mitral valve orifice.

This can cause a diastolic murmur, called an Austin Flint murmur. These effects on the mitral valve are an indicator of severe aortic regurgitation.

The LV also requires careful assessment. M-mode and 2D imaging will show LV dimensions and function. In *chronic* aortic regurgitation, volume overload leads to progressive LV dilatation but with hyperkinetic wall motion, particularly of the posterior wall and septum. LV size may be normal in *acute* severe aortic regurgitation.

Colour Doppler

Use colour Doppler to examine the jet of aortic regurgitation (**Figure 20.5**). How far the jet extends back into the LV is an unreliable indicator of severity, but assessing the width of the jet (in the parasternal long-axis view) in relation to the diameter of the LVOT is a useful guide to severity (see below). Take the measurements just below (within 1 cm of the level of) the aortic valve. Colour M-mode imaging in the parasternal long-axis view, with the cursor placed just below the aortic valve, can be a useful way to measure the width of the jet and of the LVOT. Cross-sectional imaging of the LVOT in the parasternal short-axis view allows for measurement of the aortic regurgitant jet CSA and comparison with the LVOT CSA at the same level.

Measure the width of the vena contracta (VC) – the narrowest region of colour flow at the level of the aortic valve – in the parasternal long-axis view. This also helps gauge severity. VC cannot be reliably measured if there is more than one regurgitant jet, or if the shape of the jet is irregular. If the jet is eccentric, make the measurement of VC perpendicular to the direction of the jet rather than to the orientation of the LVOT.

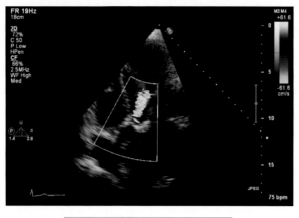

View	Apical five-chamber
Modality	Colour Doppler

Figure 20.5   Aortic regurgitation (colour Doppler).

CW and PW Doppler

Record the CW Doppler trace in the apical five-chamber view, with the probe carefully aligned with the direction of the regurgitant jet (**Figure 20.6**). An inverted trace can also be obtained from the suprasternal view. The CW Doppler trace is faint in mild aortic regurgitation, and denser in moderate or severe regurgitation. The pressure half-time of the diastolic deceleration slope, which equates to the rate of deceleration of the regurgitant jet, is a guide to severity, particularly in acute regurgitation.

PW Doppler can be used to map the extent of the regurgitant jet in the LV, by positioning the sample volume at various points in the LV (in the apical five-chamber view) and checking for regurgitant flow, although this is not a good indicator of severity.

PW Doppler can also be used to look for diastolic flow reversal in the upper descending aorta, using a suprasternal view and placing the sample volume in the descending aorta (just beyond the origin of the left subclavian artery). It is normal to have a brief reversal of aortic flow in diastole, but prominent flow reversal throughout the whole of diastole (called 'pandiastolic' or 'holodiastolic')

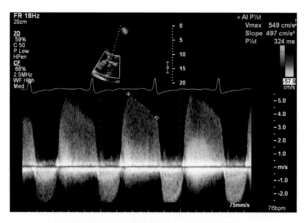

View	Apical five-chamber
Modality	CW Doppler

Figure 20.6   Aortic regurgitation (CW Doppler).

indicates severe aortic regurgitation. Measure the end-diastolic flow velocity of the flow reversal – severe regurgitation is indicated by an end-diastolic velocity of ≥ 20 cm/s. Pandiastolic flow reversal may also be seen in the abdominal aorta, where it is a specific indicator of severe aortic regurgitation.

Regurgitant volume

The volume of blood entering the LV via the mitral valve during diastole normally equals the volume of blood leaving it via the LVOT (stroke volume). In the presence of aortic regurgitation, LVOT outflow will be greater than mitral valve inflow as the systolic LVOT outflow will consist of the blood that has entered via the mitral valve plus the blood that entered the ventricle via aortic regurgitation during diastole. The difference between LVOT outflow and mitral valve inflow gives the regurgitant volume.

Although simple in principle, the measurement of regurgitant volume is difficult in practice. Firstly, the measurement is not valid if there is significant mitral regurgitation. Secondly, any error in measurement of mitral valve orifice area or LVOT diameter can have a large impact on the result. If you wish to measure regurgitant fraction, you can do so as follows:

1. In the apical four-chamber view, measure the diameter of the mitral annulus in cm, and then use this to calculate the CSA of the mitral valve in cm². This calculation makes the assumption that the mitral orifice is circular:

$$CSA_{MV} = 0.785 \times (\text{Mitral annulus diameter})^2$$

2. In the apical four-chamber view, measure the VTI of mitral valve inflow (using PW Doppler) to give VTI_{MV} in cm. It is generally easiest to place the sample volume at the valve tips (some place it at the level of the mitral valve annulus).

3. The stroke volume of the mitral valve (SV_{MV}), in mL/beat can then be calculated as follows:

$$SV_{MV} = CSA_{MV} \times VTI_{MV}$$

4. In the parasternal long-axis view, measure the diameter of the LVOT in cm, and then use this to calculate the CSA of the LVOT in cm²:

$$CSA_{LVOT} = 0.785 \times (\text{LVOT Diameter})^2$$

5. In the apical five-chamber view, measure the VTI of LVOT outflow (using PW Doppler) to give VTI_{LVOT} in cm.

6. The stroke volume of the LVOT (SV_{LVOT}), in mL/beat, can then be calculated as follows:

$$SV_{LVOT} = CSA_{LVOT} \times VTI_{LVOT}$$

7. Aortic regurgitant volume (RV) can be calculated as follows:

$$RV = SV_{LVOT} - SV_{MV}$$

8. Aortic regurgitant fraction (RF) can be calculated as follows:

$$RF = \frac{RV}{SV_{LVOT}} (\times 100 \text{ to express as a percentage})$$

Once you have calculated the aortic RV, you can also calculate the regurgitant orifice area (ROA). This is the average size of the orifice in the aortic valve, in cm², through which the regurgitation occurs during diastole, and equals the aortic RV (in mL) divided by the VTI of the aortic regurgitation Doppler trace (VTI_{AR}), measured in cm using CW Doppler:

$$ROA = \frac{RV}{VTI_{AR}}$$

Proximal isovelocity surface area assessment

The use of proximal isovelocity surface area (PISA) in the assessment of aortic regurgitation is not as common as it is for mitral regurgitation, as it is technically more challenging to obtain suitable images and the technique has not been so well-studied in relation to the aortic valve.

COMMON PITFALLS

Pitfalls in the echo assessment of aortic regurgitation include the following:

- an eccentric jet usually leads to underestimation of severity
- measuring the width of the regurgitant jet on colour Doppler too far below the aortic valve, where it tends to spread out, overestimates severity

---

Associated features

If aortic regurgitation is present:

- assess any coexistent aortic stenosis
- assess any coexistent disease affecting the other valves (as patients undergoing aortic valve surgery may also require any other valvular abnormalities to be corrected at the same time)
- assess LV dimensions and function
- assess aortic root morphology and dimensions
- if the aortic valve is bicuspid, check for the presence of coarctation of the aorta (bicuspid aortic valve and coarctation of the aorta are sometimes associated)

Severity of aortic regurgitation

Severity of aortic regurgitation can be gauged from the following (**Table 20.4**):

- Valve morphology
- LV size
- VC width
- ratio of jet width to LVOT width
- ratio of jet CSA to LVOT CSA
- jet density
- jet pressure half-time
- VTI of diastolic flow reversal in upper descending aorta
- RF
- ROA
- RV

The ratio of jet width/CSA to LVOT width/CSA is commonly used to quantify severity, but can be misleading in jets that are eccentric or have a diffuse origin. In such cases, it is generally better to use visual assessment to grade the ratio in terms of small, intermediate or large, and to use this as a gross guide to severity, than to stick slavishly to percentages. The VC width is a more reliable indicator of severity.

Table 20.4   Indicators of aortic regurgitation severity

	Mild	Moderate	Severe
2D			
Valve morphology	Normal or abnormal	–	Abnormal, flail, large coaptation defect
LV size	Normal	–	Dilated
Colour Doppler			
Vena contracta width (cm)	<0.3	0.3–0.6	>0.6
Jet width/LVOT diameter (%)	<25	25–64	≥65
Jet CSA/LVOT CSA (%)	<5	5–59	≥60
CW Doppler			
Jet density	Incomplete/Faint	Dense	Dense
Pressure half-time (ms)	>500	200–500	<200
PW Doppler			
End-diastolic velocity descending aorta (cm/s)	–	–	≥20
VTI diastolic flow reversal in upper descending aorta (cm)	Brief, early	Intermediate	Prominent holodiastolic
Multimodality			
Regurgitant fraction (%)	≤30	31–49	≥50
Regurgitant orifice area (cm²)	<0.10	0.10–0.29	≥0.30
Regurgitant volume (mL)	≤30	31–59	≥60

Abbreviations: CSA: Cross-sectional area, CW: Continuous wave, LV: Left ventricle, LVOT: Left ventricular outflow tract, PW: Pulsed-wave, VTI: Velocity time integral.
Source: Reference intervals reproduced with permission of the British Society of Echocardiography.

The pressure half-time of the diastolic deceleration slope shortens with increasing severity, as the rate of fall in aortic pressure is greater in severe regurgitation, but the half-time can also be affected by changes in LV compliance and the use of vasodilators.

MANAGEMENT OF AORTIC REGURGITATION

Echo surveillance

- Patients with severe aortic regurgitation need an echo and a cardiology review every 6–12 months, if stable and not close to needing surgery
- Patients with moderate aortic regurgitation need an echo and a cardiology review every 1–2 years
- Patients with mild-moderate aortic regurgitation need an echo every 3–5 years, and a cardiology discussion if the aortic root is dilated
- Patients with trace-mild aortic regurgitation with normal aortic valve morphology and a normal aortic root and ascending aorta does not usually need echo surveillance

Drug therapy

Patients who develop LV impairment should be treated with appropriate heart failure medication and hypertension should be well controlled. The 'pre-emptive' use of vasodilators in patients with normal LV function is unproven, but beta-blockers have a role to play in those with Marfan syndrome.

Surgery

Aortic valve surgery is indicated for symptomatic acute aortic regurgitation and in chronic aortic regurgitation when severe and symptomatic. In asymptomatic patients with severe aortic regurgitation, surgery is indicated for

- LV impairment (ejection fraction ≤50%)
- LV dilatation (end-systolic diameter >5.0 cm)
- patients needing heart surgery for other reasons (e.g., coronary artery bypass graft)

Regardless of aortic regurgitation severity, surgery is indicated for patients with aortic root disease and an aortic root diameter measuring

- ≥4.0 cm in women with low BSA, TGFBR2 mutation and severe extra-aortic features
- ≥4.5 cm in patients undergoing aortic valve surgery
- ≥4.5 cm in Marfan syndrome plus additional risk factors
- ≥5.0 cm in others with Marfan syndrome
- ≥5.0 cm in bicuspid aortic valve plus additional risk factors or coarctation
- ≥5.5 cm for all other patients

Surgery may involve aortic valve replacement or repair (where the valve is suitable), together with aortic root grafting where appropriate.

Further reading

Baumgartner H et al. Recommendations on the echocardiographic assessment of aortic valve stenosis: a focused update from the European Association of Cardiovascular Imaging and the American Society of Echocardiography. *Journal of the American Society of Echocardiography* (2017). PMID 28363204.

Ring L et al. Echocardiographic assessment of aortic stenosis: a practical guideline from the British Society of Echocardiography. *Echo Research and Practice* (2021). PMID 33709955.

Vahanian A et al. 2021 ESC/EACTS guidelines for the management of valvular heart disease. *European Heart Journal* (2022). PMID 34453165.

Zoghbi WA et al. Recommendations for noninvasive evaluation of native valvular regurgitation: a report from the American Society of Echocardiography developed in collaboration with the Society for Cardiovascular Magnetic Resonance. *Journal of the American Society of Echocardiography* (2017). PMID 28314623.

CHAPTER 21

The mitral valve

ECHO VIEWS OF THE MITRAL VALVE

The mitral valve is usually assessed in the

- Left parasternal window
  - parasternal long-axis view
  - parasternal short-axis view (mitral valve and papillary muscle levels)
- Apical window
  - apical four-chamber view
  - apical two-chamber view
  - apical three-chamber (long-axis) view

The **parasternal long-axis view** (**Figure 7.2**, p. 44) bisects the mitral valve, showing the anterior and posterior leaflets in the plane of the A2 and P2 scallops. Tilting the probe inferiorly (towards the RV inflow view) will show the A3 and P3 scallops and, eventually, the posteromedial commissure. Tilting the probe superiorly (towards the RV outflow view) will show the A1 and P1 scallops and, eventually, the anterolateral commissure.

Two-dimensional imaging shows the structure of the mitral valve and allows an assessment of leaflet thickness (normally <5 mm in diastole), calcification and mobility. You can use this view to measure antero-posterior mitral annular diameter at end-systole. A normal diameter is <38 mm in males and <36 mm in females (indexed <20.3 mm/m^2).

An M-mode study of the valve, at the level of the leaflet tips, shows the tips open widely in early diastole as blood flows from the left atrium (LA) into the left ventricle (LV), and the point at which the anterior leaflet tip reaches its most anterior position is called the E point (**Figure 21.1**). The leaflets then move back together in mid-diastole before separating once again towards the end of diastole, as a result of the extra surge of blood through the valve that accompanies atrial systole. The maximum excursion of the anterior leaflet during this phase is called the A point. The anterior leaflet then follows a straight downward line to its closure point at the onset of systole. Once you have completed the M-mode recording, use colour Doppler to assess valvular flow.

The **parasternal short-axis view** (**mitral valve level**) shows the valve 'face on' and all three scallops of both leaflets can be seen together with both mitral commissures (**Figure 7.6**, p. 48, and **Figure 21.2**). The area of the valve orifice can be measured with planimetry in this view – a normal mitral valve has an orifice area of 4.0–6.0 cm^2. Colour Doppler shows the location and extent of any valvular regurgitation. Angling the probe down to the **papillary muscle level** (**Figure 7.7**, p. 49)

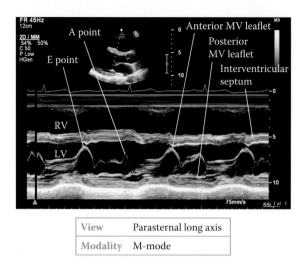

View	Parasternal long axis
Modality	M-mode

Figure 21.1 M-mode of normal mitral valve. *Abbreviations:* LV: Left ventricle, MV: Mitral valve, RV: Right ventricle.

shows both papillary muscles – anterolateral and posteromedial. Sometimes there can be three papillary muscles if one of them happens to be bifid.

The **apical four-chamber view** (**Figure 7.8**, p. 50) shows the anterior mitral leaflet (A2 and A3 scallops) adjacent to the interventricular septum and the posterior leaflet (P1) adjacent to the lateral wall, together with the anterolateral papillary muscle and its chordae.

The **apical two-chamber view** (**Figure 7.10**, p. 52) shows the anterior mitral leaflet in a 'bi-commissural view', with the P1 and P3 scallops of the posterior leaflet on either side and the A2 scallop of the anterior leaflet in the middle. Measure the bicommissural diameter from one commissure to the other in this view at end-systole. A normal bicommissural diameter is <46 mm in males and <42 mm in females (indexed <24.4 mm/m²).

The **apical three-chamber view** (**Figure 7.11**, p. 52) is similar to the parasternal long-axis view, showing the A2 and P2 scallops.

In each of the apical views, inspect the valve structure with 2D echo and assess flow with colour Doppler. The apical views permit a good alignment of continuous wave (CW) and pulsed-wave

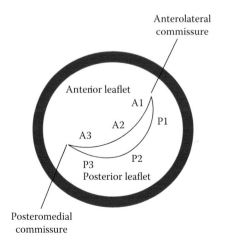

Figure 21.2 Mitral valve scallops, as seen in the parasternal short-axis view.

(PW) Doppler with the valve to assess forward (and any regurgitant) flow. Forward flow across a normal mitral valve has a pressure half-time of 40–70 ms. Additional information can also be obtained from the

- Subcostal window
  - subcostal long-axis view
  - subcostal short-axis view

The **subcostal long-axis view** provides an additional view from which the mitral valve can be examined. The **subcostal short-axis view** is seldom used to examine the mitral valve, but with appropriate angulation of the probe, it can be visualized.

Three-dimensional echo allows imaging of the whole mitral valve and can provide valuable information about the origin and size of regurgitant jets, for example by clearly demonstrating which portion of the valve is prolapsing.

MITRAL STENOSIS

Mitral stenosis is the obstruction of diastolic blood flow from the LA to the LV due to a narrowing of the mitral valve. This is almost always due to rheumatic mitral valve disease, as a consequence of rheumatic fever earlier in life.

Rheumatic valve disease can affect any of the heart valves (or several in combination), but most commonly affects the mitral valve. The characteristic feature is fusion of the mitral leaflets along their edges, starting from the mitral commissures, restricting their ability to open. The leaflet edges become thickened, although there can be thickening and/or calcification elsewhere too. As the main body of each leaflet usually remains relatively pliable, the leaflets are seen to 'dome' during diastole, with the rising LA pressure causing the leaflet body to bow forward towards the ventricle. This gives the leaflets what is described as a 'hockey stick' appearance. Rheumatic mitral stenosis also affects the chordae, causing fibrosis, shortening and calcification of the subvalvular apparatus.

Other causes of mitral stenosis are rare. These include congenital mitral stenosis, mitral annular calcification, systemic lupus erythematosus and radiation-induced valve disease. Beware of conditions that can cause obstruction of the mitral valve orifice and mimic mitral stenosis, such as left atrial myxoma, infective endocarditis with a large vegetation, ball thrombus or cor triatriatum.

MITRAL ANNULAR CALCIFICATION

Mitral annular calcification is relatively common in older patients (but can also be seen in younger patients with renal failure) and most commonly occurs in the posterior part of the mitral annulus, at the attachment point of the posterior leaflet, although rarely it can extend right round the annulus in severe cases. It is thought to be an indicator of cardiovascular risk and a marker of coronary artery disease. If annular calcification is massive, it can extend into the mitral leaflets and cause mitral stenosis. Unlike rheumatic mitral stenosis, mitral annular calcification does not affect the leaflet tips or cause fusion of the commissures.

Clinical features of mitral stenosis

The clinical features of mitral stenosis are summarized in **Table 21.1**. Most patients are female, and most will have other coexistent valve disease. Rheumatic mitral stenosis usually presents 20–40 years after an episode of rheumatic fever and is now relatively uncommon in developed countries. The onset of mitral stenosis tends to be gradual and so the symptoms can build up insidiously over a long period, but a new event (such as pregnancy or the onset of atrial fibrillation [AF]) can suddenly cause the symptoms to deteriorate. Patients usually remain asymptomatic until the

Table 21.1 Clinical features of mitral stenosis

Symptoms	Signs
Often gradual onset	Atrial fibrillation is common
Breathlessness	Malar flush ('mitral facies')
Cough	Tapping apex beat (palpable first heart sound)
Peripheral oedema	Loud first heart sound
Haemoptysis	Loud pulmonary component to second heart sound (P_2) if pulmonary hypertension present
Peripheral emboli	Opening snap
	Low pitched mid-diastolic murmur (with presystolic accentuation if in sinus rhythm)

mitral valve orifice area falls below 2.0 cm², at which point LA pressure starts to increase. As LA pressure rises, the LA starts to dilate. Pulmonary artery pressure also begins to rise and pulmonary hypertension develops. Once a patient becomes symptomatic, if left untreated, the 10-year survival is around 50%–60%.

Echo assessment of mitral stenosis

2D and M-mode

Use 2D and M-mode echo to assess the structure of the valve and the subvalvular apparatus. Be sure to describe the appearance of the mitral leaflets, mitral annulus, chordae tendineae and papillary muscles:

- Do the mitral valve leaflets appear normal? Is there evidence of rheumatic valve disease (**Figure 21.3**)?
- Does the mitral annulus appear normal? Is there annular calcification, and is this mild, moderate or severe?
- Is there any thickening of the leaflets? Is this mild, moderate or severe? Are both leaflets affected, and does this affect the tip or body of each leaflet?
- Is there any calcification of the leaflets? Is this focal or diffuse? Does the calcification affect either or both of the commissures?
- Is there fusion of one or both of the commissures?
- Are the chordae tendineae normal? Is there any chordal thickening, shortening or calcification? Does this affect the chordae to the anterior or posterior leaflet?

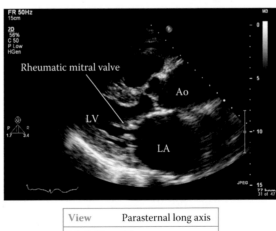

View	Parasternal long axis
Modality	2D

Figure 21.3 Rheumatic mitral valve. *Abbreviations:* Ao: Aorta, LA: Left atrium, LV: Left ventricle.

- Are the papillary muscles normal? Is there any calcification or fibrosis?
- Is mitral leaflet mobility normal or reduced? How much is it reduced (mild, moderate or severe)? Is there any doming during diastole?

In the parasternal short-axis view (at the mitral valve level), if the image quality is good enough, perform planimetry to measure the mitral orifice area. Remember that a stenosed mitral valve, when open, is funnel shaped, so be careful to ensure that you are measuring the 'funnel' at its narrowest point, i.e., the level of the leaflet tips. If you angle the probe too far upwards (towards the LA), you will overestimate the orifice area.

Once you've recorded a loop at the level of the tips, scroll the images back and forth until you find the one that shows the orifice at its widest point in mid-diastole. Take your measurement from this image, tracing around the inner edge of the leaflets – the echo machine will calculate the orifice area for you. Be careful of high gain settings, which can lead to underestimation of the mitral orifice area.

There are indirect ways of measuring mitral valve area (see below), but these can be influenced by loading conditions. Direct planimetry is therefore the 'reference standard' for grading severity.

Using M-mode in mitral stenosis, assess the following:

- Are the leaflet tips thickened?
- Is there reduced excursion of the mitral leaflets during diastole?
- Is there evidence of commissural fusion (shown by the posterior leaflet moving upwards, in the same direction as the anterior leaflet, as it opens during diastole, rather than downwards as a mirror image of the anterior leaflet)?

For rheumatic mitral stenosis, a stenotic mitral valve can be assigned a score (**Wilkins score**, see p. 215) which is assessed on the basis of leaflet mobility, valvular thickening, subvalvular thickening and valvular calcification. The Wilkins score can be used to judge the valve's suitability for percutaneous balloon mitral valvuloplasty.

An alternative to the Wilkins score is the **commissural calcification score**, in which each mitral commissure (anterolateral and posteromedial) is scored according to the degree of calcification seen on the short-axis view, with a score of 0 being given for no calcification, 1 for calcium across half a commissure and 2 for calcium across the whole commissure. The score for the two commissures is added together to give a total score of 0–4, with a score of ≥2 indicating less than a 50% probability of achieving a good haemodynamic outcome following percutaneous balloon mitral valvuloplasty.

Colour Doppler

Use colour Doppler to look for any coexistent mitral regurgitation (MR). The colour jet can also help in obtaining correct alignment of the probe for CW and PW Doppler recordings.

CW and PW Doppler

Use CW Doppler to obtain a trace of forward flow through the mitral valve (**Figure 21.4**) from an apical four-chamber view. Ignore traces obtained from ectopic beats (and the beat following an ectopic), and if the patient is in AF (as is often the case), take an average measurement from five beats.

From the trace, measure the **mean mitral valve gradient** by tracing the VTI of the mitral inflow (delineated by the 'X' markers in **Figure 21.4**, giving a mean pressure gradient of 21 mmHg). Be aware that the mean gradient is dependent not only on stenosis severity but also upon both LA and LV diastolic pressures, and is influenced by heart rate and rhythm and also by coexistent MR. When performing serial measurements over several different visits, it's important to note the patient's heart rate and rhythm each time to help gauge how comparable the measurements are.

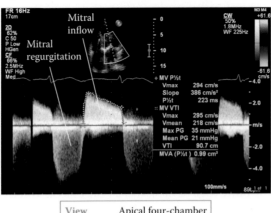

View	Apical four-chamber
Modality	CW Doppler

Figure 21.4 Severe mitral stenosis and coexistent mitral regurgitation. *Abbreviations:* MV: Mitral valve, MVA: Mitral valve area, P1/2t: Pressure half-time, PG: Pressure gradient, V_{max}: Peak velocity, V_{mean}: Mean velocity, VTI: Velocity time integral.

Because of this dependence on other factors, mean gradient is only a supportive indicator of mitral stenosis severity rather than a specific one.

Next, measure the **pressure half-time** of the mitral valve inflow by measuring the downward slope of the E wave (delineated by the '+' markers in **Figure 21.4**, giving a pressure half-time of 223 ms). Pressure half-time is a measure of the rate of fall in pressure across the valve – specifically, the time taken for the transmitral pressure gradient to fall to half of its initial peak value. The narrower the valve, the longer it takes for the pressure gradient to fall and hence the longer the pressure half-time. An echo Doppler trace displays flow velocity rather than pressure, and the mathematical relationship between pressure and flow velocity means that a fall in pressure gradient to 0.5 of its original value equates to a fall in flow velocity to 0.7 of its original value.

Studies have shown that a mitral valve area of 1 cm² has a pressure half-time of approximately 220 ms, and that the relationship between pressure half-time and valve area is linear. It is therefore possible to estimate mitral valve area from pressure half-time using the following equation:

$$\text{Mitral valve area} = \frac{220}{\text{Pressure half} - \text{Time}}$$

where the mitral valve area is measured in cm and pressure half-time in ms. In **Figure 21.4**, the pressure half-time of 223 ms gives a valve area of

$$\text{Mitral valve area} = \frac{220}{223}$$

$$\text{Mitral valve area} = 0.99 \text{ cm}^2$$

This calculated valve area can be compared with the measured area you obtained from planimetry. Pressure half-time is the least reliable of the indirect measures of mitral stenosis severity, being affected by conditions that alter compliance in the LA or LV, such as mitral or aortic regurgitation. Pressure half-time is also influenced by the acute haemodynamic changes that occur following mitral valvuloplasty (see p. 215).

Continuity equation

Mitral valve area can also be calculated using the continuity equation. This calculation relies on the volume of blood entering the LV via the mitral valve orifice during diastole (transmitral stroke volume) being equal to the volume of blood leaving the LV via the LV outflow tract (LVOT) during systole. This calculation cannot therefore be used in the presence of significant mitral or aortic regurgitation.

1. In the parasternal long-axis view, measure the diameter of the LVOT in cm, and then use this to calculate the cross-sectional area (CSA) of the LVOT in cm^2:

$$CSA_{LVOT} = 0.785 \times (LVOT\ Diameter)^2$$

2. In the apical five-chamber view, measure the velocity time integral (VTI) of LVOT outflow (using PW Doppler) to give VTI$_{LVOT}$, in cm.
3. The stroke volume of the LVOT (SV$_{LVOT}$), in mL/beat, can then be calculated as follows:

$$SV_{LVOT} = CSA_{LVOT} \times VTI_{LVOT}$$

4. This will be equal to the transmitral stroke volume (SV$_{MV}$):

$$SV_{MV} = SV_{LVOT}$$

5. In the apical four-chamber view, measure the VTI of mitral valve inflow (using PW Doppler) to give VTI$_{MV}$, in cm.
6. Mitral valve area (MVA), in cm^2, can be calculated as follows:

$$MVA = \frac{SV_{MV}}{VTI_{MV}}$$

COMMON PITFALLS

Pitfalls in the echo assessment of mitral stenosis include

- inaccurate planimetry of the mitral orifice because of suboptimal 2D image quality or heavy calcification of the mitral leaflet edges
- failure to planimeter the mitral leaflets at their tips, leading to an overestimation of orifice area
- failure to align the Doppler beam with flow through the valve during CW Doppler interrogation
- inaccurate measurement of pressure half-time due to a poor-quality mitral inflow trace
- failing to recognize that conditions affecting LA and LV compliance will affect pressure half-time
- failure to average several readings when patients are in AF

Associated features

If mitral stenosis is present,

- assess any coexistent MR
- assess any coexistent disease affecting the other valves (as patients undergoing mitral valve surgery may also require any other valvular abnormalities to be corrected at the same time)
- assess LA size – the LA dilates in mitral stenosis, and a normal LA volume is unlikely in severe mitral stenosis
- look for evidence of blood stasis in the LA, as evidenced by spontaneous echo contrast or the presence of a thrombus

- assess LV dimensions and function: Systolic function is usually normal in mitral stenosis unless other pathology is present, but mitral stenosis impairs diastolic function
- assess the right heart for evidence of pulmonary hypertension and comment on right atrial size and right ventricular size and function

Severity of mitral stenosis

Severity of mitral stenosis is quantified by valve area, which is regarded as a specific sign. Supportive indicators of severity include mean gradient and systolic pulmonary artery pressure. The method for measuring systolic pulmonary artery pressure is described in Chapter 26, p. 201).

Table 21.2 summarizes the echo indicators of mitral stenosis severity. Always state the method(s) you have used to measure mitral valve area in your report.

Management of mitral stenosis

Echo surveillance

Advise patients with asymptomatic but significant mitral stenosis to report symptoms immediately. Patients with severe mitral stenosis should have a surveillance echo and cardiology review every 6–12 months, and those with moderate stenosis every 1–2 years. Patients with mild stenosis should have an echo every 3–5 years.

Drug therapy

There is no specific drug therapy to reverse mitral stenosis, but diuretics are useful in treating breathlessness. Anticoagulation is important in those with AF and those with thrombus in the LA.

Surgery

Consider intervention for patients with clinically significant mitral stenosis (mitral valve area <1.5 cm²) if the patient is symptomatic, or if they are asymptomatic but have a high risk of decompensation, embolism or a positive stress test. If the valve is suitable, this usually takes the form of percutaneous balloon mitral valvuloplasty (PBMV, p. 215). If unsuitable for this technique, surgical intervention can be offered.

Mitral regurgitation

MR is the flow of blood from the LV back through the mitral valve during systole and can result from dysfunction of any part of the mitral valve apparatus – the leaflets, annulus, papillary muscles or chordae tendineae. MR can be classified as follows:

- *Primary MR*: due to leaflet and/or subvalvular apparatus abnormalities
  - degenerative mitral valve disease/mitral valve prolapse
  - rheumatic mitral valve disease
  - infective endocarditis
  - congenital (e.g., cleft mitral valve, which may be associated with a primum atrial septal defect)

Table 21.2   Indicators of mitral stenosis severity

	Mild	Moderate	Severe
Valve area (cm²)	1.6–2.0	1.0–1.5	<1.0
Mean gradient (mmHg)	<5.0	5–10	>10
Systolic pulmonary artery pressure (mmHg)	<30	30–50	>50

Source: Reference intervals reproduced with permission of the British Society of Echocardiography.

Table 21.3   Carpentier classification of mitral leaflet motion

Type	Leaflet motion	Description
1	Normal	• Typically, due to annular dilatation, leaflet motion itself remains normal but there is a loss of leaflet apposition which causes a failure of coaptation • Rarely, Type 1 MR can also result from leaflet perforation, for example in infective endocarditis
2	Excessive	• Typically, due to leaflet prolapse, although excessive leaflet motion can also result from papillary muscle rupture
3a	Restricted (Systole and diastole)	• Leaflet restriction in both systole and diastole is most often the result of rheumatic mitral leaflet thickening and fusion, although it can also be seen in post-inflammatory states and also following radiotherapy
3b	Restricted (Systole only)	• Leaflet restriction in systole only is seen when the leaflet is tethered as a result of LV dysfunction, such as ischaemic tethering, or when the LV is globally dilated (see Box **Ischaemic Mitral Regurgitation**)

- *Secondary MR*: when abnormalities of the LV and/or LA disrupt normal mitral valve function, sometimes termed 'functional' MR
  - LA dilatation (e.g., atrial fibrillation)
  - LV dilatation (e.g., dilated cardiomyopathy)

The mechanism of MR can be described according to the Carpentier classification, which categorizes the mechanism of MR based upon mitral valve leaflet motion (**Table 21.3**).

Identifying the underlying mechanism of MR is a crucial element of the echo assessment of MR, as this will guide the subsequent management strategy.

ISCHAEMIC MITRAL REGURGITATION

Ischaemic MR occurs due to a change in LV structure and function (but where the mitral valve itself remains structurally normal) as a result of myocardial ischaemia. Moderate or severe chronic ischaemic MR in the months or years after a myocardial infection is associated with an increased risk of heart failure and death.

Broadly speaking, two patterns of ischaemic MR are recognized:

- in **symmetric** ischaemic MR, there is global LV dilatation leading to displacement of both papillary muscles, mitral annular dilatation and a consequent failure of mitral leaflet coaptation. A central jet of MR results
- in **asymmetric** ischaemic MR, abnormal motion of the inferolateral LV wall causes displacement of the posteromedial papillary muscle, with subsequent displacement of the posterior mitral leaflet and tethering of the secondary chordae of the anterior leaflet, which results in a posteriorly directed jet of MR

Ischaemic MR is a chronic problem and is therefore distinct from the **acute** MR that can occur in acute myocardial infarction as a result of the rupture of a papillary muscle, leading to flailing of the affected leaflet segments (the attached portion of ruptured muscle can usually be seen swinging between atrium and ventricle on its chordal attachments), often with disastrous clinical consequences for the patient. For further information on the complications of acute myocardial infarction, see page 124.

Clinical features of mitral regurgitation

The clinical features of MR are summarized in **Table 21.4**. Chronic MR places a volume overload on the LV, which, with time, dilates and becomes increasingly impaired, leading to an increase in LA pressure, at which point the patient develops symptoms. Pulmonary hypertension can ensue.

Table 21.4   Clinical features of mitral regurgitation (MR)

Symptoms	Signs
May be asymptomatic	Atrial fibrillation may be present
Symptoms of heart failure – breathlessness, orthopnoea, paroxysmal nocturnal dyspnoea, fatigue	Displaced apex beat (as a result of left ventricular dilatation)
Symptoms may be insidious (chronic MR) or abrupt (acute MR)	Pansystolic murmur, heard at apex and radiating to axilla
Symptoms may also indicate the aetiology (e.g., myocardial infarction, infective endocarditis)	Mid–late systolic click followed by late systolic murmur (mitral valve prolapse)
	Signs of heart failure in advanced (or acute) cases

Infective endocarditis and papillary muscle or chordal rupture can cause acute MR, in which the abrupt volume overload increases the LV filling pressure and can lead to acute pulmonary oedema.

Echo assessment of mitral regurgitation

2D and M-mode

Use 2D and M-mode echo to assess the structure of the valve and the sub valvular apparatus, and also of the LA and LV, with the aim of identifying the mechanism of MR. Be sure to describe the appearance of the mitral leaflets, mitral annulus, chordae tendineae and papillary muscles:

- Do the mitral valve leaflets appear normal? Is there evidence of rheumatic valve disease, or of myxomatous degeneration?
- Does the mitral annulus appear normal? Is the annulus dilated? Is there annular calcification, and is this mild, moderate or severe?
- Is there any thickening of the leaflets? Is this mild, moderate or severe? Are both leaflets affected, and does this affect the tip or body of each leaflet?
- Is there any calcification of the leaflets? Is this focal or diffuse? Does the calcification affect either or both of the commissures?
- Are the chordae tendineae normal? Is there any chordal elongation or rupture? Does this affect the chordae to the anterior or posterior leaflet?
- Are the papillary muscles normal? Is there any rupture or partial rupture?
- Is mitral leaflet mobility normal, or is it excessive or restricted? If it is restricted, is this during systole only, or throughout systole and diastole?
- Is there any leaflet prolapse (see the box **Mitral Valve Prolapse**)? Which leaflet scallops are affected?
- Is there a coaptation defect? How large is the defect, and where is it located?
- Are there any vegetations? Where are they located? Are they mobile and/or pedunculated? What are their dimensions?
- Is there any evidence of an abscess or a mass? Where is it located? What are its dimensions?

MITRAL VALVE PROLAPSE

Diagnose MVP when

- any part of either leaflet moves >2 mm behind the plane of the mitral annulus in the parasternal long-axis view
- the coaptation point of the leaflets moves behind the annular plane in the apical four-chamber view

The population prevalence of MVP is around 2%. In addition to MR, MVP has also been associated with autonomic dysfunction (Barlow's syndrome) with symptoms including palpitations and syncope. In describing MVP, comment on

- the leaflet scallops that are affected (most commonly P2)
- the extent of any MR, and the direction of the MR jet

A **flail leaflet** usually results from rupture of a chordae tendineae or papillary muscle, and it should be distinguished from MVP. The tip of a flail leaflet will point upwards into the atrium, whereas the tip of a prolapsing leaflet continues to point downwards towards the ventricle.

Colour Doppler

Use colour Doppler to examine the jet of MR in the parasternal (**Figure 21.5**) and apical views. Describe

- how far the MR jet extends back into the LA – in the apical view, trace the area of the jet and of the LA
- the position of the jet in relation to the mitral leaflets (e.g., central jet, or evidence of regurgitation through a leaflet perforation)
- the direction of travel of the MR jet (**Figure 21.6**) within the atrium (central, anteriorly directed, posteriorly directed) and whether it impinges on the atrial wall or flows retrogradely up a pulmonary vein. Eccentric jets are usually directed *away from* the abnormal leaflet (e.g., anterior leaflet prolapse gives rise to a posteriorly directed jet)

Central jets can appear more severe than they really are on colour Doppler because of entrainment – blood cells along the sides of the jet are drawn along with the regurgitant blood. Conversely, eccentric jets that impinge on the LA wall can appear less severe than they are, because they cannot entrain blood cells on the side of the jet that hits the wall.

Measure the width of the vena contracta (VC) – the narrowest region of colour flow at the level of the mitral valve – in whichever views where all three components of the MR jet (the flow convergence, vena contracta and jet expansion) are clearly seen. Because the MR jet tends to be elliptical in secondary MR, it is important to average the VC measurements from two (approximately) orthogonal views – typically, the apical four-chamber and apical two-chamber views. The measurement of VC helps gauge severity even if the jet is eccentric, but it cannot be used to assess the severity of multiple regurgitant jets.

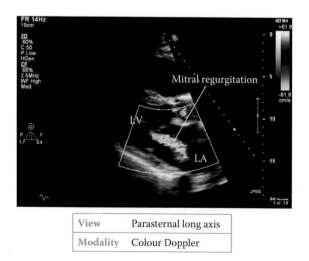

View	Parasternal long axis
Modality	Colour Doppler

Figure 21.5   Mitral regurgitation. *Abbreviations:* LA: Left atrium, LV: Left ventricle.

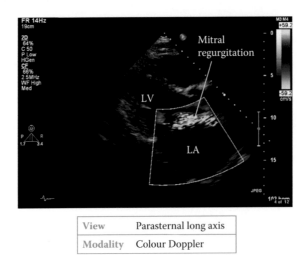

View	Parasternal long axis
Modality	Colour Doppler

Figure 21.6   Mitral valve prolapse with eccentric (anterior) jet of mitral regurgitation. *Abbreviations:* LA: Left atrium, LV: Left ventricle.

It is important to use appropriate (and consistent) colour gain settings for these assessments to avoid under/overestimating severity. For measurement of jet area and VC width, a Nyquist limit setting of 50–60 cm/s is usually appropriate.

CW and PW Doppler

Record the CW Doppler trace in the apical four-chamber view, with the probe carefully aligned with the direction of the MR jet (**Figure 21.7**). The CW Doppler trace is faint in mild MR, and denser in moderate or severe MR. The velocity of the MR jet is usually high (e.g., 5 m/s) and, in chronic MR, remains high throughout systole. By contrast, in acute MR, the jet velocity starts to fall towards the end of systole, as the pressure gradient between the ventricle and the LA equalizes more rapidly than it does in chronic MR: A triangular waveform suggests torrential or acute severe MR. The LA (and LV) is usually non-dilated in acute MR as it has not had time to dilate.

PW Doppler can be performed at end-expiration to obtain a VTI of mitral valve inflow and LVOT outflow (which are necessary for calculation of MR volume; see below). A ratio between mitral valve inflow VTI and LVOT outflow VTI of >1.4 is consistent with severe MR.

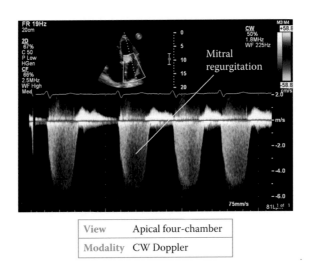

View	Apical four-chamber
Modality	CW Doppler

Figure 21.7   Mitral regurgitation.

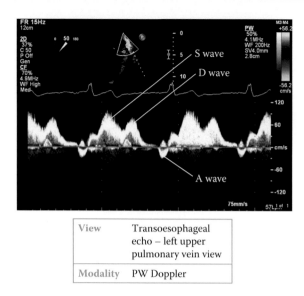

View	Transoesophageal echo – left upper pulmonary vein view
Modality	PW Doppler

Figure 21.8 Normal pulmonary vein flow (transoesophageal echo).

LA pressure rises with the increasing MR severity, which in turns leads to a higher early diastolic flow velocity (E wave). An E wave velocity >1.5 m/s is consistent with severe MR (in the absence of mitral stenosis or high-flow states), whereas a dominant A wave makes severe MR very unlikely.

PW Doppler can also be used to assess flow, where possible, in the pulmonary veins. The pulmonary veins are reasonably easy to assess with transoesophageal echo, but somewhat harder with transthoracic echo. It is however usually possible to locate one or the other of the right pulmonary veins in the corner of the LA, adjacent to the interatrial septum, in the apical four-chamber view. Place the PW Doppler sample volume 1 cm into the pulmonary vein and obtain a recording at end-expiration (**Figure 21.8**). Normally, the systolic (S) wave is larger than the diastolic (D) wave: If the D wave is larger, then there is blunting of forward flow in the pulmonary vein; if the S wave is inverted, there is systolic flow reversal (indicative of severe MR).

Proximal isovelocity surface area assessment

The use of proximal isovelocity surface area (PISA) has been well-validated in the assessment of MR and is the recommended indictor for quantifying MR severity.

The principle behind PISA is that blood flowing towards a circular orifice converges to form a series of hemispheric shells, each of which gets smaller and faster as it approaches the orifice. If the aliasing velocity (Nyquist limit) of the echo machine is adjusted, it can be made to match the velocity of blood flow in the 'shells' – there will be a blue–red interface at the point in the series of shells where aliasing occurs, and at that position, the velocity of blood flow equals the aliasing velocity you have selected (**Figure 21.9**). Knowing the velocity of blood flow at that point, and calculating the surface area of the relevant hemisphere, you can calculate MR flow rate:

1. Using colour Doppler in the apical four-chamber view, narrow down the sector width and minimize the depth before zooming in on the location of the regurgitant jet through the mitral valve. Adjust the aliasing velocity by adjusting the zero point on the colour flow scale until you see a clear hemisphere of converging blood flow on the ventricular side of the valve, usually at a setting of 20–40 cm/s. There should be a clear interface between red- and blue-coloured flow, and the velocity of blood flow at this point equals the aliasing velocity (in cm/s).

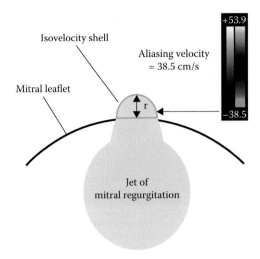

Figure 21.9 The proximal isovelocity surface area (PISA) method uses the surface area of a hemispheric 'shell' of uniform velocity and the aliasing velocity to calculate the regurgitant flow rate. *Abbreviation:* r: Shell radius).

2. Measure the radius (r) of this hemisphere by taking a measurement from the edge of the hemisphere (i.e., the red–blue interface) to the centre of the valve orifice. Use this to calculate PISA, the surface area of this hemisphere, in cm^2:

$$PISA = 2\pi r^2$$

3. The MR flow rate, in mL/s, can be calculated as follows:

$$MR\ flow\ rate = PISA \times Aliasing\ velocity$$

4. Next, use CW Doppler to measure the maximum velocity of the MR jet (MR V_{max}) in cm/s and also trace the mitral regurgitant VTI_{MR} (in cm). Take your measurement from a beat with a similar R–R interval to the one you used to measure the PISA. You can use colour M-mode to check when PISA is at its largest extent, and use this to help guide when to measure MR V_{max} on CW Doppler, particularly when the MR is not holosystolic but occurs in early or late systole. Use MR V_{max} to calculate effective regurgitant orifice area (EROA) in cm^2:

$$EROA = \frac{MR\ Flow\ rate}{MR\ V_{max}}$$

5. Finally, use the measured VTI_{MR} and the calculated EROA to calculate the MR volume in mL:

$$MR\ volume = EROA \times VTI_{MR}$$

If MR is not holosystolic, for example in mitral valve prolapse (where it tends to occur principally in late systole), then EROA tends to overestimate MR severity, and in this situation, it is recommended that MR volume is used to gauge severity, rather than EROA.

Do not use the PISA technique if a clear symmetrical hemisphere cannot be obtained or if the jet of MR is eccentric.

Regurgitant volume

The volume of blood entering the LV via the mitral valve during diastole normally equals the volume of blood leaving the LV via the LVOT (stroke volume) in systole. In the presence of MR, LVOT outflow will be less than mitral valve inflow as the LVOT outflow will be missing the regurgitant volume of blood that has re-entered the LA. The difference between mitral valve inflow and LVOT outflow gives the MR volume.

As with any assessment of valvular regurgitant volume, any error in the measurement of mitral valve orifice area or LVOT diameter can have a large impact on the result. Calculation of regurgitant volume is not appropriate if there is significant coexistent aortic regurgitation.

To measure MR volume:

1. In the apical four-chamber view, measure the diameter of the mitral annulus in cm in mid-diastole, and then use this to calculate the CSA of the mitral valve in cm². This calculation makes the assumption that the mitral orifice is circular:

$$CSA_{MV} = 0.785 \times (\text{Mitral annulus diameter})^2$$

2. In the apical four-chamber view, measure the VTI of mitral valve inflow (using PW Doppler) to give VTI_{MV}, in cm. It is generally easiest to place the sample volume at the valve tips (some place it at the level of the mitral valve annulus).

3. The stroke volume of the mitral valve (SV_{MV}), in mL/beat, can then be calculated as follows:

$$SV_{MV} = CSA_{MV} \times VTI_{MV}$$

4. In the parasternal long-axis view, measure the diameter of the LVOT in cm, and then use this to calculate the CSA of the LVOT in cm²:

$$CSA_{LVOT} = 0.785 \times (\text{LVOT diameter})^2$$

5. In the apical five-chamber view, measure the VTI of LVOT outflow (using PW Doppler) to give VTI_{LVOT}, in cm.

6. The stroke volume of the LVOT (SV_{LVOT}), in mL/beat, can then be calculated as follows:

$$SV_{LVOT} = CSA_{LVOT} \times VTI_{LVOT}$$

7. MR volume can be calculated as follows:

$$\text{MR volume} = SV_{MV} - SV_{LVOT}$$

8. MR fraction can be calculated as follows:

$$\text{MR fraction} = \frac{\text{MR volume}}{SV_{MV}} \ (\times 100 \text{ to express as a percentage})$$

Once you have calculated the MR volume, you can also calculate the regurgitant orifice area (ROA). This is the average size of the orifice in the mitral valve, in cm², through which the MR occurs during systole, and equals the MR volume (in mL) divided by the VTI of the MR Doppler trace (VTI_{MR}), measured in cm using CW Doppler:

$$ROA = \frac{RV}{VTI_{MR}}$$

Associated features

If MR is present,

- assess any coexistent mitral stenosis

- assess any coexistent disease affecting the other valves (as patients undergoing mitral valve surgery may also require any other valvular abnormalities to be corrected at the same time)
- assess LA size
- assess LV dimensions and function
- assess the right heart for evidence of pulmonary hypertension and comment on the right atrial and ventricular size.

COMMON PITFALLS

Pitfalls in the echo assessment of MR include

- measuring MR jet area or VC width on colour Doppler with inappropriate colour gain settings
- underestimating the severity of eccentric jets on colour Doppler
- failure to align the Doppler beam with regurgitant flow during CW Doppler interrogation
- inaccurate measurement of mitral valve orifice area or LVOT diameter when calculating RV
- trying to calculate RV when there is coexistent aortic regurgitation
- using the PISA method to assess eccentric jets
- failure to average several readings when the patient is in AF

Severity of mitral regurgitation

Table 21.5 summarizes the echo indicators of mitral regurgitation severity.

Table 21.5   Indicators of mitral regurgitation severity

	Mild	Moderate	Severe
2D			
Mitral leaflets	Normal	–	Abnormal, flail, restriction, perforation or wide coaptation defect
LA size (chronic primary MR)	Normal	–	Dilated
LV size (chronic primary MR)	Normal	–	Dilated (but normal size does not rule out severe MR)
Colour Doppler			
Ratio of jet area to LA area (%)	Small, brief	20–50	Large, >50
Flow convergence	None, brief, small	Intermediate	Large and holosystolic
Vena contracta width (cm)	<0.3	0.30–0.69	≥0.7
Biplane vena contracta width (cm)	<0.3	0.30–0.79	≥0.8
PISA radius at Nyquist 40 cm/s (cm)	<0.3	0.4–1.0	>1.0
CW and PW Doppler			
CW Doppler	Faint, partial, parabolic	Intermediate	• Similar density to forward flow • Triangular waveform suggests torrential or acute severe MR
Dominant MV inflow wave (cm/s)	A wave	Variable	E wave >1.5
MV inflow VTI/LVOT VTI	<1	–	>1.4
Pulmonary vein systolic flow	Dominance	Blunting	Flow reversal
Multimodality			
Regurgitant orifice area (cm²)	<0.20	0.20–0.39	≥0.40
Regurgitant volume (mL/beat)	<30	30–59	≥60
Regurgitant fraction (%)	<30	30–49	≥50

Source: Reference intervals reproduced with permission of the British Society of Echocardiography.

Management of mitral regurgitation

Echo surveillance

Asymptomatic patients with severe MR (and normal LV function) need a cardiology review every 6 months and an echo every 6–12 months. Urgent review is needed if the LV ejection fraction is ≤60%, the LV systolic diameter is approaching 45 mm or there is severe LV volume dilatation, or if the MR is due to a flail leaflet, the PA systolic pressure is >50 mmHg, or there is severe MR with an LA volume ≥60 mL/m² (in sinus rhythm). Cardiology review is also needed if there is development of symptoms or new atrial fibrillation.

Those with moderate MR (and normal LV function) need a cardiology review and echo every 1–2 years. For those with mild MR, an echo is required every 3–5 years if there is mild prolapse, but no follow-up is usually needed if the mitral valve is structurally normal.

Drug therapy and surgery

Drug therapy does not alter the course of primary MR, and surgery should be considered for severe primary MR when accompanied by any of the following:

- symptoms
- LV dilatation (by volume, or LV end-systolic diameter ≥40 mm)
- LV systolic dysfunction (defined as LVEF ≤60%)
- pulmonary hypertension (systolic pulmonary artery pressure >50 mmHg)
- LA volume ≥60 mL/m² (in sinus rhythm)
- flail leaflet

Where patients require mitral valve surgery, valve repair is, where feasible, generally considered superior to valve replacement. The more complex the mitral valve lesions, the more challenging the valve repair. For some patients, transcatheter intervention (e.g., MitraClip™) may be appropriate to improve symptoms.

For secondary MR, mitral valve surgery may improve symptoms but has not been shown to alter prognosis. The focus is therefore on medical therapy as appropriate (e.g., treatment of heart failure), with surgery generally reserved for those with symptoms despite optimal medical therapy or for those already undergoing cardiac surgery for another indication.

MITRAL REGURGITATION AND 3D ECHO

Three-dimensional echo can be extremely useful in assessing mitral valve disease and in planning surgery (see Chapter 13). It offers more accurate visualization and measurement of valve orifice area in mitral stenosis and better assessment of the geometry of the mitral valve apparatus in assessing the cause of MR. Combining 3D echo with colour Doppler is helpful in determining the origin and direction of MR jets.

Further reading

Robinson S et al. The assessment of mitral valve disease: a guideline from the British Society of Echocardiography. *Echo Research and Practice* (2021). PMID 34061768.

Vahanian A et al. 2021 ESC/EACTS Guidelines for the management of valvular heart disease. *European Heart Journal* (2022). PMID 34453165.

Zoghbi WA et al. Recommendations for Noninvasive Evaluation of Native Valvular Regurgitation: a report from the American Society of Echocardiography Developed in Collaboration with the Society for Cardiovascular Magnetic Resonance. *Journal of the American Society of Echocardiography* (2017). PMID 28314623.

CHAPTER 22

The right ventricle

The right heart tends to be a relatively neglected part of the standard transthoracic echo study, because

- much of the right heart lies behind the sternum, making it difficult to image using ultrasound
- the anatomy and orientation of the right heart is relatively complex compared with the left
- the right ventricle (RV) is trabeculated, which makes accurate measurements difficult

Nonetheless, an assessment of RV dimensions and function is an essential part of the standard echo study, not only to detect primary RV disorders but also because RV size and function can reveal a great deal about disorders affecting other parts of the heart (e.g., pulmonary hypertension, atrial septal defect).

The RV can be best seen in the:

- parasternal long-axis view (**Figure 7.2**, p. 44)
- parasternal RV inflow view (**Figure 7.3**, p. 45)
- parasternal RV outflow view (**Figure 7.4**, p. 46)
- parasternal short-axis view (at the aortic valve level) (**Figure 7.5**, p. 47)
- parasternal short-axis view (at the mitral valve level) (**Figure 7.6**, p. 48)
- parasternal short-axis view (at the papillary muscle level) (**Figure 7.7**, p. 49)
- RV-focused apical view (p. 53)
- subcostal long-axis view (**Figure 7.12**, p. 54)

To obtain an optimal view of the right ventricle, the standard apical four-chamber view should be adjusted to centre the right heart on the screen while keeping the *left* ventricular apex at the top of the image sector. The left ventricular outflow tract should *not* be visible. The transducer should be rotated to maximize the RV basal diameter. This view is known as the 'RV-focused' or 'modified' apical view, and this view should be used for all RV measurements made from the apical window to reduce the risk of foreshortening (which tends to exaggerate RV size).

An RV assessment includes:

- RV dimensions
- cavity size
- wall thickness
- global systolic function
- regional systolic function
- RV masses or thrombus (Chapter 32)

DOI: 10.1201/9781003304654-22

RIGHT VENTRICULAR DIMENSIONS

An initial evaluation of whether the RV is dilated can be made in the apical four-chamber view by measuring the basal diameters of both the RV and the LV at end-diastole. An RV/LV basal diameter ratio of >0.66 is suggestive of RV dilatation.

However, because of its complex morphology, a more detailed assessment of the RV size should be undertaken by obtaining RV diameters from several different points. Use 2D imaging to take measurements at **end-diastole** as follows:

- Parasternal long-axis view (**Figure 22.1**)
  - RVOT proximal diameter – perpendicularly from the junction between the interventricular septum and aortic valve to the RVOT wall
- Parasternal short-axis view – at the aortic valve level (**Figure 22.2**)
  - RVOT1 proximal diameter – from the anterior aortic wall to the RVOT wall
  - RVOT2 distal diameter – just proximal to the pulmonary valve
- RV-focused apical view (**Figure 22.3**)
  - RVD1 basal RV diameter – the maximal diameter in the basal third of the RV
  - RVD2 mid-RV diameter – at the level of the LV papillary muscles
  - RVD3 RV long-axis (base-to-apex) length – from the plane of the tricuspid annulus to the RV apex

The measurement of RV and RVOT dimensions is an important element in the assessment of arrhythmogenic right ventricular cardiomyopathy (p. 233).

The reference intervals for RV and RVOT dimensions are listed in **Table 22.1**.

The RV end-diastolic area is measured in the RV-focused apical view, tracing around the endocardial border to obtain an outline of the cavity area. The area measurement should be indexed for body surface area. The reference intervals for RV end-diastolic area are given in **Table 22.2**.

The thickness of the RV wall is ideally measured, at end-diastole, using a zoomed subcostal view. RV hypertrophy is indicated by a wall thickness of >5 mm and commonly indicates RV pressure overload (but may also be seen in hypertrophic and infiltrative cardiomyopathies).

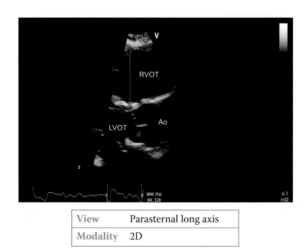

View	Parasternal long axis
Modality	2D

Figure 22.1   Measurement of RVOT proximal diameter (red line) in the parasternal long-axis view at end-diastole. *Abbreviations:* Ao: Aortic root, LVOT: Left ventricular outflow tract, RVOT: Right ventricular outflow tract.

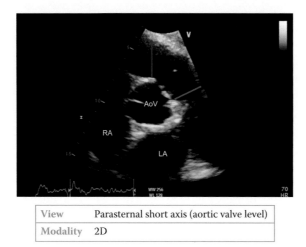

View	Parasternal short axis (aortic valve level)
Modality	2D

Figure 22.2   Measurement of RVOT1 (red line) and RVOT2 (blue line) diameters in the parasternal short-axis view. *Abbreviations:* AoV: Aortic valve, LA: Left atrium, RA: Right atrium.

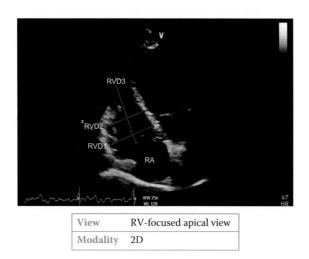

View	RV-focused apical view
Modality	2D

Figure 22.3   Measurement of RV dimensions RVD1, RVD2 and RVD3 in the RV-focused apical view. *Abbreviations:* LV: Left ventricle, RA: Right atrium.

Table 22.1   Reference intervals for RV and RVOT dimensions

	Male	Female
Parasternal long-axis view		
RVOT proximal diameter (mm)	25–43	22–40
Parasternal short-axis view		
RVOT1 proximal diameter (mm)	24–44	20–42
RVOT2 distal diameter (mm)	16–29	14–28
RV-focused apical view		
RVD1 basal RV diameter (mm)	26–47	22–43
RVD2 mid-RV diameter (mm)	19–42	17–35
RVD3 long-axis RV diameter (mm)	55–87	51–80

Abbreviations: RV: Right ventricle, RVOT: Right ventricular outflow tract.
Source: Reference intervals reproduced with permission of the British Society of Echocardiography.

Table 22.2   Reference intervals for RV end-diastolic area

	Male	Female
RV end-diastolic area indexed (cm²/m²)	≤13.6	≤12.6

Abbreviation: RV: Right ventricle.
Source: Reference intervals reproduced with permission of the British Society of Echocardiography.

Although RV volume can be estimated using area–length or Simpson's rule methods, as for the LV, the more complex geometry of the RV means that simplifying assumptions have to be made about RV morphology. Volume calculations obtained via 2D echo are therefore used infrequently. Three-dimensional echo permits a more comprehensive evaluation of RV volumes and the calculation of RV ejection fraction (RVEF). Broadly speaking, an RVEF ≥45% obtained by 3D echo usually indicates normal RV systolic function, although some centres use age- and sex-specific values.

RIGHT VENTRICULAR SYSTOLIC FUNCTION

The assessment of RV function is often made qualitatively, using 'eyeball' assessment of the RV contractility from several different views. Inspect the RV carefully for evidence of regional wall motion abnormality (normokinesia, hypokinesia, akinesia, dyskinesia) and describe the region(s) affected (RV anterior wall, RV lateral wall, RV inferior wall, RV apex, interventricular septum [IVS], RVOT anterior wall).

A more quantitative approach to RV function can also be taken, using one or more of the following parameters:

- fractional area change
- tricuspid annular plane systolic excursion
- RV S′
- RV index of myocardial performance (RIMP)

Fractional area change

To calculate RV fractional area change:

1. In the RV-focused apical view, trace the RV endocardium to obtain an area measurement (in cm²) at end-diastole and end-systole.

2. RV fractional area change can then be calculated (as a percentage) follows:

$$\text{RV fractional area change} = \frac{\text{End-diastolic area} - \text{End-systolic area}}{\text{End-diastolic area}} \; (\times 100 \text{ to express as a percentage})$$

Reference ranges are given in **Table 22.3**. It's important to remember than RV fractional area change does not include the RVOT and therefore only gives a 'selective' impression of RV systolic function.

Table 22.3   Reference intervals for RV systolic function

	Male	Female
Fractional area change (%)	≥30	≥35
TAPSE (mm)	≥17	≥17
RV S′ (cm/s)	≥9	≥9

Abbreviations: RV: Right ventricle, TAPSE: Tricuspid annular plane systolic excursion.
Source: Reference intervals reproduced with permission of the British Society of Echocardiography.

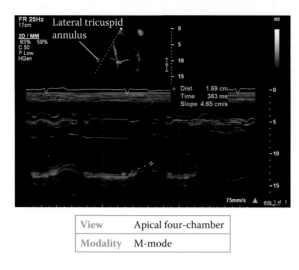

View	Apical four-chamber
Modality	M-mode

Figure 22.4   Measurement of tricuspid annular plane systolic excursion.

Tricuspid annular plane systolic excursion

Tricuspid annular plane systolic excursion (TAPSE) is a simple and well-validated method of assessing RV function. The underlying principle is based on measuring how much the lateral tricuspid annulus moves vertically during systole – the more impaired the RV, the less the annular displacement seen. A normal TAPSE is ≥17 mm.

To measure TAPSE:

1. Obtain an RV-focused apical view of the RV.
2. Using M-mode, place the cursor so that it passes through the lateral tricuspid annulus. Obtain an M-mode trace.
3. Measure the vertical displacement of the lateral tricuspid annulus from the M-mode trace (**Figure 22.4**).

Right ventricular S′

Right ventricular S′ is measured using tissue Doppler imaging of the lateral tricuspid annulus during systole. Normal RV long-axis systolic function is indicated by an RV S′ ≥9 cm/s. There is normally a close correlation between the RV S′ and TAPSE findings, i.e., if one of these parameters is in the normal range, then the other should be too, and vice versa.

RV index of myocardial performance

The RV index of myocardial performance (RIMP, also known as the Tei index) is a measure of myocardial function that takes into account both systolic and diastolic function. It can be measured using tissue Doppler or pulsed-wave (PW) Doppler, but the tissue Doppler method is preferred as all the measurements are made from a single heartbeat. To calculate RIMP:

1. Use tissue Doppler in the *standard* apical four-chamber view to obtain a trace at the lateral tricuspid annulus.
2. Measure the time interval from the tricuspid valve closure to opening (TCO) by measuring the interval from the end of the tricuspid valve A′ wave to the start of the following E′ wave.

3. Measure the ejection time (ET) of the right ventricle which is the duration of the S' wave.

4. Calculate RIMP from

$$RIMP = \frac{TCO - ET}{ET}$$

A RIMP >0.54 (when measured by tissue Doppler, or >0.43 when measured by PW Doppler) is indicative of RV dysfunction.

RIGHT VENTRICULAR DIASTOLIC FUNCTION

Diastolic function of the RV is not commonly assessed in everyday clinical practice. Nonetheless, it is possible to gain valuable insights into RV diastolic function using several echo parameters. The British Society of Echocardiography advocates a four-step approach to the evaluation of RV diastolic function:

1. Assess right heart and IVC dimensions, as significant RV diastolic dysfunction is unlikely if the right-sided chambers are non-dilated with normal wall thickness and a normal IVC.

2. Perform PW Doppler of tricuspid inflow, measuring E and A velocities, E/A ratio and E deceleration time. Restrictive RV physiology is indicated by
   a. E/A ratio >2.1
   b. E deceleration time <120 ms

3. Perform tissue Doppler at the lateral tricuspid annulus, measuring RV isovolumic relaxation time (IVRT), e', a' and e'/a' ratio. Abnormal RV physiology is indicated by
   a. E/a' ratio <1
   b. E/e' ratio >6
   c. RV IVRT >73 ms

4. Perform PW Doppler of hepatic vein flow. Abnormal RV physiology is indicated by
   a. hepatic vein S/D ratio <1
   b. hepatic vein (S/[S + D] × 100) <55
   c. Prominent inspiratory reversal

VOLUME AND PRESSURE OVERLOAD

Assessing the IVS in the parasternal short-axis view can provide useful information about the RV haemodynamics. Normally septal motion is dominated by the LV, and the septum bulges towards the RV in the short-axis views. If the RV is overloaded, this septal bulge starts to flatten, and in the short-axis views, this gives the LV a 'D' shape rather than its usual circular appearance. In the presence of chronic RV **volume** overload (e.g., severe tricuspid regurgitation), the RV is dilated and the septum is pushed towards the LV in diastole. In RV pressure overload (e.g., severe pulmonary hypertension), the RV is hypertrophied and the septum is pushed towards the LV in systole. Coexistent volume and pressure overload will flatten the septum in both systole and diastole.

The **LV eccentricity** index can be used to quantify these changes in the RV. In the parasternal short-axis view, at the papillary muscle level, the LV septo-lateral cavity diameter is measured across the LV cavity at right angles to the interventricular septum (**Figure 22.5**). The LV antero-posterior diameter is then measured at right angles to the first measurement, to give two perpendicular cavity diameters which are then expressed as a ratio (of the antero-posterior diameter to the septo-lateral diameter). The measurements are taken at end-systole and at end-diastole. Normal individuals have a circular LV cavity and therefore have a ratio of 1 in both systole and diastole. In RV volume overload, the flattening of the septum in diastole means that the septo-lateral LV diameter becomes smaller than the antero-posterior diameter, and a diastolic ratio >1.1 is considered abnormal. In RV pressure overload, the ratio is >1.1 in both diastole *and* systole.

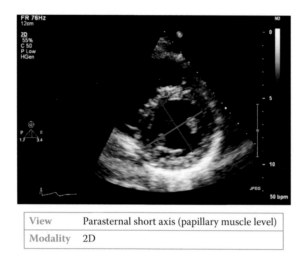

View	Parasternal short axis (papillary muscle level)
Modality	2D

Figure 22.5 Measurement of LV septo-lateral (red line) and antero-posterior (blue line) cavity diameters in order to calculate the LV eccentricity index in the assessment of RV volume and pressure overload.

Further reading

Lang RM et al. Recommendations for cardiac chamber quantification by echocardiography in adults: an update from the American Society of Echocardiography and the European Association of Cardiovascular Imaging. *Journal of the American Society of Echocardiography* (2015). PMID 25559473.

Park JB et al. Quantification of right ventricular volume and function using single-beat three-dimensional echocardiography: a validation study with cardiac magnetic resonance. *Journal of the American Society of Echocardiography* (2016). PMID 26969137.

Zaidi A et al. Echocardiographic assessment of the right heart in adults: a practical guideline from the British Society of Echocardiography. *Echo Research & Practice* (2020). PMID 32105053.

CHAPTER 23

The right atrium

The right atrium (RA) receives venous blood returning from the upper body (via the superior vena cava [SVC]), the lower body (via the inferior vena cava [IVC]) and also from the myocardium (via the coronary sinus). It can best be seen in the:

- parasternal RV inflow view (**Figure 7.3**, p. 45)
- parasternal short-axis view (aortic valve level) (**Figure 7.5**, p. 47)
- apical four-chamber view (**Figure 7.8**, p. 50)
- subcostal view (**Figure 7.12**, p. 54)

When studying the RA, assess and describe the

- RA size
- RA pressure
- embryological remnants
  - crista terminalis
  - Eustachian valve
  - Chiari network
- presence or absence of masses (tumour/thrombus)
- presence or absence of a pacing wire or venous catheter

RIGHT ATRIAL SIZE

Assessment of RA size can be challenging in view of the difficulty that can be encountered in imaging it clearly. In an apical four-chamber view, you can simply 'eyeball' the relative sizes of the left and right atria. The RA is normally no larger than the left – if it is larger, it is dilated.

RA size can be assessed using liner, area or volumetric approaches. Linear measurements are made in the apical four-chamber view at end-systole: Measure the RA minor axis from the lateral wall of the RA to the interatrial septum (perpendicular to the RA major axis, **Figure 23.1**). The normal range (indexed to body surface area) for the RA major axis is 24 ± 3 mm/m^2 for males and 25 ± 3 mm/m^2 for females. For the minor axis, the normal range is 19 ± 3 mm/m^2 for both sexes.

For an area measurement, perform planimetry of the RA in the apical four-chamber view. A dilated RA is indicated by an area >22 cm^2 (indexed >11 cm^2/m^2) for males and >19 cm^2 (indexed >11 cm^2/m^2) for females.

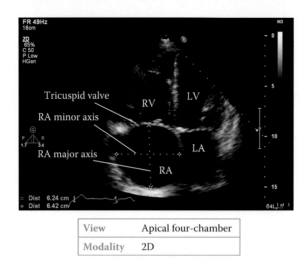

View	Apical four-chamber
Modality	2D

Figure 23.1 Measurement of right atrial dimensions. *Abbreviations:* LA: Left atrium, LV: Left ventricle, RA: Right atrium, RV: Right ventricle.

Calculation of RA volume can be made on 2D echo from the apical four-chamber view by using a single-plane area–length method or the method of disks summation, with a normal range of 25 ± 7 mL/m^2 for males and 21 ± 6 mL/m^2 for females. RA volumes can also be measured using 3D echo, although the measured values tend to be slightly higher than for volumes calculated from 2D measurements.

RA dilatation can result from RA pressure overload (e.g., pulmonary hypertension, restrictive cardiomyopathy, tricuspid stenosis), RA volume overload (e.g., tricuspid regurgitation, atrial septal defect) and chronic atrial fibrillation.

ESTIMATED RIGHT ATRIAL PRESSURE

The accuracy of estimating RA pressure using echo is generally poor. Indeed, published data show an accuracy of around 34% when estimated right atrial pressure (eRAP) measurements made by echo are compared with invasive RAP measurements. For this reason, contemporary pulmonary hypertension guidelines have demoted the importance of eRAP (for use in the calculation of systolic pulmonary arterial pressure) and now place more emphasis on peak tricuspid regurgitation velocity.

However, with this caveat in mind, if you wish to obtain an eRAP using echo, then you can attempt to do so by assessing the inferior vena cava (IVC). Measure the IVC diameter in both expiration and inspiration, within 1–2 cm of its junction with the right atrium, using the subcostal window (**Figure 23.2**). Take two measurements: One during normal breathing, and one during an inspiratory 'sniff'. Calculate the IVC collapsibility index as follows:

$$\text{Collapsibility index} = \frac{\text{Minimum IVC diameter during sniff}}{\text{Maximum IVC diameter during normal breathing}} \times 100$$

Normally the IVC measures <2.1 cm in diameter and decreases by >50% in inspiration. The data in **Table 23.1** will allow you to place an approximate value on eRAP. For example, if the IVC measures 2.8 cm in expiration and 1.8 cm in inspiration, a reduction of 36%, the eRAP would be 10–20 mmHg.

Another indicator of eRAP is simply the RA size, which is usually normal when RAP is ≤10 mmHg, but becomes dilated at pressures above this (and, in general, the higher the RAP, the greater the dilatation). Pulmonary hypertension guidelines regard an RA area (at end-systole) of >18 cm^2

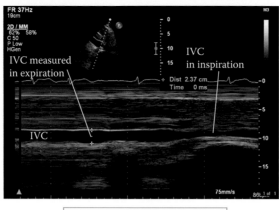

View	Subcostal (IVC view)
Modality	M-mode

Figure 23.2   Measurement of inferior vena cava (IVC) diameter.

Table 23.1   Estimation of right atrial pressure (eRAP)

IVC size (cm)	IVC collapsibility index	eRAP (mmHg)
≤2.1	>50%	3 (0–5)
≤2.1	<50%	8 (5–10)
>2.1	<50%	15 (10–20)

Abbreviation: IVC: Inferior vena cava.

as a suggestive 'additional' echo feature of pulmonary hypertension. Similarly, the hepatic veins become increasingly dilated as RAP rises above 15 mmHg.

EMBRYOLOGICAL REMNANTS

Echocardiography can reveal a number of embryological remnants in the right atrium that are sometimes mistaken for pathological findings by the unwary.

The **crista terminalis** is a fibromuscular ridge that represents the junction between the sinus venosus and the primitive right atrium in the embryo. In the adult it can be seen as a vertical ridge running along the posterolateral wall. On echo, it can be mistaken for a mass, thrombus or vegetation.

Where the IVC enters the RA, there is often an embryological remnant, the **Eustachian valve**, which in fetal life directs oxygenated blood away from the tricuspid valve and towards the foramen ovale. The Eustachian valve can remain prominent in adult life and is a normal finding but, like the crista terminalis, can be mistaken for a pathological lesion.

Similarly, a **Chiari network** is a fetal remnant and appears as a web-like structure extending into the RA with an attachment near the RA–IVC junction. It is reportedly present in around 4.6% of the population as a normal variant.

Usually neither a prominent Eustachian valve nor a Chiari network is of any clinical significance, although there is some evidence that either remnant in combination with a patent foramen ovale may increase the risk of paradoxical (right-to-left) embolism.

RIGHT ATRIAL MASSES

Cardiac tumours and thrombi are described in Chapter 32. Renal cell carcinoma can extend from the kidney all the way up the IVC and into the RA.

Further reading

Humbert M et al. 2022 ESC/ERS guidelines for the diagnosis and treatment of pulmonary hypertension. *European Heart Journal* (2022). PMID 36017548.

Lang RM et al. Recommendations for cardiac chamber quantification by echocardiography in adults: an update from the American Society of Echocardiography and the European Association of Cardiovascular Imaging. *Journal of the American Society of Echocardiography* (2015). PMID 25559473.

Lang RM et al. Imaging assessment of the right atrium: anatomy and function. *European Heart Journal – Cardiovascular Imaging* (2022). PMID 35079782.

Magnino C et al. Inaccuracy of right atrial pressure estimates through inferior vena cava indices. *American Journal of Cardiology* (2017). PMID 28912040.

Zaidi A et al. Echocardiographic assessment of the right heart in adults: a practical guideline from the British Society of Echocardiography. *Echo Research & Practice* (2020). PMID 32105053.

CHAPTER 24

The tricuspid valve

As outlined in Chapter 2, the tricuspid valve has three cusps, called anterior, posterior and septal. There are also three papillary muscles which, in a similar way to the mitral valve, are attached to the cusps via chordae tendineae.

The tricuspid valve can be best seen in

- parasternal RV inflow view (**Figure 7.3**, p. 45)
- parasternal short-axis view (at the aortic valve level) (**Figure 24.1**)
- RV-focused apical view (p. 53)
- subcostal view (**Figure 7.12**, p. 54)

TRICUSPID STENOSIS

Tricuspid stenosis is most commonly a consequence of previous rheumatic fever, and it almost invariably occurs together with mitral stenosis (indeed, it is important not to 'miss' coexistent tricuspid stenosis in patients undergoing surgery for mitral stenosis). Rheumatic thickening of the tricuspid leaflets tends to be subtler than that of the mitral leaflets and so is harder to spot. Rarer causes of tricuspid stenosis include

- carcinoid syndrome
- Ebstein's anomaly (Chapter 33)
- 'functional' tricuspid stenosis as a result of obstruction of the valve by a large RA tumour, thrombus or vegetation

Patients may present with fatigue, peripheral oedema or symptoms relating to an underlying cause (e.g., flushing in carcinoid syndrome) or coexistent condition (e.g., mitral stenosis). Physical signs include a prominent 'a' wave in the JVP, a tricuspid opening snap and a diastolic murmur at the left sternal edge.

Echo assessment of tricuspid stenosis

2D and M-mode

Use 2D and M-mode echo to assess the structure of the valve:

- Is the tricuspid valve normal, rheumatic or myxomatous?
- Is there evidence of Ebstein's anomaly?
- Are the valve leaflets (anterior, posterior, septal) normal? Is there thickening, and does this affect the tips or the body of the leaflet(s)?

DOI: 10.1201/9781003304654-24

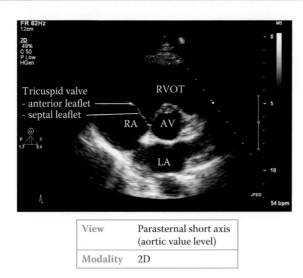

View	Parasternal short axis (aortic value level)
Modality	2D

Figure 24.1 Normal tricuspid valve. *Abbreviations:* LA: Left atrium, RA: Right atrium, AV: Aortic valve, RVOT: Right ventricular outflow tract.

- Is there commissural fusion?
- Is there leaflet calcification, and is this focal (anterior, posterior, septal) or diffuse?
- Is leaflet mobility normal or reduced? How much is it reduced?
- How well do the leaflets coapt? Is there any doming or prolapse of the leaflets?
- Is there any evidence of papillary muscle rupture?
- Are there any tricuspid valve vegetations or abscesses?
- Is the tricuspid annulus normal, dilated or calcified?

Colour Doppler

Use colour Doppler to look for any coexistent tricuspid regurgitation (TR). The colour jet can also help in obtaining correct alignment of the probe for continuous wave (CW) and pulsed-wave (PW) Doppler recordings.

CW and PW Doppler

Use Doppler to record forward flow through the tricuspid valve from an RV-focused apical view and using a sweep speed of 100 mm/s. Ignore traces obtained from ectopic beats (and the beat following an ectopic), and if the patient is in atrial fibrillation, average the measurements taken from several beats. From the trace, measure the mean pressure gradient (trace the velocity time integral (VTI) of the tricuspid inflow) and the pressure half-time.

SEVERITY OF TRICUSPID STENOSIS

Severe tricuspid stenosis can be identified quantitatively by measuring the

- mean pressure gradient
- pressure half-time
- valve area (by continuity equation)

Mean pressure gradient and pressure half-time are measured using CW and PW Doppler as above. Be aware that the pressure half-time is difficult to measure at heart rates >100/min.

Table 24.1   Indicators of severe tricuspid stenosis

	Severe
Mean pressure gradient (mmHg)	≥5
Pressure half-time (ms)	≥190
Valve area by continuity equation (cm²)	<1

Source: Reference intervals reproduced with permission of the British Society of Echocardiography.

You might recall from Chapter 21 that in mitral stenosis, the mitral valve area can be estimated by dividing 220 by the mitral pressure half-time (p. 160). This method is less well-validated in tricuspid stenosis, although some have suggested estimating the tricuspid valve area using the tricuspid pressure half-time as follows:

$$\text{Tricuspid valve area }\left(\text{cm}^2\right) = \frac{190}{\text{Tricuspid pressure half-time (ms)}}$$

However, guidelines recommend that in tricuspid stenosis, the tricuspid valve area should be calculated using the continuity equation (as long as there is no significant valvular regurgitation). To calculate this, you need to measure

- stroke volume (in mL) in the right (or left) ventricular outflow tract
- VTI (in cm) of the tricuspid inflow

The calculation is then as follows:

$$\text{Tricuspid valve area }\left(\text{cm}^2\right) = \frac{\text{Stroke volume (mL)}}{\text{Tricuspid valve VTI (cm)}}$$

Table 24.1 summarizes the echo indicators of severe tricuspid stenosis.

TRICUSPID REGURGITATION

TR is the flow of blood from the RV back through the tricuspid valve during systole. TR can result from dysfunction of the tricuspid valve apparatus (primary TR) or from anatomical abnormalities affecting the valve's supporting structures (secondary TR). A trace amount of TR, in the absence of any structural heart disease, is a common finding in around 70% of normal individuals.

Significant primary TR can be the result of

- rheumatic valve disease
- infective endocarditis
- myxomatous degeneration
- Ebstein's anomaly
- carcinoid syndrome
- some serotoninergic drugs

The presence of a pacing wire that passes through the tricuspid valve can also lead to a degree of TR by preventing full closure of the valve leaflets.

Secondary TR occurs with RA or RV dilatation/remodelling, for instance with RV volume overload or the atrial dilatation that can occur in persistent atrial fibrillation.

Significant TR can cause symptoms and signs of right-sided heart failure, with a prominent V wave in the jugular venous pressure, peripheral oedema, ascites and a distended pulsatile liver.

> **CARCINOID SYNDROME AND THE HEART**
>
> Carcinoid tumours are rare and usually arise in the gastrointestinal system. If they metastasize, they can produce the carcinoid syndrome, in which secretion of vasoactive substances such as 5-hydroxytryptamine causes flushing, diarrhoea and bronchospasm. These substances can also affect the heart, leading to the development of fibrous endocardial plaques, typically on the right-sided valves and chambers. The tricuspid and pulmonary valve leaflets characteristically become shortened and thickened (but without commissural fusion, in contrast to rheumatic tricuspid valve disease), leading to stenosis and/or regurgitation and ultimately right heart failure.

Echo assessment of tricuspid regurgitation

2D and M-mode

Use 2D and M-mode echo to assess the structure of the valve as described for tricuspid stenosis (above). In mild TR, the tricuspid leaflets are usually normal or just mildly abnormal. With severe TR, there are usually severe leaflet lesions such as flailing, restriction, perforation or a wide coaptation deficit. Remember to look at the whole valve apparatus (tricuspid annulus, papillary muscles and chordae), not just the leaflets.

Using the RV-focused apical view, measure the septal-lateral annular dimension at end-diastole (**Figure 24.2**). Reference intervals are

- normal tricuspid annular dimension 28 ± 5 mm
- significantly dilated annular dimension >40 mm (or >21 mm/m^2)

In the same view, measure the tricuspid valve tenting height and tenting area at end-systole (**Figure 24.3**). In the evaluation of secondary TR, a tenting area >1 cm^2 indicates that it is likely to be more than mild. In relation to tricuspid valve surgery, a tenting height >0.76 cm and a tenting area >1.6 cm^2 predict significant residual TR.

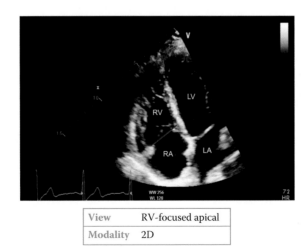

View	RV-focused apical
Modality	2D

Figure 24.2   Measurement of the septal-lateral annular dimension (red line). *Abbreviations:* LA: Left atrium, RA: Right atrium, LV: Left ventricle, RV: Right ventricle.

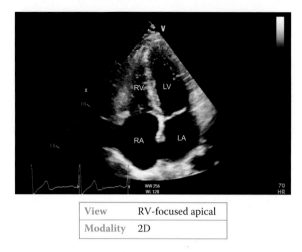

View	RV-focused apical
Modality	2D

Figure 24.3 Measurement of the tricuspid valve tenting height (blue line) and tenting area (red triangle). *Abbreviations:* LA: Left atrium, RA: Right atrium, LV: Left ventricle, RV: Right ventricle.

Colour Doppler

Use colour Doppler to examine the jet of TR in the parasternal and apical (**Figure 24.4**) views. Describe

- the extent of the TR jet within the RA (trace the colour flow area in the RV-focused apical view)
- the direction of travel of the TR jet within the atrium (central or directed towards the interatrial septum or the RA free wall)
- the position of the TR jet in relation to the tricuspid leaflets (e.g., central jet, or evidence of regurgitation through a leaflet perforation)

Trace the area of the TR jet (a colour flow area of >10 cm² indicates severe TR) and calculate the ratio between the colour flow area and RA area (a ratio >50% indicates severe TR).

Gauge the relative size of the flow convergence zone – a large zone seen throughout systole is indicative of severe TR. Measure the width of the vena contracta (VC) – the narrowest region of colour

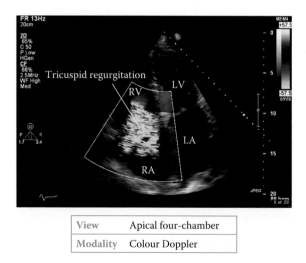

View	Apical four-chamber
Modality	Colour Doppler

Figure 24.4 Severe tricuspid regurgitation. *Abbreviations:* LA: Left atrium, RA: Right atrium, LV: Left ventricle, RV: Right ventricle.

flow at the level of the tricuspid valve – in the RV-focused apical view and with the Nyquist limit set at 50–60 cm/s.

CW and PW Doppler

Record the CW Doppler trace with the probe carefully aligned with the direction of the regurgitant jet (**Figure 24.5**). The CW Doppler trace is faint in mild TR but denser in moderate or severe TR. Look at the contour of the regurgitant jet – in mild TR, the shape of the waveform is parabolic; but in severe TR, the shape becomes more triangular with an early peak. Measure the TR peak velocity (TR V_{max}) and also the VTI of the TR jet.

Use PW Doppler to assess the tricuspid valve inflow and measure the E and A wave velocities. Also use PW Doppler to assess the hepatic vein flow, ideally in the central hepatic vein, in the subcostal window (**Figure 24.6**). Hepatic vein flow is normally directed towards the RA throughout the

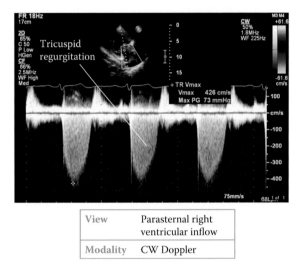

View	Parasternal right ventricular inflow
Modality	CW Doppler

Figure 24.5 Moderate tricuspid regurgitation (TR), showing measurement of peak velocity (TR V_{max}). *Abbreviation:* PG: Pressure gradient.

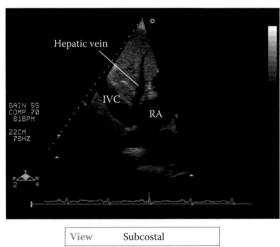

View	Subcostal
Modality	2D

Figure 24.6 Hepatic veins. *Abbreviations:* IVC: Inferior vena cava, RA: Right atrium.

cardiac cycle, with the systolic component being predominant. Systolic hepatic vein flow becomes blunted in moderate TR and reversed in severe TR.

Proximal Isovelocity Surface Area assessment

The proximal isovelocity surface area (PISA) principle can be used for TR as for mitral regurgitation (Chapter 21):

1. Using colour Doppler in the RV-focused apical view, narrow down the sector width and minimize the depth before zooming in on the location of the TR jet through the tricuspid valve. Adjust the aliasing velocity by adjusting the zero point on the colour flow scale in the direction of the TR jet until you see a clear hemisphere of converging blood flow on the ventricular side of the valve, usually at a setting of 20–40 cm/s. There should be a clear interface between red- and blue-coloured flow, and the velocity of blood flow at this point equals the aliasing velocity (in cm/s).

2. Measure the radius (r) of this hemisphere by taking a measurement from the edge of the hemisphere (i.e., the red–blue interface) to the centre of the valve orifice. Use this to calculate PISA, the surface area of this hemisphere, in cm²:

$$PISA = 2\pi r^2$$

3. The regurgitant flow rate, in mL/s, can be calculated from the PISA (in cm²) and the aliasing velocity (in cm/s):

$$Regurgitant\ flow\ rate = PISA \times Aliasing\ velocity$$

4. Using the calculated regurgitant flow rate (in mL/s) and the measured TR V_{max} (in cm/s) measured using CW Doppler, calculate the effective regurgitant orifice area (EROA) in cm² using

$$EROA = \frac{Regurgitant\ flow\ rate}{TR\ V_{max}}$$

5. Finally, you can calculate the regurgitant volume (in mL) using the calculated EROA (in cm²) and the measured VTI (in cm) using

$$Regurgitant\ volume = EROA \times VTI$$

For the purposes of estimating severity, it is sufficient just to measure the PISA radius. A radius >0.9 cm (measured at a Nyquist limit of 28 cm/s) indicates severe TR. Do not use the PISA technique if a clear symmetrical hemisphere cannot be obtained or if the jet of TR is eccentric.

3D echo

Where available, 3D echo permits a more comprehensive assessment of tricuspid valve anatomy and in particular allows for a more detailed evaluation of the mechanism and severity of TR. When measured with 3D echo, the normal tricuspid annular area is 8.6 ± 2.0 cm², and the normal tricuspid annular perimeter measures 10.5 ± 1.2 cm. When measured using 3D echo, an EROA of >0.4 cm² or a VC area of >0.4 cm² indicates severe TR.

Associated features

If TR is present,

- assess any coexistent tricuspid stenosis
- assess any coexistent disease affecting the other valves (as patients undergoing tricuspid valve surgery may also require any other valvular abnormalities to be corrected at the same time)

- assess the size of the RA, RV and IVC – these chambers are usually dilated if TR is severe
- assess RV function
- look for evidence of pulmonary hypertension (Chapter 26)

Severity of tricuspid regurgitation

Severity of TR can be assessed from the

- tricuspid leaflet morphology
- colour flow area
- colour flow area/RA area
- flow convergence zone
- VC width
- PISA radius
- EROA (by PISA)
- regurgitant volume (by PISA)
- CW Doppler jet density/Contour
- tricuspid valve E velocity
- tricuspid valve E/A ratio
- RV/RA/IVC size
- hepatic vein flow

The approach to measuring each of these parameters has been discussed above, and **Table 24.2** summarizes how each of these parameters correlates with TR severity.

Table 24.2   Indicators of tricuspid regurgitation severity

	Mild	Moderate	Severe
Tricuspid leaflets	Normal, mildly abnormal		Severe lesions
Colour flow area (cm²)	<5	5–10	>10
Colour flow area/RA area (cm²)	Small, narrow, central		Large, >50%
Flow convergence zone	Not seen/Transient	Intermediate	Large holosystolic
Vena contracta width (cm)	<0.3	0.3–0.69	≥0.7
PISA radius at Nyquist 28 cm/s (cm)	<0.5	0.5–0.9	>0.9
EROA by PISA (mL)	<0.20	0.20–0.39	≥0.40
Regurgitant volume by PISA (mL)	<30	30–44	≥45
CW Doppler jet density	Faint	Intermediate	Dense
CW Doppler jet contour	Parabolic	Variable	Triangular confirms severe TR
Tricuspid valve E velocity	Variable	Variable	≥1 m/s
Tricuspid valve E/A ratio	Variable	Variable	≥1
RV size (chronic primary TR)	Normal	Normal	Usually dilated
RA size (chronic primary TR)	Normal	Normal	Dilated
IVC diameter (cm)	Variable	Variable	<21 mm with >50% inspiratory collapse *unlikely* in severe TR
Hepatic vein flow	Systolic dominance	Systolic blunting	Systolic flow reversal

Abbreviations: CW: Continuous wave, EROA: Effective regurgitant orifice area, IVC: Inferior vena cava, PISA: Proximal isovelocity surface area, RA: Right atrium, RV: Right ventricle.

Source: Reference intervals reproduced with permission of the British society of echocardiography.

Further reading

Arsalan M et al. Tricuspid regurgitation diagnosis and treatment. *European Heart Journal* (2017). PMID 26358570.

Go YY et al. The conundrum of tricuspid regurgitation grading. *Frontiers in Cardiovascular Medicine* (2018). PMID 30474032.

Lancellotti P et al. Recommendations for the echocardiographic assessment of native valvular regurgitation: an executive summary from the European Association of Cardiovascular Imaging. *European Heart Journal – Cardiovascular Imaging* (2013). PMID 23733442.

Zaidi A et al. Echocardiographic assessment of the tricuspid and pulmonary valves: a practical guideline from the British Society of Echocardiography. *Echo Research and Practice* (2020). PMID 33339003.

Zoghbi WA et al. Recommendations for noninvasive evaluation of native valvular regurgitation: a report from the American Society of Echocardiography developed in collaboration with the Society for Cardiovascular Magnetic Resonance. *Journal of the American Society of Echocardiography* (2017). PMID 28314623.

CHAPTER 25

The pulmonary valve

As we saw in Chapter 2, the pulmonary valve lies between the right ventricular outflow tract (RVOT) and the pulmonary artery. The valve itself is structurally similar to the aortic valve, albeit with thinner cusps (owing to the lower right-sided pressures). The three cusps are called anterior, left and right.

The pulmonary valve can be best seen in the

- parasternal right ventricular (RV) outflow view (**Figure 7.4**, p. 46)
- parasternal short-axis view (at the aortic valve level) (**Figure 7.5**, p. 47)
- subcostal short-axis view

Beyond the pulmonary valve, it is possible to visualize the main pulmonary artery ('pulmonary trunk'), sometimes to the point of its bifurcation into left and right pulmonary arteries (often best seen in the parasternal RV outflow view). In the parasternal short-axis view, measure the diameter of the main pulmonary artery during diastole in between the pulmonary valve and the pulmonary artery bifurcation, approximately 1 cm distal to the valve (**Figure 25.1**). The main pulmonary artery is considered dilated if the diameter is >25 mm.

PULMONARY STENOSIS

Pulmonary stenosis is most commonly a congenital defect, often presenting in infancy or childhood, although it can also result from the previous rheumatic fever or from the carcinoid syndrome (Chapter 24).

Patients are often asymptomatic and are diagnosed when an incidental heart murmur is found during examination. Symptomatic patients may have fatigue, breathlessness, presyncope/syncope, symptoms of RV dysfunction or symptoms relating to an underlying cause (e.g., flushing in carcinoid syndrome), or cyanosis (when there is a coexistent right-to-left shunt). Physical signs include a widely split second heart sound and an ejection systolic murmur in the pulmonary area, and in severe stenosis, there may be evidence of RV hypertrophy.

Echo assessment of pulmonary stenosis

2D and M-mode

Use 2D echo to assess the pulmonary valve and surrounding structures:

- Is it a tricuspid pulmonary valve, or is it bicuspid or dysplastic?
- Is there any thickening or calcification of the cusps? Is this diffuse or focal? If focal, which area of each cusp is affected?

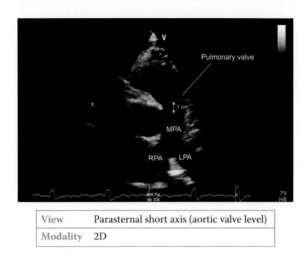

View	Parasternal short axis (aortic valve level)
Modality	2D

Figure 25.1 Measurement of main pulmonary artery diameter (red line), 1 cm distal to the pulmonary valve. *Abbreviations:* LPA: Left pulmonary artery, MPA: Main pulmonary artery, RPA: Right pulmonary artery.

- Is cusp mobility normal or reduced? How much is it reduced?
- Is there any systolic doming of the cusps?
- Is there any evidence of subvalvular or supravalvular stenosis? Is there any stenosis in the branch pulmonary arteries?
- Are there any vegetations or masses attached to the valve?
- Is there any thrombus (pulmonary embolism) visible in the main pulmonary artery or its branches?

Although it is possible to obtain an M-mode recording of the motion of the individual pulmonary valve cusps in the parasternal short-axis view, this is seldom necessary in everyday practice.

Colour Doppler

Use colour Doppler to map any regurgitant blood flow proximal to the pulmonary valve:

- Is there any pulmonary regurgitation?
- Which part of the valve does it arise from?
- How extensive is it?

CW and PW Doppler

Use CW Doppler to obtain a trace of forward flow through the pulmonary valve (**Figure 25.2**). Obtain traces from the parasternal right ventricular outflow view and the parasternal short-axis view (aortic valve level).

The CW Doppler trace will give peak transpulmonary velocity (V_{max}) which relates to peak transpulmonary pressure gradient (ΔP_{max}) via the simplified Bernoulli equation:

$$\Delta P_{max} = 4 \times V_{max}^2$$

If peak velocity in the RVOT is >1.0 m/s, use the full Bernoulli equation for greater accuracy:

$$\Delta P_{max} = 4 \times \left(V_2^2 - V_1^2 \right)$$

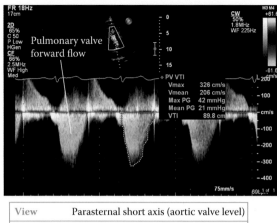

View	Parasternal short axis (aortic valve level)
Modality	CW Doppler

Figure 25.2   Moderate pulmonary stenosis. *Abbreviations:* PG: Pressure gradient, PV: Pulmonary valve, V_{max}: Peak velocity, V_{mean}: Mean velocity, VTI: Velocity time integral.

where V_2 is the peak transpulmonary velocity, assessed by CW Doppler, and V_1 is the peak RVOT velocity, assessed by PW Doppler.

The mean transpulmonary pressure gradient (ΔP_{mean}) can be obtained by tracing the Doppler envelope, from which the echo machine can calculate a mean value by averaging the instantaneous gradients throughout the trace. Calculation of the pulmonary valve effective orifice area is seldom necessary; but if it is required, then the continuity equation can be used (as for aortic stenosis, see Chapter 20).

If you suspect subvalvular or supravalvular stenosis, use PW Doppler to assess blood flow at different levels above and below the valve to detect where the main flow acceleration occurs.

Associated features

Pulmonary stenosis is often associated with other congenital heart disorders, and so look carefully for any other structural heart defects (e.g., tetralogy of Fallot). In addition,

- assess any coexistent pulmonary regurgitation
- assess any coexistent tricuspid valve disease (carcinoid syndrome can affect both tricuspid and pulmonary valves)
- assess RV dimensions and function. Obstruction to RV outflow by the pulmonary valve raises RV pressure, leading to RV hypertrophy and subsequently dilatation and impaired function
- assess pulmonary artery dimensions (pulmonary artery dilatation is a common finding in pulmonary stenosis)

Severity of pulmonary stenosis

Severity of pulmonary stenosis can be quantified by the pulmonary valve V_{max} (**Table 25.1**).

Table 25.1   Indicators of pulmonary stenosis severity

	Mild	Moderate	Severe
Peak velocity (m/s)	<3	3–4	>4

Source: Reference intervals reproduced with permission of the British Society of Echocardiography.

PULMONARY REGURGITATION

Pulmonary regurgitation is the flow of blood from the pulmonary artery back through the pulmonary valve during diastole. A trace amount of pulmonary regurgitation, in the absence of any structural heart disease, is present in around 75% of normal individuals. More significant pulmonary regurgitation can be the result of

- previous pulmonary valvuloplasty/valvotomy
- repaired tetralogy of Fallot
- rheumatic valve disease
- pulmonary artery dilatation (e.g., in pulmonary hypertension)
- idiopathic dilatation of the pulmonary annulus
- infective endocarditis
- carcinoid syndrome
- congenital absence of one or more cusps

Pulmonary regurgitation can be classified as primary (due to abnormal cusps, most commonly as a result of congenital heart disease and pulmonary valvuloplasty/valvotomy) or secondary (where the cusps themselves are normal, most often seen in pulmonary hypertension). Significant pulmonary regurgitation leads to RV volume overload and can cause symptoms and signs of right-sided heart failure.

Echo assessment of pulmonary regurgitation

2D and M-mode

Use 2D and M-mode echo to assess the structure of the valve as described for pulmonary stenosis (above).

Colour Doppler

Use colour Doppler to examine the jet of pulmonary regurgitation and describe the jet size. In mild pulmonary regurgitation, the jet width just below the pulmonary valve is narrow and the jet is usually <1.0 cm in length. In severe pulmonary regurgitation, the jet usually occupies >65% of the RVOT width. In addition, measure the vena contracta of the proximal regurgitant jet and compare this to the pulmonary valve annulus diameter: A ratio of >0.7 usually indicates severe regurgitation.

Be aware that in severe pulmonary regurgitation, there may be rapid equalization of the pulmonary artery and RV diastolic pressures that can lead to a 'brief' colour jet, which is challenging to assess.

CW and PW Doppler

Record a CW Doppler trace with the probe carefully aligned with the direction of the regurgitant jet (**Figure 25.3**). The CW Doppler trace is faint in mild pulmonary regurgitation and denser in moderate or severe regurgitation.

Look at the contour of the regurgitant jet – in mild pulmonary regurgitation, the deceleration rate of the jet is slow, becoming steeper with more severe degrees of regurgitation (although this is also affected by decreased RV compliance). A pressure half-time of <100 ms and a deceleration time of <260 ms are indicative of severe pulmonary regurgitation. Measure the duration of pulmonary regurgitation and express this as a ratio of total diastolic time to give the Doppler PR index: A value of <0.77 suggests severe pulmonary regurgitation.

Use PW Doppler to look for evidence of diastolic flow reversal in the branch pulmonary arteries: If present, this has been reported to have an 87% sensitivity and specificity for severe pulmonary regurgitation. You can also use PW Doppler to assess the VTI of forward flow in the RVOT

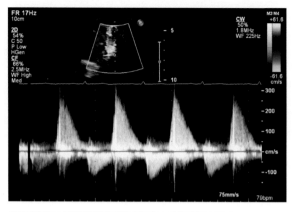

View	Parasternal short axis (aortic valve level)
Modality	CW Doppler

Figure 25.3   Severe pulmonary regurgitation.

(in the parasternal view) and also in the LVOT (in the apical five-chamber view). The ratio of $RVOT_{VTI}/LVOT_{VTI}$ increases with the increasing severity of pulmonary regurgitation. Measurement of the peak velocity of the jet of pulmonary regurgitation allows calculation of pulmonary artery diastolic pressure (p. 205).

Regurgitant volume and fraction

Calculation of pulmonary regurgitant volume and fraction by echocardiography is fraught with difficulty and highly prone to technical error. For this reason, it is generally better avoided.

Associated features

If pulmonary regurgitation is present,

- assess any coexistent pulmonary stenosis
- assess any coexistent disease affecting the other valves
- assess RV dimensions and function – the RV may become dilated due to volume overload if pulmonary regurgitation is severe
- assess flow in the pulmonary artery (diastolic flow reversal indicates severe pulmonary regurgitation)
- look for evidence of pulmonary hypertension (Chapter 26)

Severity of pulmonary regurgitation

Severity of pulmonary regurgitation can be assessed by

- jet size
- jet width/RVOT ratio
- vena contracta/PV annulus ratio
- CW jet density
- pressure half-time
- PR deceleration time
- Doppler PR index
- branch PA flow reversal
- $RVOT_{VTI}/LVOT_{VTI}$ ratio

Table 25.2 Indicators of pulmonary regurgitation severity

	Mild	Moderate	Severe
Jet size	Narrow, <1.0 cm in length	Intermediate	Wide, large
Jet width/RVOT (%)			>65
Vena contracta/PV annulus (%)	<50		>70
CW jet density	Faint		Dense
Pressure half-time (ms)			<100
PR deceleration time (ms)			<260
Doppler PR index			<0.77
Branch PA flow reversal	Absent	Absent	Present
RVOT$_{VTI}$/LVOT$_{VTI}$	↑	↑↑	↑↑↑

Abbreviations: CW: Continuous wave, LVOT: Left ventricular outflow tract, PA: Pulmonary artery, PR: Pulmonary regurgitation, PV: Pulmonary valve, RVOT: Right ventricular outflow tract, VTI: Velocity time integral.

Source: Reference intervals reproduced with permission of the British Society of Echocardiography.

The approach to measuring each of these parameters has been discussed above, and **Table 25.2** summarizes how each of these parameters correlates with pulmonary regurgitation severity.

Further reading

British Society of Echocardiography (2022). https://www.bsecho.org/common/Uploaded%20files/Education/Posters/PUA006-Valve-disease-assessment-poster_print-ready.pdf

Vahanian A et al. 2021 ESC/EACTS Guidelines for the management of valvular heart disease. *European Heart Journal* (2022). PMID 34453165.

Zaidi A et al. Echocardiographic assessment of the tricuspid and pulmonary valves: a practical guideline from the British Society of Echocardiography. *Echo Research & Practice* (2020). PMID 33339003.

Zoghbi WA et al. Recommendations for noninvasive evaluation of native valvular regurgitation: a report from the American Society of Echocardiography developed in collaboration with the Society for Cardiovascular Magnetic Resonance. *Journal of the American Society of Echocardiography* (2017). PMID 28314623.

CHAPTER 26

Pulmonary hypertension

Pulmonary hypertension refers to an increase in blood pressure within the pulmonary vasculature. It is defined haemodynamically as a mean pulmonary artery pressure ≥25 mmHg at rest. Note that the haemodynamic definition refers to *mean* pulmonary artery pressure, not to the pulmonary artery systolic pressure, and the definition is based on cardiac catheter studies.

Historically, the role of echo in pulmonary hypertension used to centre on using echo to estimate pulmonary artery systolic pressure using a combination of the tricuspid regurgitation (TR) peak velocity and an estimation of right atrial (RA) pressure. However, this approach carries significant pitfalls and the correlation between echo and catheter-based measurements is generally poor.

For this reason, contemporary guidelines take a different and more pragmatic approach, using echo to grade the *probability* of pulmonary hypertension being present, rather than trying to calculate the actual pulmonary artery pressures. A standard echo report will therefore indicate whether there is a low, intermediate or high probability of pulmonary hypertension. Confirmation of the diagnosis requires right heart cardiac catheterization.

However, there are situations when estimating the actual pulmonary artery pressure is reasonable, such as when assessing patients with left-sided valvular disease, or when performing serial follow-up studies in an individual patient. This is because some treatment guidelines make use of absolute pulmonary artery pressure values in their decision-making algorithms. Therefore, this chapter will also describe the methods for estimating pulmonary artery systolic and diastolic pressure for those occasions when it is applicable to do so.

CAUSES OF PULMONARY HYPERTENSION

Pulmonary hypertension results from an increased resistance to blood flow through the pulmonary vasculature. The World Health Organization categorizes the causes of pulmonary hypertension into five groups:

Group 1: Pulmonary arterial hypertension (e.g., idiopathic, hereditary, drug- or toxin-induced, connective tissue disease, shunts in congenital heart disease)

Group 2: Pulmonary hypertension due to left heart disease (e.g., valvular disease, left ventricular systolic or diastolic dysfunction)

Group 3: Pulmonary hypertension due to lung disease (e.g., chronic obstructive pulmonary disease, interstitial lung disease, sleep apnoea)

Group 4: Chronic thromboembolic pulmonary hypertension (chronic pulmonary embolism)

Group 5: Unclear and/or multifactorial causes (e.g., sarcoidosis, vasculitis)

DOI: 10.1201/9781003304654-26

Pulmonary hypertension can also be subdivided into

- pre-capillary pulmonary hypertension (in which the pulmonary capillary wedge pressure is normal, i.e., ≤15 mmHg)
- post-capillary pulmonary hypertension (in which the pulmonary capillary wedge pressure is increased, i.e., >15 mmHg)

Post-capillary pulmonary hypertension is seen in pulmonary hypertension due to left heart disease. Pre-capillary pulmonary hypertension is seen in all the other causes, except in Group 5 where pre- and/or post-capillary causes may be present.

It is important to be aware of the potential causes of pulmonary hypertension, so that a search can be made for clues to the underlying cause whenever a suspicion of pulmonary hypertension is detected on echo.

CLINICAL FEATURES OF PULMONARY HYPERTENSION

The clinical features of pulmonary hypertension are summarized in **Table 26.1**. In addition to symptoms and signs related to the pulmonary hypertension itself, the patient may also have clinical features specific to the underlying cause.

GRADING THE PROBABILITY OF PULMONARY HYPERTENSION

Grading the probability of pulmonary hypertension on echo begins with the measurement, where feasible, of the TR peak velocity, TR V_{max}, using colour Doppler in whichever view the TR can be visualized optimally. The highest velocity should be chosen (if the patient has atrial fibrillation, then five beats should be averaged). If TR is severe and 'free-flowing', then the TR V_{max} may be underestimated and it is important to highlight this in your report.

Normally the TR V_{max} is <2.8 m/s. If the TR V_{max} is >3.4 m/s, then you can immediately conclude that there is a **high probability** of pulmonary hypertension.

If the TR V_{max} is ≤3.4 m/s, or if TR is not present, then you need to assess additional echo indicators before you can draw conclusions about the probability of pulmonary hypertension (**Figure 26.1**). These indicators are grouped into three categories:

- Ventricular indicators
    - right ventricle (RV)/left ventricle (LV) basal diameter ratio >1.0
    - flattening of the interventricular septum
- Pulmonary artery indicators
    - right ventricular outflow tract (RVOT) acceleration time <105 ms and/or mid-systolic notching
    - early diastolic pulmonary regurgitation (PR) velocity >2.2 m/s
    - pulmonary artery diameter >25 mm

Table 26.1   Clinical features of pulmonary hypertension

Symptoms	Signs
Symptoms are often of very gradual onset	Elevated jugular venous pressure
Breathlessness	Parasternal heave
Fatigue	Loud pulmonary component to second heart sound (P2)
Cough	Tricuspid regurgitation
Dizziness and syncope	Peripheral oedema
Peripheral oedema	Ascites

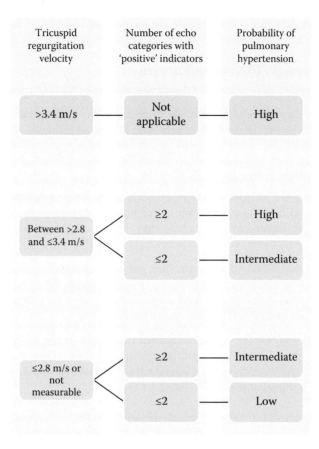

Figure 26.1   Grading the probability of pulmonary hypertension using tricuspid regurgitation velocity and additional echo indicators.

- Inferior vena cava (IVC)/RA indicators
  - IVC diameter >21 mm with decreased inspiratory collapse
  - RA area >18 cm² at end-systole

Ventricular indicators

The RV/LV basal diameter ratio is measured in the 'standard' apical four-chamber view at end-diastole. A ratio >1.0 is indicative of RV dilatation.

Flattening of the interventricular septum can be assessed using the LV eccentricity index, which is the ratio between the antero-posterior diameter and the septo-lateral diameter of the LV (as described on p. 178). This can be measured in both systole and diastole, and for the purposes of pulmonary hypertension assessment, an LV eccentricity index >1.1 is abnormal in systole (or in systole and diastole).

Pulmonary artery indicators

In the parasternal short-axis view (at the aortic valve level), perform pulsed-wave (PW) Doppler just proximal to the pulmonary valve at end-expiration. Measure the RVOT acceleration time from the onset of flow to the peak flow velocity. An RVOT acceleration time <105 ms is an indicator of pulmonary hypertension, as is the presence of a mid-systolic notch.

In the same view (or the parasternal RV outflow view), align a continuous wave (CW) cursor with the PR jet, if present, and measure the peak early diastolic velocity. A value of >2.2 m/s is an indicator of pulmonary hypertension.

The pulmonary artery diameter is measured in the parasternal short-axis view (at the aortic valve level) at end-diastole, and a diameter >25 mm is abnormal (**Figure 25.1**, p. 196).

Inferior vena cava (IVC)/RA indicators

In the apical four-chamber view, trace the RA area at end-systole. An RA area >18 cm^2 is abnormal.

In the subcostal view, use 2D and/or M-mode to measure the IVC diameter and assess how it changes with a 'sniff'. An IVC diameter >21 mm with decreased inspiratory collapse (<50% with a sniff) is abnormal.

Using multiple indicators

Once you've measured the indicators described above, you are now in a position to draw conclusions about the likelihood of pulmonary hypertension. As we saw earlier, if the TR V$_{max}$ is >3.4 m/s, then you can immediately conclude that there is a **high probability** of pulmonary hypertension.

If the TR V$_{max}$ is between >2.8 and ≤3.4 m/s, then you need to count up how many of the three 'categories' contain positive indicators for pulmonary hypertension. If two or more categories contain abnormal parameters, then there is a **high probability** of pulmonary hypertension; if not, then there is an **intermediate probability** of pulmonary hypertension.

If the TR V$_{max}$ is ≤2.8 m/s (or is not measurable), then you need to count up how many of the three 'categories' contain positive indicators for pulmonary hypertension. If two or more categories contain abnormal parameters, then there is an **intermediate probability** of pulmonary hypertension; if not, then there is a **low probability** of pulmonary hypertension.

Estimating pulmonary artery systolic pressure

As already discussed, the echo estimation of an *absolute* pulmonary artery pressure measurement can be unreliable and that is why contemporary echo guidelines focus on grading the probability of pulmonary hypertension. However, some clinical guidelines still incorporate an absolute value for pulmonary artery systolic pressure in the decision-making process, for instance, in the management of valve disease. For this reason, there can be circumstances where an absolute measurement needs to be made.

The technique that is commonly used for measuring pulmonary artery systolic pressure (PASP) relies upon the presence of TR. As with the probability-based approach already described, you can assess TR using CW Doppler in the

- parasternal RV inflow view (**Figure 7.3**, p. 45)
- parasternal short-axis view (aortic valve level) (**Figure 7.5**, p. 47)
- RV-focused apical view (p. 53)

Using CW Doppler, measure the peak velocity of *regurgitant* flow through the tricuspid valve (TR V$_{max}$) in m/s. It is a good idea to assess the tricuspid regurgitation in as many of the above views as possible and to use the highest value (or, if atrial fibrillation is present, to calculate the mean of five consecutive values). If it's difficult to obtain a clear spectral Doppler trace using CW Doppler, the use of agitated saline bubble contrast can enhance the tricuspid regurgitation jet.

Figure 24.5 (p. 190) shows a CW doppler trace of a TR jet with a TR V$_{max}$ of 4.26 m/s. The TR is driven by, and therefore reflects, the pressure gradient between the right ventricular systolic pressure (RVSP) and the RA pressure (RAP), and this pressure gradient can be calculated using the simplified Bernoulli equation:

$$RVSP - RAP = 4 \times \left(TR\,V_{max}\right)^2$$

For example, if the peak velocity of the TR jet is 4.26 m/s, then

$$RVSP - RAP = 4 \times (4.26)^2$$

$$RVSP - RAP = 4 \times 18.15$$

$$RVSP - RAP = 73 \text{ mmHg}$$

Now that you know the pressure *difference* between the RV and the RA, the next step is to estimate the *actual* systolic pressure in the RV, and to do that you need to know what the RAP is. The estimation of RAP from the IVC diameter has been described earlier in Chapter 23 (p. 182). If the assessment of the IVC gives an estimated RAP of 15 mmHg, then, continuing with our example from above,

$$RVSP - RAP = 73 \text{ mmHg}$$

$$RVSP = 73 \text{ mmHg} + RAP$$

$$RVSP = 73 + 15 \text{ mmHg}$$

$$RVSP = 88 \text{ mmHg}$$

The patient therefore has an estimated RVSP of approximately 88 mmHg. Assuming there is no significant pulmonary stenosis, the RVSP is approximately equal to the pulmonary artery systolic pressure (PASP):

$$PASP = RVSP$$

$$PASP = 88 \text{ mmHg}$$

(If there *is* coexistent pulmonary stenosis, then the RVSP will be higher than the PASP, and the difference will be equal to the peak pressure gradient across the stenosis.)

Pulmonary artery diastolic pressure

You don't often need to estimate pulmonary artery diastolic pressure (PADP). However, should you wish to do so, you can use the following method (which relies on the presence of pulmonary regurgitation). You can assess pulmonary regurgitation using CW Doppler in the

- parasternal RV outflow view (**Figure 7.4**, p. 46)
- parasternal short-axis view (aortic valve level) (**Figure 7.5**, p. 47)

Using CW Doppler, measure the end-diastolic velocity of *regurgitant* flow through the pulmonary valve (end-diastolic PR velocity) in m/s. The pulmonary regurgitation is driven by, and therefore reflects, the diastolic pressure gradient between the pulmonary artery (PADP) and the right ventricle (RVDP), and this pressure gradient can be calculated using the simplified Bernoulli equation:

$$PADP - RVDP = 4 \times (\text{End-diastolic PR velocity})^2$$

For example, if the end-diastolic velocity of the pulmonary regurgitation jet is 1.1 m/s, then

$$PADP - RVDP = 4 \times (1.1)^2$$

$$PADP - RVDP = 4 \times 1.2$$

$$PADP - RVDP = 4.8 \text{ mmHg}$$

Now you know the end-diastolic pressure *difference* between the pulmonary artery and the RV. The next step is to estimate the *actual* diastolic pressure in the RV, and this is taken to be the same as the RA pressure (estimated using the IVC technique, as outlined in Chapter 23). For example, if the IVC is normal, then the RAP would be estimated at 3 mmHg, and so the RVDP would be 3 mmHg too. Continuing with our example,

$$PADP - RVDP = 4.8 \text{ mmHg}$$

$$PADP = 4.8 \text{ mmHg} + RVDP$$

$$PADP = 4.8 + 3 \text{ mmHg}$$

$$PADP = 7.8 \text{ mmHg}$$

The patient therefore has a PADP of approximately 8 mmHg.

Associated features

If pulmonary hypertension is present, include a careful search for potential causes in your echo study, for example,

- mitral and/or aortic valve disease
- left-to-right shunts (e.g., ASD, VSD)
- LV dysfunction
- pulmonary emboli

You must also look for, and report upon, any consequences of pulmonary hypertension:

- pulmonary artery dilatation
- pulmonary and/or tricuspid regurgitation
- RV dilatation and impairment
- RA dilatation

Further reading

Augustine DX et al. Echocardiographic assessment of pulmonary hypertension: a guideline protocol from the British Society of Echocardiography. *Echo Research and Practice* (2018). PMID 30012832.

Galiè N et al. 2015 ESC/ERS guidelines for the diagnosis and treatment of pulmonary hypertension: the joint task force for the diagnosis and treatment of pulmonary hypertension of the European Society of Cardiology (ESC) and the European Respiratory Society (ERS): Endorsed by: Association for European Paediatric and Congenital Cardiology (AEPC), International Society for Heart and Lung Transplantation (ISHLT). *European Heart Journal* (2016). PMID 26320113.

Humbert M et al. 2022 ESC/ERS guidelines for the diagnosis and treatment of pulmonary hypertension. *European Respiratory Journal* (2022). PMID 36028254.

CHAPTER 27

Heart valve repair and replacement

Valvular heart disease can be treated in a variety of ways:

- valve replacement, in which a valve is implanted surgically or percutaneously to replace an abnormal (regurgitant or stenotic) valve. These valves can be
  - *mechanical* – the valve is constructed using artificial materials
  - *biological* – the valve contains biological material, either derived from a natural valve or fashioned from pericardium
- valve repair, in which a regurgitant valve is corrected surgically, preserving the original valve rather than replacing it
- percutaneous techniques, which include percutaneous balloon valvuloplasty (in which a stenotic valve is 'stretched' with a balloon) and transcatheter mitral valve repair

Each year over 16,000 people in the UK undergo heart valve repair or replacement, and surveillance scans account for a significant proportion of the overall echo workload. It is important to be aware of the different valvular procedures that patients undergo, as patients will require an initial baseline echo study to confirm the success of the procedure, and in many cases will need longer-term surveillance scans to monitor their valve for any subsequent structural valve deterioration (SVD).

Following valve surgery, a pre-discharge echo is usually performed to check for any major post-operative concerns such as valve dehiscence or cardiac tamponade. However, it is important to schedule a full 'baseline' echo study 6–8 weeks post-discharge. This allows time for any post-operative anaemia to resolve (which would otherwise cause a hyperdynamic high-output state, affecting quantitative measurements) and for left ventricular function to improve, as well as making the scan more comfortable for the patient once their chest wound has healed.

Before undertaking an echo assessment following valve repair or replacement, it is essential to know the details of the procedure that was undertaken and, where applicable, the type of valve implanted. The request form must therefore include

- the type of valve (e.g., biological, mechanical) and its specific name (e.g., Bjork–Shiley)
- the size of valve replacement (which is its internal diameter, stated in mm)
- the date of implantation
- current clinical details (e.g., new diastolic murmur)
- a specific question to be addressed (e.g., valve dehiscence?)

Details of the type of valve can usually be obtained from the original operation note. Normal reference intervals for individual replacement valves can usually be obtained from the manufacturer or via online resources such as the British Society of Echocardiography's EchoCalc app.

DOI: 10.1201/9781003304654-27

ECHO ASSESSMENT OF MECHANICAL VALVES

A mechanical valve consists of three parts – the **sewing ring** (which is like the 'annulus' of the valve, used by the surgeon to sew the valve into position), the **occluder** (the moving part of the valve which opens and closes during the cardiac cycle) and the **retaining mechanism** (which is attached to the sewing ring and holds the occluder in position).

There are three types of mechanical valves (**Figure 27.1**):

- *Bileaflet valves*: in which two semicircular disc occluders open and close on hinges – these are the most commonly used type
- *Tilting disc valves*: in which a single disc occluder tilts within its retaining mechanism
- *Ball and cage valves*: consisting of a silastic ball occluder which can move up and down within the cage-like retaining mechanism – this was the earliest type of mechanical valve, introduced during the 1960s, and is seldom seen now

The advantage of mechanical valves is their long-term durability (although some earlier valves were prone to catastrophic failure). The main disadvantage of mechanical valves is that, because they are constructed from artificial materials, they can be a source of thrombus formation. Patients with mechanical valves, therefore, require lifelong anticoagulation with drugs such as warfarin, which can be a major drawback, particularly in patients at risk of bleeding or women of childbearing age who wish to become pregnant.

Mechanical valve structure

Mechanical valves can be challenging to assess on echo because of the reverberation caused by the materials in the valve (**Figure 27.2**). Mitral replacement valves are usually best assessed from the apical window and aortic replacement valves from the apical and parasternal windows. Transoesophageal echo (TOE) can help, particularly for replacement valves in the mitral position, providing good resolution of the left atrium and the mitral valve. TOE is less useful for imaging mechanical aortic valves, particularly when a mechanical mitral valve is also present.

As far as possible, examine the structure of the mechanical valve, asking the following questions:

- Is the valve well-seated, or does it appear to be 'rocking'? A rocking replacement valve indicates separation ('dehiscence') of the valve's sewing ring from the rest of the heart – look carefully for associated paravalvular regurgitation. Valve dehiscence may indicate infective endocarditis and requires urgent clinical evaluation.
- Is there a normal range of movement of the valve occluder(s)? Occluder motion can be obstructed by thrombus or pannus (endothelial overgrowth around the valve). Obstruction to occluder opening causes stenosis, while obstruction to occluder closure causes regurgitation.
- Are there any masses associated with the valve, and are the masses mobile or immobile? Pannus is an immobile mass, whereas thrombus or vegetations are usually (but not always) mobile.

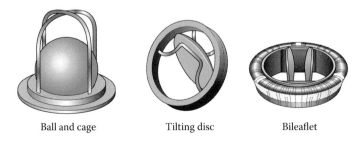

Ball and cage   Tilting disc   Bileaflet

Figure 27.1 Types of mechanical heart valves.

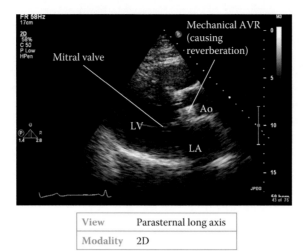

View	Parasternal long axis
Modality	2D

Figure 27.2 Normal mechanical aortic valve replacement (AVR). *Abbreviations:* Ao: Aorta, LA: Left atrium, LV: Left ventricle.

Pannus typically occurs 5 years or more post-surgery, although it has been found as early as 6 months post-surgery. Thrombus or vegetations can occur at any time. Replacement valve masses usually require a TOE study for full characterization.

Sometimes very small bubbles are seen near a mechanical valve just as its occluder closes (**Figure 27.3**). These microbubbles are caused by cavitation of blood by the occluder, and are regarded as a harmless finding.

If the replacement valve cannot be imaged adequately, state this in your report so that appropriate alternative imaging can be arranged.

Mechanical valve function

Forward flow

For mechanical valves in the aortic position, assess forward flow by measuring

● peak velocity

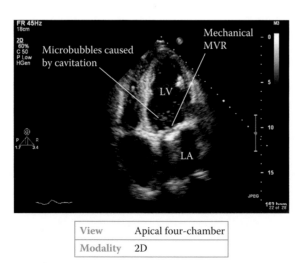

View	Apical four-chamber
Modality	2D

Figure 27.3 Normal mechanical mitral valve replacement (MVR) showing cavitation. *Abbreviations:* LA: Left atrium, LV: Left ventricle.

- mean gradient
- effective orifice area (EOA)

For replacement aortic valves, EOA is measured using the continuity equation (p. 143). Be particularly careful when measuring the left ventricular outflow tract (LVOT) diameter – it is important to be sure that you're measuring the true LVOT diameter, and not the diameter of the replacement valve itself. When measuring the velocity time integral of flow in the LVOT using pulsed-wave (PW) Doppler, it is important to place the PW sample volume 0.5–1.0 cm proximal to the valve (if it's too close to the valve, it may lie within the region of subvalvular flow acceleration).

For replacement valves in the mitral position, assess peak velocity and mean gradient; EOA is not routinely used. Do not use the pressure half-time method to estimate replacement mitral valve EOA (although a rise in pressure half-time is an indicator of valve obstruction).

Bear in mind that the flow through a mechanical valve tends to be very different to that through a native valve. For instance, forward flow through a bileaflet disc valve will consist of three individual jets. Careful Doppler interrogation is necessary to ensure that you identify the true peak velocity.

The reference intervals of forward flow parameters for replacement valves vary according to the type and size of the valve concerned, and tables of normal values can be obtained either from the valve's manufacturer or by referring to published tables (e.g., via the EchoCalc app).

Obstruction to forward flow occurs if motion of the valve occluder is obstructed (by thrombus, pannus, vegetations or mechanical failure), so that the occluder cannot open properly, or if there is subvalvular or supravalvular obstruction from pannus formation. Inspect the valve carefully to assess the occluder motion where possible. If obstruction occurs intermittently, a prolonged period of Doppler interrogation may be required.

High forward flow velocities also occur in high-output states (such as anaemia), and it can also be the result of measuring the central jet in the bileaflet valves ('central jet artifact'). High velocities can also be seen in 'patient–prosthesis mismatch'. This term is used to describe a normally functioning replacement valve that has an effective orifice area that is disproportionately small for the patient's body size, leading to high velocity flow through it.

Patient–prosthesis mismatch can affect both mechanical and biological replacement valves, and the key to diagnosis is to show that the valve replacement is opening normally, but that its indexed EOA is small relative to the patient's body surface area.

For replacement valves in the aortic position, an indexed EOA of 0.66–0.85 cm^2/m^2 indicates moderate patient–prosthesis mismatch and of $\leq$0.65 cm^2/m^2 indicates severe mismatch. For patients with a body mass index $\geq$30 kg/m^2, the threshold values in moderate mismatch are 0.56–0.7 cm^2/m^2 and in severe mismatch are $\leq$0.55 cm^2/m^2.

For replacement valves in the mitral position, an indexed EOA of 0.91–1.2 cm^2/m^2 indicates moderate patient–prosthesis mismatch and of $\leq$0.9 cm^2/m^2 indicates severe mismatch. For patients with a body mass index $\geq$30 kg/m^2, the threshold values in moderate mismatch are 0.76–1.0 cm^2/m^2 and in severe mismatch are $\leq$0.75 cm^2/m^2.

It can be challenging to demonstrate normal cusp or occluder opening on transthoracic echo, and this is sometimes easier to assess by transoesophageal echo (or using fluoroscopy for mechanical valves).

Regurgitant flow

A small amount of regurgitation is normal for replacement mechanical valves. There is an initial regurgitant flow as the occluder closes and blood is pushed backwards by it. Then, once the occluder is closed, there is a further regurgitant flow which is intended to 'wash' over the replacement valve and reduce the risk of thrombus formation. These normal regurgitant jets are usually small – the precise timing, extent and location of the regurgitant jet(s) depend on the type of valve – as well as symmetrical and brief.

Abnormal regurgitation through the orifice of the replacement valve may occur if the occluder fails to close properly, either because closure is obstructed (e.g., by thrombus, vegetations or pannus) or because of mechanical failure of the occluder itself. Regurgitation through a replacement valve orifice is called **transvalvular regurgitation**. Regurgitation may also occur around the valve, due to dehiscence of part of the sewing ring – this is **paravalvular regurgitation**. Use colour Doppler to examine the location and extent of any abnormal regurgitation and describe it as fully as possible. Regurgitation from mitral replacement valves can be difficult to see with transthoracic echo and a TOE study may be required.

Follow-up of mechanical valves

If the baseline echo is unremarkable, mechanical valves don't usually require further 'routine' follow-up scans unless there is a clinical cause for concern – this might result from new symptoms (e.g., dyspnoea), changing clinical signs (e.g., a change in heart murmur), a clinical event (e.g., an embolic event) or a suspicion of infective endocarditis. However, if a patient has had a mechanical mitral valve replacement, it is prudent to perform an echo after 5 years to check for tricuspid regurgitation or right ventricular dysfunction (unless they underwent simultaneous tricuspid valve repair).

ECHO ASSESSMENT OF BIOLOGICAL VALVES

As with a mechanical valve, biological valves contain a sewing ring which the surgeon uses to sew the valve into position. From the sewing ring projects a framework consisting of a number of struts, commonly called stents, to which the valve leaflets are attached. These stents take up space and thus can cause a degree of obstruction to blood flow through the valve. Valves which lack this supporting framework, called 'stentless valves', offer a greater orifice area (for the same overall size of valve), reducing the gradient across the replacement valve.

There are three types of biological valves:

- *Xenograft valves*: in which the valve is fashioned from a porcine valve or from bovine pericardium
- *Homograft valves*: which are human valves obtained from cadavers
- *Autograft valves*: in which a patient's own pulmonary valve is used to replace their aortic valve (and the pulmonary valve is itself replaced with a xenograft or homograft valve) – this is known as the Ross procedure

Transcatheter aortic valve implantation (TAVI) is a form of biological valve replacement that is implanted percutaneously rather than surgically, most commonly in the treatment of aortic stenosis (although some can now be implanted for aortic regurgitation, and some are used as valve-in-valve implants inside failing replacement valves).

Unlike mechanical valves, biological valves do not require long-term anticoagulation. However, they do not have the durability of mechanical valves and hence require monitoring for signs of SVD. SVD can occur as a result of gradual fibrosis and calcification of the valve, causing stenosis or regurgitation.

Biological valve structure

Stentless biological valves can look very similar to native valves on echo. For stented valves, the stents can be very obvious (**Figures 27.4** and **27.5**) and can cause shadowing of the ultrasound beam.

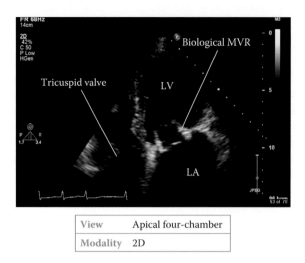

View	Apical four-chamber
Modality	2D

Figure 27.4 Normal biological mitral valve replacement (MVR). *Abbreviations:* LA: Left atrium, LV: Left ventricle.

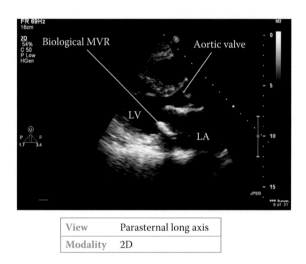

View	Parasternal long axis
Modality	2D

Figure 27.5 Normal biological mitral valve replacement (MVR). *Abbreviations:* LA: Left atrium, LV: Left ventricle.

Examine the structure of the biological valve, asking the following questions:

- Is the valve well-seated, or does it appear to be 'rocking'? As for mechanical valves, a rocking biological valve indicates dehiscence of the sewing ring, so check for associated paravalvular regurgitation.
- Do the valve leaflets appear thin and mobile? Biological valve leaflets become fibrotic and calcified with time, developing a thickened appearance on echo with reduced mobility.
- Are there any masses associated with the valve (pannus, thrombus, vegetations)?
- If the replacement valve cannot be imaged adequately, state this in your report so that appropriate alternative imaging can be arranged.

Biological valve function

Forward flow

As with mechanical valves, biological valves have a smaller effective orifice area than the native valves they replace (although less so with stentless valves). As time passes, biological valve leaflets tend to become deformed as a result of fibrosis, and this can result in stenosis, with an increase in the gradient across the valve (and a decrease in the EOA).

For biological valves in the aortic position, assess forward flow by measuring the

- peak velocity
- mean gradient
- EOA (calculated using the continuity equation)

When calculating EOA of a TAVI valve, it is particularly important to ensure that LVOT flow is measured using PW Doppler with the sample volume positioned in the LVOT *proximal* to the valve stent – if measured within the stent, the valve's EOA will be overestimated.

For replacement valves in the mitral position, assess the peak velocity and mean gradient, but EOA is not routinely used.

The reference intervals of replacement valve forward flow parameters vary according to the type and size of the valve concerned. The assessment of abnormally high flow velocities is undertaken in essentially the same way as for mechanical valves, as outlined earlier in this chapter.

Regurgitant flow

Around 10% of normal biological replacement valves have a trivial or mild degree of transvalvular regurgitation. Abnormal transvalvular regurgitation may occur if the valve has developed fibrocalcific degeneration (so examine the leaflets carefully for evidence of thickening), or if there has been acute leaflet rupture. Paravalvular regurgitation may occur around the valve due to dehiscence of part of the sewing ring (**Figure 27.6**), as for mechanical valves.

Use Doppler interrogation to examine the location and extent of any abnormal regurgitation and describe it as fully as possible. Grading the severity of regurgitation for replacement valves is done in the same way as for native valves.

Follow-up of biological valves

For biological valves, routine echo surveillance is required because there is a much greater likelihood of developing SVD as the biological valve becomes fibrosed and calcified over time. Several factors influence the likelihood of developing SVD, including

- valve design
- valve position

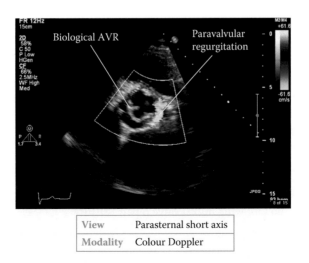

View	Parasternal short axis
Modality	Colour Doppler

Figure 27.6   Biological aortic valve replacement (AVR) with paravalvular regurgitation.

- patient–prosthesis mismatch
- clinical factors
  - patient age
  - systemic hypertension
  - diabetes
  - renal dysfunction
  - smoking
  - high body mass index

SVD is commoner in stented valves than in stentless valves, and biological valves implanted in the mitral position are more likely to undergo SVD (40% at 10 years) than those in the aortic position (<10% at 10 years). SVD is more likely to occur sooner in valves that show evidence of patient–prosthesis mismatch.

There is considerable variation between different guidelines regarding the timing of echo surveillance for biological valves. The British Heart Valve Society and the British Society of Echocardiography have examined the available guidelines and come up with practical guidance of their own. Each patient with a replacement valve should have an individualized surveillance plan documented in their casenotes that takes into account any risk factors for SVD:

- for patients with a biological valve of proven longevity (e.g., Edwards Perimount) in the aortic position, who were aged 60 or over at the time of implantation, echo surveillance can begin 10 years after implantation and performed annually thereafter
- for patients with a biological valve in the mitral or tricuspid positions, or those with an aortic xenograft implanted below the age of 60, or who have major risk factors for SVD (see above), echo surveillance can begin 5 years after implantation and performed annually thereafter
- for patients with a new design of biological valve, or who have undergone a transcatheter aortic valve implantation or a Ross procedure, surveillance echo should be undertaken annually from the time of implantation

It is important to remember that these recommended screening intervals only apply if the baseline echo shows normal function of the valve replacement post-implantation, and there are no other significant abnormalities (e.g., aortic dilatation, significant left ventricular dysfunction) that merit echo surveillance in their own right.

VALVE REPAIR

Mitral valve repair is, where feasible, the preferred surgical option for mitral regurgitation with better long-term outcomes than valve replacement. The operation usually involves resection of a wedge of redundant mitral tissue and, where necessary, inserting an annuloplasty ring to reinforce the mitral annulus and repairing/replacing damaged chordae tendineae. An alternative technique is the so-called Alfieri or 'edge-to-edge' repair, in which the central points of the two mitral leaflets are sutured together to create a double-orifice mitral valve.

Echo assessment of valve repair

When performing an echo following mitral valve repair (**Figure 27.7**), assess

- mitral valve morphology, looking in particular at leaflet mobility and for the presence of an annuloplasty ring and/or repaired/replaced chordae
- mitral valve flow, looking for evidence of stenosis or regurgitation as for a native valve

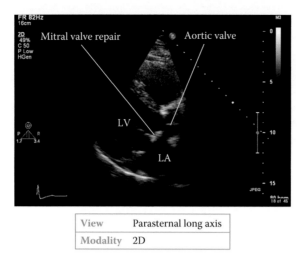

View	Parasternal long axis
Modality	2D

Figure 27.7   Normal mitral valve repair. *Abbreviations:* LA: Left atrium, LV: Left ventricle.

PERCUTANEOUS TECHNIQUES

Percutaneous techniques for valvular intervention include percutaneous balloon mitral valvuloplasty (PBMV) and percutaneous mitral valve repair. Transcatheter aortic valve implantation (TAVI) has been discussed earlier in this chapter.

Percutaneous balloon mitral valvuloplasty

PBMV is a technique in which a balloon is passed to the heart via a femoral vein and a deliberate puncture is made in the interatrial septum to allow access to the left atrium. The balloon is then passed across the stenosed mitral valve and inflated to relieve the stenosis. The technique works primarily through commissural splitting, and it is important to assess the mitral valve (and particularly the commissures) to select patients most likely to benefit from this procedure.

Echo assessment for PBMV is formalized in the Wilkins score, which grades the valve's suitability according to four criteria, each of which is scored 1–4:

- leaflet mobility (mobile = 1; immobile = 4)
- valvular thickening (normal [<5 mm thick]) = 1; severe thickening [>8–10 mm] = 4)
- sub-valvular thickening (minimal thickening = 1; thickening of all chordal structures = 4)
- valvular calcification (no bright echoes = 1; extensive brightness = 4)

A total score >8 indicates a low probability of successful PBMV. Full assessment will entail a TOE.

An alternative to the Wilkins score is the commissural calcification score, in which each mitral commissure (anterolateral and posteromedial) is scored according to the degree of calcification seen on the short-axis view. A score of 0 is given for no calcification, 1 for calcium across half a commissure and 2 for calcium across the whole commissure. The score for the two commissures is added together to give a total score of 0–4. A score of ≥2 indicates less than a 50% probability of achieving a good haemodynamic outcome following PBMV.

Patients not suitable for PBMV include those with

- significant mitral regurgitation
- bilateral commissural calcification
- thrombus on the interatrial septum, protruding into the atrial cavity or obstructing the mitral orifice

The presence of unilateral commissural calcification or thrombus in the left atrial appendage is a relative contraindication to PBMV.

Following PBMV, assess the mitral valve carefully for any residual stenosis or for the development of regurgitation and for any residual atrial septal defect. Note that mitral valve pressure half-time is *not* a reliable way to assess mitral stenosis in the 72 hours following PBMV. During this period, the improvement in transmitral flow following the procedure causes an increase in left atrial (and a decrease in left ventricular) compliance, which affects pressure half-time measurements. Once chamber compliance has stabilized after 72 hours, pressure half-time can be used once again.

PERCUTANEOUS MITRAL VALVE REPAIR

A number of percutaneous techniques have been developed for mitral valve repair in mitral regurgitation, but one of the most commonly used is the MitraClip procedure. This procedure uses a 'clip' device (which reaches the mitral valve via the venous circulation and a trans-septal puncture) to anchor the A2 and P2 scallops of the anterior and posterior mitral leaflets together, thus creating a 'double orifice' mitral valve.

During a MitraClip procedure, TOE guidance is used to help position the device correctly. Following the procedure, the extent of any residual mitral regurgitation is assessed. This can prove challenging, as the presence of a double-orifice mitral valve means that many of the quantitative techniques that are normally used to assess the mitral regurgitation severity cannot be reliably applied. Semi-quantitative estimation of colour Doppler jet dimensions is often used instead, and 3D echo can be particularly helpful.

Further reading

Baumgartner H et al. 2017 ESC/EACTS guidelines for the management of valvular heart disease. *European Heart Journal* (2017). PMID 28886619.

Bilkhu R et al. Patient–prosthesis mismatch following aortic valve replacement. *Heart* (2019). PMID 30846522.

Chambers JB. The echocardiography of replacement heart valves. *Echo Research and Practice* (2016). PMID 27600454.

Chambers JB et al. Appropriateness criteria for the use of cardiovascular imaging in heart valve disease in adults: a European Association of Cardiovascular Imaging report of literature review and current practice. *European Heart Journal – Cardiovascular Imaging* (2017). PMID 28586420.

Chambers JB et al. Indications for echocardiography of replacement heart valves: a joint statement from the British Heart Valve Society and British Society of Echocardiography. *Echo Research and Practice* (2019). PMID 30763277.

Lancellotti P et al. Recommendations for the imaging assessment of prosthetic heart valves: a report from the European Association of Cardiovascular Imaging endorsed by the Chinese Society of Echocardiography, the Inter-American Society of Echocardiography, and the Brazilian Department of Cardiovascular Imaging. *European Heart Journal – Cardiovascular Imaging* (2016). PMID 27143783.

Otto CM et al. 2020 ACC/AHA guideline for the management of patients with valvular heart disease: executive summary: a report of the American College of Cardiology/American Heart Association Joint Committee on Clinical Practice Guidelines. *Circulation* (2021). PMID 33332149.

Zoghbi WA et al. Recommendations for evaluation of prosthetic valves with echocardiography and Doppler ultrasound. *Journal of the American Society of Echocardiography* (2009). PMID 19733789.

CHAPTER 28

Endocarditis

Endocarditis refers to inflammation of the endocardium, the inner layer of the heart (including the heart valves). Endocarditis can be

- infective (e.g., bacterial, fungal)
- non-infective (e.g., Libman–Sacks endocarditis in systemic lupus erythematosus)

INFECTIVE ENDOCARDITIS

Although infective endocarditis is uncommon (fewer than 10 cases per 100,000 population every year), it is nevertheless a serious and dangerous condition, with a mortality of around 20% even with treatment. Transthoracic echo (TTE) is the recommended first-line imaging modality in patients with suspected infective endocarditis. In addition to its role in establishing the diagnosis of endocarditis, echo can provide information about pre-existing abnormalities, help to identify complications, assist in prognostication and predict embolic risk.

Infective endocarditis starts with organisms reaching the endocardium either via a bacteraemia or directly via surgery or device placement. The organisms adhere to a region of endocardium that has a predisposing abnormality, such as an area that has been damaged by turbulent blood flow. Clumps of platelets, fibrin and red blood cells tend to aggregate on such damaged endocardium, and microorganisms can adhere to and then colonize these clumps. This leads to the characteristic lesion in endocarditis – the vegetation.

Left untreated, infective endocarditis can also cause local tissue destruction (e.g., valvular regurgitation) and can lead to abscess and/or fistula formation.

The single most common causative organism is *Staphylococcus aureus*; other commonly encountered organisms are listed in **Table 28.1**.

Table 28.1 Common causes of infective endocarditis

Bacterial	*Staphylococcus aureus*
	Streptococcus viridans
	Streptococcus intermedius
	Pseudomonas aeruginosa
	HACEK organisms
	Bartonella
	Coxiella burnetii
Fungal	*Candida*
	Aspergillus
	Histoplasma

Clinical features of infective endocarditis

The clinical features of infective endocarditis (**Table 28.2**) can be subtle and sometimes will have been present for several weeks, so a high index of suspicion is needed to avoid missing the diagnosis. Be particularly alert to the possibility of infective endocarditis in those at risk (see above) and/ or those with a history of invasive procedures or intravenous drug use.

Modified Duke criteria

The diagnosis of endocarditis can be made using the modified Duke criteria, which divides the clinical features into major and minor criteria. Echo evidence of endocardial involvement forms one of the major criteria, as indicated by

- oscillating intracardiac mass (vegetation)
- cardiac abscess
- new partial dehiscence of a replacement heart valve

The vegetation may be located on a heart valve, on a valve's supporting structure, in the path of a jet (see box **Jet Lesions**), or on implanted material.

Blood cultures are also a major diagnostic criterion, and at least three sets should be taken from different sites at different times. Always perform an echo study in any patient with a positive blood culture for *S. aureus* or for *Candida*, in view of the likelihood of infective endocarditis with these organisms and the particularly serious consequences that can result. Blood cultures may be negative, even in the presence of infective endocarditis, because of the prior antibiotic treatment or the presence of fastidious (difficult to culture) organisms.

JET LESIONS

Vegetations occur most commonly on heart valves. However, they can also occur anywhere where a high-velocity jet of blood flow ('jet lesion') occurs between a high-pressure and low-pressure chamber, impinging on the endocardium and potentially resulting in endothelial injury and establishing a focus for infection. Examples include the high-velocity jets found in ventricular septal defect (VSD) or persistent ductus arteriosus (PDA).

Echo assessment of infective endocarditis

TTE is the recommended first-line imaging investigation in suspected infective endocarditis, and is ideally performed within 24 hours, but consider TOE in cases where the TTE is negative or inconclusive (particularly if the clinical suspicion of infective endocarditis is high), or where there is suspected endocarditis on a replacement heart valve or intracardiac device. Indeed, TOE should be considered in most adult patients with suspected infective endocarditis, even when the TTE is

Table 28.2   Clinical features of infective endocarditis

Symptoms	Signs
Fever	Fever
Fatigue	Heart murmur
Anorexia	Splinter haemorrhages
Weight loss	Janeway lesions
Flu-like symptoms	Osler's nodes
	Roth spots
	Peripheral emboli

positive, as it is more effective in evaluating local complications such as abscess. However, in isolated right-sided native valve endocarditis, where there has been a good quality transthoracic study with unequivocal echo findings, it is not usually necessary to proceed to a TOE.

Where the clinical suspicion of infective endocarditis is high, but an initial scan has been negative, a repeat TTE/TOE within 5–7 days is appropriate (or even sooner in the case of *S. aureus* infection). It is important to note that a negative echo (even TOE) does *not* rule out a diagnosis of infective endocarditis and it is prudent to include a comment to this effect, when appropriate, in your echo report.

Perform a full echo study and note any structural abnormalities that predispose to infective endocarditis, such as

- acquired valvular disease, including stenosis or regurgitation
- replacement heart valves
- structural congenital heart disease, including surgically corrected or palliated conditions (except isolated atrial septal defect and fully repaired VSD or PDA, and endothelialized closure devices)
- hypertrophic cardiomyopathy
- previous infective endocarditis

Look carefully for any features of infective endocarditis:

- vegetations
- valvular destruction
- abscess
- fistula

A full assessment of the left and right ventricles is required, because heart failure is the commonest complication of endocarditis and the most common reason for surgery. The development of heart failure in endocarditis is usually a consequence of severe valvular regurgitation, although it can also be seen with fistulas or, rarely, with valve obstruction. It's essential that echo be undertaken as soon as symptoms or signs of heart failure occur, to identify the cause and to assess the patient's hemodynamic status.

Vegetations

The characteristic echo appearance of a vegetation is of an echogenic mass, irregular in shape, attached to the 'upstream' side of a valve leaflet (i.e., the atrial side in the case of the mitral and tricuspid valves, and the ventricular side for the aortic and pulmonary valves). Vegetations can be attached to any part of the valve, but most commonly at the coaptation line. Vegetations move with the leaflet but in a more chaotic ('oscillating') manner. It is common for a vegetation to prolapse through the valve as it opens.

Vegetations vary in size, often being just a few millimetres in diameter but sometimes reaching 2–3 cm. Vegetations resulting from fungal infections (e.g., *Candida*, *Aspergillus*) are usually much bigger than bacterial vegetations, and they can be so big that they are mistaken for a cardiac tumour. Fungal endocarditis is rare and is more likely to occur in patients who are immunosuppressed.

In order of decreasing frequency, the valves affected by infective endocarditis are the mitral (**Figure 28.1**), aortic, tricuspid and pulmonary. More than one valve can be affected. Right heart endocarditis is much commoner in patients who are intravenous drug users, and can also occur in association with right-sided devices such as pacemaker leads.

If vegetations are present, describe their:

- location (which valve(s) and which parts of the valve are affected)
- mobility (e.g., immobile, oscillating)
- size

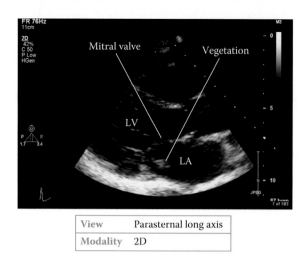

View	Parasternal long axis
Modality	2D

Figure 28.1   Vegetation on mitral valve. *Abbreviations:* LA: Left atrium, LV: Left ventricle.

Because infective endocarditis usually occurs on a valve that is already abnormal, you must also describe any underlying valvular disease as well as looking for any evidence that the infection is causing valvular destruction (see below).

PITFALLS IN THE ECHO ASSESSMENT OF VEGETATIONS

TTE can, at best, detect vegetations down to a minimum size of 2 mm (and is known to miss the majority of vegetations <5 mm). The superior image quality of transoesophageal echo (TOE) makes it more sensitive and specific than TTE, particularly in cases of replacement valve endocarditis and in the detection of abscesses. TTE has an overall sensitivity in detecting native valve vegetations of 70%, whereas the sensitivity of TOE is 96%.

Infective endocarditis commonly occurs on a heart valve that is already abnormal, and a pre-existing abnormality (e.g., myxomatous mitral valve disease, nodular aortic cusp thickening) can be mistaken for vegetations or can make the recognition of existing vegetations more difficult. Patients who are left with sterile vegetations following a previously treated episode of endocarditis can pose a difficult diagnostic challenge.

Cardiac tumours and thrombi can also be mistaken for vegetations (and vice versa). Benign structures that can be mistaken for vegetations include Lambl's excrescences and the Eustachian valve (see Chapter 32). Remember too that not all vegetations are infective in nature (p. 260).

Valvular destruction

Infective endocarditis can cause valvular destruction, leading to regurgitation either through distorting normal valve closure or through perforation of a valve leaflet (**Figure 28.2**). Assess and describe valvular regurgitation as for native valvular regurgitation, as outlined in Chapters 20, 21, 24 and 25. Valvular stenosis as a result of infective endocarditis is much rarer, and usually results from obstruction of the valve orifice by a large vegetation.

Abscess

A valvular infection can spread to involve surrounding tissues, particularly in replacement valve endocarditis. On echo, an abscess appears as an echolucent or echodense area in the valve annulus or surrounding tissues. TTE only has a sensitivity of around 50% for abscess detection, so it's possible to miss an abscess. TOE is significantly better, with a sensitivity of 90%. Both modalities have a similar specificity for abscess detection, at around 90%.

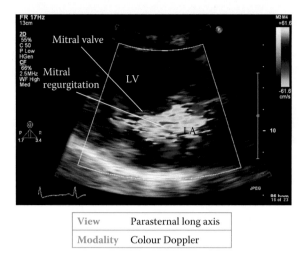

View	Parasternal long axis
Modality	Colour Doppler

Figure 28.2   Mitral regurgitation as a result of infective endocarditis. *Abbreviations:* LA: Left atrium, LV: Left ventricle.

Abscesses occur more commonly around the aortic valve (or in association with replacement valves) than the mitral valve, although an aortic root abscess can sometimes spread to affect the anterior mitral valve leaflet. A mitral valve abscess typically affects the posterior annulus, appearing on echo as a thickened and echodense region.

If an abscess is present, describe its

- location (which valve is affected, and where the abscess lies in relation to the valve)
- size

Fistula

Fistulas are uncommon, seen in around 1%–2% of endocarditis cases overall, although they occur more commonly in cases where an abscess has been identified. An aortic root abscess (or pseudoaneurysm) may rupture into a neighbouring chamber (usually the right ventricle, but sometimes one of the atria) to form an abnormal communication or fistula. Fistulas can be multiple.

A fistula can be demonstrated using colour Doppler and continuous wave (CW) Doppler to show abnormal flow arising in the aortic root and flowing through the fistula. Describe where the fistula arises and which chambers it connects. Also describe its haemodynamic effects, such as consequent chamber dilatation and/or dysfunction.

Replacement valve endocarditis

Replacement valve endocarditis accounts for around 20% of infective endocarditis cases and occurs in 2%–3% of patients within the first 12 months of a valve replacement (and 0.5% of patients per year thereafter). It can affect both mechanical and biological replacement valves, and it is the most severe form of endocarditis, with an in-hospital mortality rate of 20%–40%.

Replacement valve endocarditis can be challenging to diagnose, particularly with mechanical valves. Imaging of the valve itself is often suboptimal because of shadowing and reverberation of the echo signal by the replacement valve. Furthermore, mechanical valve infections typically occur at the sewing ring and tend to be associated with fewer vegetations but a higher incidence of perivalvar complications such as abscesses or fistulas. Look carefully for any signs of dehiscence ('splitting open') of the sewing ring around the valve, allowing regurgitant blood flow around the replacement valve (paravalvular regurgitation).

The sensitivity of TTE for detecting vegetations on replacement valves is ≈50%. A TOE study is therefore recommended to obtain better resolution of the replacement valve and any associated abnormalities. Replacement valve endocarditis is difficult to treat with antibiotics alone and early redo surgery is usually required, particularly in the first 12 months after the valve was first implanted.

Prognostic echo indicators

Echo also provides useful information for prognosis, which can be valuable when triaging patients at presentation. Imaging features that indicate a higher risk of death or the need for urgent surgery include large vegetations, impaired left ventricular systolic function, periannular complications, severe left-sided valvular regurgitation or severe replacement valve dysfunction, pulmonary hypertension, and indicators of elevated diastolic pressures such as premature mitral valve closure.

Echo can also help to predict which patients are at increased risk of embolic events and, therefore, identify which patients are most likely to benefit from early surgical intervention. An embolic event can cause major morbidity, such as disability due to stroke, but it is also associated with a much higher risk of death.

There are four echo features that have been shown to correlate with the risk of embolism:

- vegetation size
- vegetation mobility
- whether the vegetation is located on the mitral valve
- whether the vegetations affect multiple valves

To assess vegetation size, the vegetation needs to be measured in multiple planes to find the maximal length. If there happen to be multiple vegetations, then the largest value is the one that matters. The risk of embolism steadily increases with increasing vegetation size, and the threshold for surgery depends upon the clinical status of the patient.

For all patients with left-sided endocarditis, very large vegetations (greater than 30 mm in size) are a class IIa indication for urgent surgery. Vegetations over 15 mm in size are a class IIb indication. For patients with vegetations measuring 10 mm or more, surgery is indicated if the operative risk is low and there has already been an embolic event despite appropriate antibiotic therapy, or if there is severe valve stenosis or regurgitation.

Vegetation mobility can be described using a four-point scale of absent mobility, low mobility, moderate mobility and severe mobility. The more mobile the vegetation, the higher the embolic risk. Mobility is said to be absent if there is a fixed vegetation with no detectable independent motion. However, because vegetations are oscillatory structures, the truly 'absent' mobility is rarely seen. Mobility is low if there is a vegetation with a fixed base but a mobile free edge. Moderate mobility refers to a pedunculated vegetation that remains within the same chamber throughout the cardiac cycle. Severe mobility means a prolapsing vegetation that crosses the coaptation plane of the leaflets during the cardiac cycle.

Embolism is more common with mitral valve endocarditis, and also if multiple valves are affected.

Management of infective endocarditis

The treatment of infective endocarditis usually requires a prolonged (4–6 week) course of antibiotics, chosen where possible according to the antibiotic sensitivities of the causative organism. Cardiac surgery is necessary in about half of patients with infective endocarditis. Ideally, in stable patients, surgery should be performed only once the infection has been successfully treated with antibiotics to minimize the risk of recurrent infection. However, it is not always possible to delay surgery if patients are unstable or at high risk of complications (e.g., embolization).

Consider early surgery for

- haemodynamic instability/heart failure as a result of acute aortic or mitral regurgitation or valve obstruction
- persistent infection (fever and bacteraemia despite treatment with appropriate antibiotics for 7–10 days)
- development of a perivalvular abscess, false aneurysm or fistula
- infective endocarditis on a replacement valve
- fungal infections
- difficult to treat organisms (e.g., *Brucella*)
- high embolic risk

Follow-up echo

With effective treatment of infective endocarditis, the vegetations may gradually shrink and become less mobile. The sudden disappearance of a vegetation between studies raises a suspicion that the vegetation has broken free and embolized elsewhere.

Perform an up-to-date TTE if there is a suboptimal response to treatment or if complications are suspected, and a TTE study should also be undertaken following completion of antimicrobial treatment to assess the cardiac and valve structure and function. In the absence of any clinical concerns, however, it is not necessary to perform routine 'monitoring' echo studies during the course of antimicrobial treatment.

Following a successful course of treatment, patients should have a baseline transthoracic echo at the completion of antimicrobial therapy, and then go on to have serial surveillance scans at 1 month, 3 months, 6 months and 12 months during the first year. Even when an episode of infective endocarditis has been fully treated, (sterile) vegetations may remain visible on echo. This can make the diagnosis of recurrent infection challenging in patients who have suffered an episode of endocarditis previously – clinical evidence of active infection, particularly on blood cultures, is the key to diagnosis in such cases.

NON-INFECTIVE ENDOCARDITIS

Not all vegetations occur as a result of infection, a fact that emphasizes the importance of taking a patient's clinical history (and in particular the results of blood cultures) into account when making a diagnosis of infective (versus non-infective) endocarditis.

Non-infective endocarditis has also been termed non-bacterial thrombotic endocarditis (NBTE) or, historically, marantic endocarditis. The vegetations that occur are sterile, and are composed mainly of fibrin and platelets. Non-infective endocarditis can result from

- trauma to the valve leaflets (e.g., from an intracardiac catheter)
- circulating immune complexes
- vasculitis
- hypercoagulability
- mucin-producing adenocarcinomas

Non-infective endocarditis occurring in systemic lupus erythematosus is called Libman–Sacks endocarditis (also known as 'verrucous' endocarditis), and in this condition, the vegetations mainly consist of immune complexes and mononuclear cells. The mitral and aortic valves are most commonly affected, although just about any part of the endocardium can be involved. The vegetations are usually small, irregular and immobile (compared with the vegetations in infective endocarditis). Libman–Sacks endocarditis is usually asymptomatic, but can present with valvular regurgitation or, less commonly, stenosis. There is also a risk of embolization, although this is uncommon.

Further reading

Afonso L et al. Echocardiography in infective endocarditis: state of the art. *Current Cardiology Reports* (2017). PMID 29071426.

Durack DT et al. New criteria for diagnosis of infective endocarditis: utilization of specific echocardiographic findings. Duke Endocarditis Service. *American Journal of Medicine* (1994). PMID 8154507.

Habib G et al. 2015 ESC guidelines for the management of infective endocarditis: the task force for the management of infective endocarditis of the European Society of Cardiology (ESC). Endorsed by: European Association for Cardio-Thoracic Surgery (EACTS), the European Association of Nuclear Medicine (EANM). *European Heart Journal* (2015). PMID 26320109.

Rajani R et al. Infective endocarditis: a contemporary update. *Clinical Medicine* (2020). PMID 31941729.

Xie P et al. An appraisal of clinical practice guidelines for the appropriate use of echocardiography for adult infective endocarditis: the timing and mode of assessment (TTE or TEE). *BMC Infectious Diseases* (2021). PMID 33478412.

CHAPTER 29

The cardiomyopathies

CLASSIFICATION OF CARDIOMYOPATHIES

In 2006, the American Heart Association (AHA) proposed a scheme in which cardiomyopathies are defined as 'a heterogeneous group of diseases of the myocardium associated with mechanical and/or electrical dysfunction that usually (but not invariably) exhibit inappropriate ventricular hypertrophy or dilatation and are due to a variety of causes that frequently are genetic. Cardiomyopathies either are confined to the heart or are part of generalized systemic disorders, often leading to cardiovascular death or progressive heart failure-related disability.'

According to the AHA classification, cardiomyopathies can be classified as primary (mainly or only affecting the heart) or secondary (where the cardiomyopathy is part of a wider multisystem disorder):

- Primary cardiomyopathies:
  - genetic (e.g., hypertrophic cardiomyopathy [HCM], arrhythmogenic right ventricular cardiomyopathy [ARVC], left ventricular non-compaction [LVNC])
  - acquired (e.g., post-myocarditis, stress-induced [Takotsubo], peripartum, tachycardia-induced)
  - mixed (e.g., dilated cardiomyopathy [DCM], restrictive cardiomyopathy)
- Secondary cardiomyopathies:
  - infiltrative (e.g., amyloidosis)
  - storage (e.g., haemochromatosis, Fabry disease)
  - toxicity (e.g., drugs)
  - endomyocardial (e.g., endomyocardial fibrosis)
  - inflammatory (e.g., sarcoidosis)
  - endocrine (e.g., diabetes mellitus, acromegaly)
  - cardiofacial (e.g., Noonan syndrome)
  - neuromuscular/neurological (e.g., Friedreich ataxia)
  - nutritional deficiencies (e.g., beriberi, scurvy)
  - autoimmune/collagen (e.g., systemic lupus erythematosus)
  - electrolyte imbalance
  - consequence of cancer therapy (e.g., anthracyclines)

The echo assessment of any cardiomyopathy requires a detailed study with a particular emphasis on chamber morphology, dimensions and function (including ventricular systolic and diastolic function), as outlined in Chapters 16–18 and 22, together with a full assessment of valvular function. In addition, you will need to look for the specific features relating to the cardiomyopathy in question. This chapter describes the key features of the cardiomyopathies most likely to be encountered in everyday practice.

DILATED CARDIOMYOPATHY

DCM is characterized by dilatation and systolic impairment of the left ventricle (LV) in the absence of known abnormal loading conditions or significant coronary artery disease, and is sometimes accompanied by dilatation of the right ventricle (RV). DCM affects between 1 in 250 and 1 in 500 of the general population, and it can be idiopathic or can result from a number of conditions, including

- myocarditis
- alcohol
- prolonged tachycardia (tachycardia-induced cardiomyopathy)
- pregnancy (peripartum cardiomyopathy)

Familial DCM is also recognized, defined by the presence of DCM in two or more first- or second-degree relatives, or autopsy-proven DCM in a first-degree relative who has suffered a sudden death <50 years of age. DCM is also seen in X-linked diseases such as Becker and Duchenne muscular dystrophies. DCM without an identifiable cause is called idiopathic DCM.

Echo features

The echo assessment of DCM includes a comprehensive assessment of

- LV dimensions and function (Chapters 16–18)
- RV dimensions and function (Chapter 22)
- left atrial (LA) dimensions (Chapter 19)
- right atrial dimensions (Chapter 23)
- valvular function (Chapters 20, 21, 24, 25)

In the presence of a dilated LV, an ejection fraction of <45% is a diagnostic criterion for idiopathic DCM once secondary causes have been excluded. The LV becomes more spherical in DCM, and this can be measured using the sphericity index, which is the ratio between the length (mitral annulus to apex) and width (mid-cavity) of the LV, assessed in the apical four-chamber view. Sphericity index can be measured at end-diastole and at end-systole, and in normal subjects in >1.5 but approaches 1 in DCM. An abnormal sphericity index has been shown to predict an adverse prognosis.

Examples of DCM are shown in **Figures 29.1** and **29.2**.

STRESS-INDUCED CARDIOMYOPATHY

Stress-induced cardiomyopathy is also known as apical ballooning cardiomyopathy or Takotsubo ('octopus bottle') cardiomyopathy, named after the characteristic shape of the LV seen in this condition. It accounts for 1%–2% of patients suspected of having acute coronary syndrome, and is most commonly seen in post-menopausal women. It is classically triggered by extreme emotional or clinical stress, which leads to ballooning of the LV apex through mechanisms which remain unclear, although sympathetic overdrive, catecholamines and microvascular dysfunction may all play a role. Patients present with chest pain and/or heart failure with ECG changes suggestive of an anterior myocardial infarction (but in the absence of coronary artery disease). In most cases, echo shows systolic apical ballooning of the LV (with basal hyperkinesis), although other geometric variants are recognized. Treatment is supportive with appropriate drug therapy for LV dysfunction. Most patients recover, although mortality is as high as 8% in some studies.

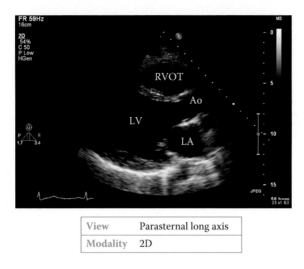

View	Parasternal long axis
Modality	2D

Figure 29.1 Dilated cardiomyopathy. *Abbreviations:* Ao: Aorta, LA: Left atrium, LV: Left ventricle, RVOT: Right ventricular outflow tract.

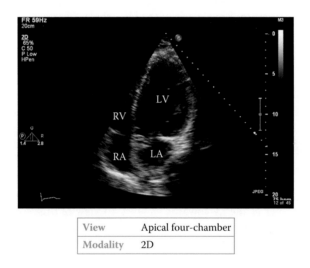

View	Apical four-chamber
Modality	2D

Figure 29.2 Dilated cardiomyopathy. *Abbreviations:* LA: Left atrium, LV: Left ventricle, RA: Right atrium, RV: Right ventricle.

HYPERTROPHIC CARDIOMYOPATHY

HCM is an autosomal dominant condition affecting 1 in 500 of the population and is a common cause of sudden cardiac death, particularly in the young. The condition is defined by a wall thickness ≥15 mm in one or more LV myocardial segments that is not solely the result of abnormal loading conditions.

If the hypertrophy is located in the LV outflow tract (LVOT), it may obstruct the flow of blood out of the LV into the aorta – this is hypertrophic *obstructive* cardiomyopathy (HOCM). Another common pattern is apical hypertrophy, which gives the LV cavity a characteristic 'ace of spades' appearance.

Transthoracic echo is part of the initial evaluation of all patients with suspected HCM, and it should be repeated in clinically stable patients every 1–2 years to assess LV hypertrophy, LV function, dynamic LVOT obstruction and mitral regurgitation. A change in clinical status should prompt an earlier follow-up echo study.

Echo should also be included in the screening of family members. Screening is recommended for all first-degree relatives of a patient with HCM. Note that the diagnostic wall LV thickness when screening first-degree relatives is ≥13 mm, rather than the ≥15 mm that is applied more generally.

Echo features

In HCM, the LV is hypertrophied in the absence of an underlying cause such as hypertension, aortic stenosis or coarctation of the aorta. In an echo study for HCM, look for the following features:

- LV wall thickness
- LV systolic and diastolic function (Chapters 16–18)
- evidence of flow obstruction (subaortic, intracavity)
- systolic anterior motion of the anterior mitral valve leaflet
- mitral regurgitation

LV morphology

In HCM, the LV is non-dilated; indeed, the LV cavity is usually small. Assess LV morphology and dimensions looking carefully at wall thickness (**Figure 29.3**). If hypertrophy is present, examine its distribution carefully using multiple views of the LV – short-axis views at several levels are particularly useful.

Describe the pattern of the hypertrophy, reporting not just the wall thickness in the hypertrophied region but also how it compares to wall thickness in normal regions. Four principal patterns are recognized:

- sigmoid septal, with maximal wall thickness in the basal anteroseptum
- reverse curvature, with maximal wall thickness in the mid-inferoseptum
- apical, with maximal wall thickness at the apex
- neutral, with maximal wall thickness in the anterior wall

Wall thickness in apical HCM sometimes does not reach the conventional threshold of 15 mm because of the natural taper of the LV towards its apex. In view of this, some define apical HCM when there is a ratio of 1.3:1 between apical wall thickness and basal wall thickness.

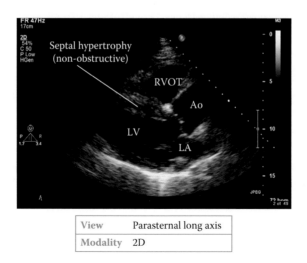

View	Parasternal long axis
Modality	2D

Figure 29.3   Asymmetrical septal hypertrophy in hypertrophic cardiomyopathy. *Abbreviations:* Ao: Aorta, LA: Left atrium, LV: Left ventricle, RVOT: Right ventricular outflow tract.

Measure wall thickness in the parasternal short-axis view:

- In the basal LV, of the septum, anterior wall, lateral wall and inferior wall
- In the mid-LV, of the septum, anterior wall, lateral wall and inferior wall
- In the apical LV, of the septum, anterior wall, lateral wall and inferior wall

Historically, an LV wall thickness of ≥15 mm was thought to indicate HCM. However, more recent genetic studies have shown that HCM can cause milder degrees of hypertrophy. Severe hypertrophy (an LV wall thickness ≥30 mm) is a risk factor for sudden cardiac death.

Assess LV systolic and diastolic function as described in Chapters 16–18, including tissue Doppler imaging and global longitudinal strain as appropriate. Assess LA dimensions, which are usually increased. LA diameter, measured at end-systole in the parasternal long-axis view, is a parameter in the risk calculator for sudden cardiac death.

Look carefully at the LV apex, which can become aneurysmal in the presence of apical HCM. This can be a substrate for apical thrombus. Consider the use of echo contrast if appropriate.

Measure RV wall thickness at end-diastole in the parasternal long-axis and subcostal views. RV hypertrophy is present if the RV wall thickness is >5 mm, and this is seen in around 20% of cases. Check for evidence of RV outflow tract obstruction and of tricuspid regurgitation, screening also for evidence of pulmonary hypertension.

Flow obstruction

Assess flow in the LV, looking for any evidence of obstruction (increased flow velocity). Obstruction is most often subaortic, due to systolic anterior motion of the mitral valve leaflets (see below) causing obstruction to flow in the LVOT, but obstruction can sometimes be mid-ventricular. Perform colour Doppler to look for evidence of turbulent flow in the LVOT or LV cavity, and use continuous wave (CW) Doppler in the apical five-chamber view to measure any LVOT gradient. You can also use pulsed-wave (PW) Doppler to assess flow in different regions of the LVOT, to distinguish between gradients caused by asymmetrical hypertrophy and any gradient across the aortic valve. Look carefully for evidence of early aortic valve closure.

LVOT obstruction is characteristically dynamic, with the rate of increase in flow velocity rising as the velocity increases – this gives the spectral Doppler trace a characteristic 'sabre-shaped' appearance (**Figure 29.4**). LVOT obstruction may not be present at rest, but can occur with provocation.

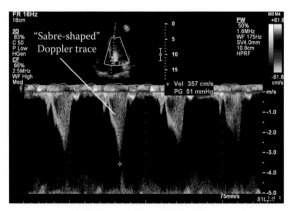

View	Apical five-chamber
Modality	PW Doppler

Figure 29.4   Dynamic left ventricular outflow tract obstruction in hypertrophic obstructive cardiomyopathy. *Abbreviations:* PG: Pressure gradient, Vel: Velocity.

For this reason, it is important to try to provoke LVOT obstruction during the echo study by measuring flow velocities during a Valsalva manoeuvre and in a sitting and standing position. HCM can then be categorized according to the type of obstruction:

- *Resting obstruction*: gradient ≥30 mmHg at rest
- *Latent obstruction*: gradient <30 mmHg at rest, but ≥30 mmHg with provocation
- *Non-obstructive*: gradient <30 mmHg at rest and with provocation

Systolic anterior motion

Inspect the mitral valve for structural abnormalities and look carefully for systolic anterior motion (SAM) of the mitral valve leaflets (**Figure 29.5**). SAM is caused by accelerated flow in the LVOT, causing a Venturi effect that 'drags' the anterior leaflet towards the septum (causing the leaflet tip to make contact with the septum) during systole. This opens the mitral valve, leading to an eccentric (posteriorly directed) jet of mitral regurgitation into the LA. Assess the degree of mitral regurgitation (Chapter 21).

SAM is not unique to HCM, and can also be seen with concentric LVH, with hyperdynamic LV function, and following mitral valve repair.

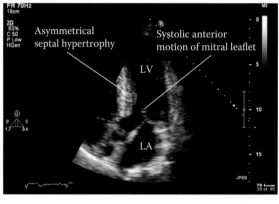

View	Apical five-chamber
Modality	2D

Figure 29.5   Systolic anterior motion in hypertrophic obstructive cardiomyopathy.

REPORT CONCLUSIONS IN HYPERTROPHIC CARDIOMYOPATHY

The choice of words is very important when writing your report for a HCM echo study, as an incorrect diagnosis of HCM (or a missed diagnosis) can have significant consequences. The British Society of Echocardiography recommend the following phrases:

- "Consistent with HCM" when there is unequivocal evidence of HCM on the study.
- "Raises the possibility of HCM" when there is uncertainty about the findings.
- "Wall thickness is normal" when a screening scan reveals no LVH.

FABRY DISEASE

Fabry disease (also known as Anderson–Fabry disease) is an X-linked lysosomal storage disorder in which glycosphingolipids accumulate in and damage various organs, including the heart. Echo features include

- concentric LV hypertrophy
- global LV hypokinesia with or without dilatation
- RV free wall thickening
- thickened mitral and tricuspid valve leaflets

Always consider a diagnosis of Fabry disease in patients with unexplained LV hypertrophy.

LEFT VENTRICULAR NON-COMPACTION CARDIOMYOPATHY

Left ventricular non-compaction (LVNC) is a cardiomyopathy caused by a failure of the normal compaction or 'condensation' process that occurs in the LV myocardium during intrauterine life. The end result is an LV that is heavily trabeculated with deep recesses between the trabeculae. This can cause systolic and/or diastolic dysfunction, and can predispose the patient to thromboembolism and arrhythmias. In most cases LVNC is familial (autosomal dominant), and sometimes occurs in families where there is a history of DCM or HCM, indicating that it may be a morphological variant of these conditions.

Echo features

Jenni et al. (2001) have described diagnostic criteria for LVNC based upon four echo features:

1. The LV myocardium is two-layered, with a thin (compacted) epicardial layer and a much thicker (non-compacted) endocardial layer that is trabecular with deep endocardial spaces. Measure the ratio between the thickness of the non-compacted (N) and compacted (C) layers at end-systole; in LVNC, this ratio is characteristically >2.

2. The non-compacted myocardium is predominantly seen at the apical level and at the mid-ventricular level in the inferior and lateral walls. For the purposes of describing LVNC, a 9-segment LV model is used (rather than the usual 16- or 17-segment model) with a single apical segment and four mid and basal segments (anterior, septal, lateral and inferior).

3. Colour Doppler shows deep perfusion of the inter-trabecular recesses.

4. Other than the abnormalities already described, there should (by definition) be no other cardiac abnormalities.

A number of echo experts have expressed concern about the 'over-diagnosis' of non-compaction cardiomyopathy, and it is certainly the case that quite marked trabeculation of the LV is sometimes seen in cases of LV hypertrophy and this can be mislabelled as non-compaction. A diagnosis of non-compaction should therefore be made with care, and the use of echo contrast agents can often be helpful in clarifying the endocardial appearances.

RESTRICTIVE CARDIOMYOPATHY

In restrictive cardiomyopathy, the LV is not dilated. However, the LV may be hypertrophied and its diastolic function is impaired, causing myocardial 'stiffness'. Restrictive cardiomyopathy is most commonly secondary to

- myocardial infiltration, as seen in amyloidosis, haemochromatosis or sarcoidosis
- endomyocardial fibrosis (including Loeffler syndrome)
- scleroderma
- post-radiotherapy

Primary (idiopathic) restrictive cardiomyopathy is rare.

Echo features

A full evaluation of the LV is required, looking in particular at the following:

- LV dimensions, wall thickness and mass
- LV systolic function (usually normal)
- LV diastolic function (impaired)

See Chapters 16–18 for details on how to evaluate the LV. The LV cavity size may be normal or small. The LV wall thickness may be normal, but if there is concentric LV wall thickening (in the absence of hypertrophic cardiomyopathy or increased afterload), then consider myocardial infiltration – cardiac amyloidosis is usually associated with >12 mm LV wall thickening, particularly in the transthyretin form of amyloid.

The LV myocardium may appear echo-reflective and 'speckled' in amyloid infiltration, and the endocardium is echo-reflective in endomyocardial fibrosis. Restrictive cardiomyopathy may also involve the RV and both atria are usually significantly dilated as a consequence of elevated ventricular filling pressures.

LV systolic function is usually normal or only mildly impaired initially, although it may become more significantly impaired in end-stage restrictive cardiomyopathy. A reduction in LV longitudinal function may be seen before a fall in ejection fraction, and speckle tracking echo is particularly useful in cardiac amyloidosis, revealing a reduction in global longitudinal strain but with apical sparing (Chapter 12). This is clearly seen in 'bull's-eye' maps of segmental longitudinal strain, where the characteristic red colour-coding that denotes apical sparing is described as the 'cherry on top' pattern (**Figure 29.6**).

In cardiac amyloid, small pericardial and pleural effusions may be present, and there may be thickening not only of the LV myocardium but also of the RV free wall (≥5 mm), of the interatrial septum and of the heart valves. However, although mild valvular dysfunction may be present, it is unusual to see severe valvular dysfunction as a result of amyloid.

The distinction between restrictive cardiomyopathy and constrictive pericarditis can be challenging. The distinguishing features of the two conditions are listed in **Table 30.5** (p. 242).

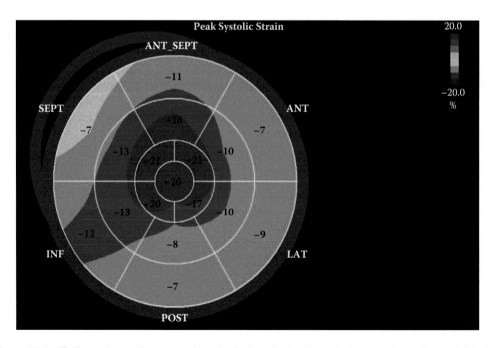

Figure 29.6 'Bull's-eye' map of segmental longitudinal strain showing apical sparing in cardiac amyloidosis.

ARRHYTHMOGENIC RIGHT VENTRICULAR CARDIOMYOPATHY

Arrhythmogenic RV cardiomyopathy or dysplasia (ARVC or ARVD) is a rare hereditary cardiomyopathy, primarily affecting the RV, in which there is loss of myocytes and replacement with fatty/fibrous tissue. ARVC affects between 1 in 1000 and 1 in 5000 of the general population. Patients may present with ventricular arrhythmias; sudden cardiac death may occur.

The diagnosis of ARVC is based upon the identification of a number of so-called 'major' and 'minor' criteria across several categories (global or regional dysfunction and structural alterations, tissue characterization, repolarization abnormalities, depolarization/conduction abnormalities, arrhythmias and family history). Full details of the diagnostic criteria can be found in the paper by Marcus et al. (2010).

Echo features

Echo has a key role to play in the diagnosis of ARVC by facilitating the assessment of global or regional dysfunction and structural alterations.

A 'major' echo criterion is defined by

- regional RV akinesia, dyskinesia or aneurysm
- *and* one of the following (measured at end-diastole):
  - RVOT diameter ≥ 32 mm (or ≥ 19 mm/m^2 indexed for body surface area) in parasternal long-axis view
  - RVOT diameter ≥ 36 mm (or ≥ 21 mm/m^2 indexed for body surface area) in parasternal short-axis view
- *or* fractional area change $\leq 33\%$ in *apical* four-chamber view

A 'minor' echo criterion is defined by

- regional RV akinesia or dyskinesia
- *and* one of the following (measured at end diastole):
  - RVOT diameter ≥ 29 to <32 mm (or ≥ 16 to <19 mm/m^2 indexed for body surface area) in parasternal long-axis view
  - RVOT diameter ≥ 32 to <36 mm (or ≥ 18 to <21 mm/m^2 indexed for body surface area) in parasternal short-axis view
- *or* fractional area change $>33\%$ to $\leq 40\%$ in *apical* four-chamber view

An echo assessment for suspected ARVC must therefore include an assessment of the RV for evidence of regional akinesia, dyskinesia or aneurysm, plus careful measurement of the RVOT diameter and/or RV fractional area change. For more detailed information on echo assessment of the RV, see Chapter 22. The RV is always involved in ARVC, but there may be LV abnormalities in >30% of cases. The echo findings can sometimes be subtle, making the diagnosis of ARVC challenging. Several tests, including cardiac magnetic resonance imaging and endomyocardial biopsy, may be needed to establish the diagnosis.

Further reading

Agha AM et al. Role of cardiovascular imaging for the diagnosis and prognosis of cardiac amyloidosis. *Open Heart* (2018). PMID 30305910.

Ghadri JR et al. International Expert Consensus Document on Takotsubo Syndrome (Part I): Clinical Characteristics, Diagnostic Criteria, and Pathophysiology. *European Heart Journal* (2018). PMID 29850871.

Jenni R et al. Echocardiographic and pathoanatomical characteristics of isolated left ventricular non-compaction: a step towards classification as a distinct cardiomyopathy. *Heart* 2001. PMID 11711464.

Marcus FI et al. Diagnosis of arrhythmogenic right ventricular cardiomyopathy/dysplasia: proposed modification of the task force criteria. *European Heart Journal* (2010). PMID 20172912.

Maron BJ et al. Contemporary definitions and classification of the cardiomyopathies. *Circulation* (2006). PMID 16567565.

Mathew T et al. Diagnosis and assessment of dilated cardiomyopathy: a guideline protocol from the British Society of Echocardiography. *Echo Research and Practice* (2017). PMID 28592613.

Ommen SR et al. 2020 AHA/ACC guideline for the diagnosis and treatment of patients with hypertrophic cardiomyopathy: executive summary: a report of the American College of Cardiology/American Heart Association Joint Committee on Clinical Practice Guidelines. *Circulation* (2020). PMID 33215938.

Turvey L et al. Transthoracic echocardiography of hypertrophic cardiomyopathy in adults: a practical guideline from the British Society of Echocardiography. *Echo Research and Practice* (2021). PMID 33667195.

The British Society of Echocardiography (www.bsecho.org) has published several useful protocols relating to the echo assessment of cardiomyopathies:

- The echocardiographic assessment of the right ventricle with particular reference to arrhythmogenic right ventricular cardiomyopathy
- A guideline protocol for the assessment of restrictive cardiomyopathy.

CHAPTER 30

The pericardium

ECHO APPEARANCES OF THE NORMAL PERICARDIUM

The pericardium is visible in each of the standard imaging planes of the heart and should therefore be examined in each view. As the normal pericardium is thin (1–2 mm), it is not prominent on echo, but may appear as a thin bright line around the heart. The trace of pericardial fluid that is normally present may be visible as a thin black line separating the two layers of the serous pericardium (**Figure 30.1**).

Use 2D echo to inspect the pericardium in as many views as possible and describe its appearance:

- Does the pericardium appear normal or abnormal?
- Is there thickening of the pericardium?
- Is there pericardial calcification?
- Is there a pericardial effusion? Describe its appearance. How big is it, where is it located and what are its haemodynamic effects?
- Is there evidence of pericardial constriction? What are the haemodynamic effects?
- Are there any pericardial masses?

PERICARDIAL EFFUSION

Any process that causes inflammation or injury to the pericardium can result in a pericardial effusion (**Table 30.1**).

Echo assessment of pericardial effusion

Pericardial or pleural?

First of all, be sure what you are assessing. At first glance pericardial and pleural effusions can appear similar on echo, but there are important distinguishing features. Use 2D echo in the parasternal long-axis view to assess where the effusion lies in relation to the descending aorta. A pericardial effusion will extend just up to the gap in between the left atrium (LA) and the *front* of the descending aorta (**Figure 30.2**). In contrast, a pleural effusion extends *behind* the aorta and around the LA (**Figure 30.3**). However, bear in mind that some patients will have coexistent pericardial *and* pleural effusions.

2D and M-mode

Use 2D echo to assess the extent of the effusion – is it circumferential, filling the entire pericardium, or localized? If localized, record where the effusion lies in relation to the atria and/or ventricles. Very

DOI: 10.1201/9781003304654-30

Table 30.1   Causes of pericardial effusion

Infection	Viral
	Bacterial (particularly tuberculosis)
Malignant	Primary spread from a local tumour (e.g., lung, breast)
	Distant metastasis (e.g., melanoma)
Inflammatory	Dressler's syndrome (after myocardial infarction)
	Uraemia (renal failure)
	Collagen vascular diseases (e.g., rheumatoid arthritis, systemic lupus erythematosus)
	Post–cardiac surgery
	Post-radiotherapy
Injury/Trauma	Post-cardiac surgery
	Aortic dissection
	Blunt or direct chest trauma
Idiopathic	

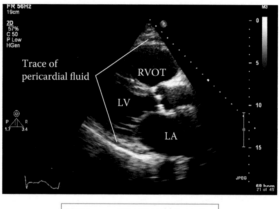

View	Parasternal long axis
Modality	2D

Figure 30.1   Trace of pericardial fluid (normal). *Abbreviations:* LA: Left atrium, LV: Left ventricle, RVOT: Right ventricular outflow tract.

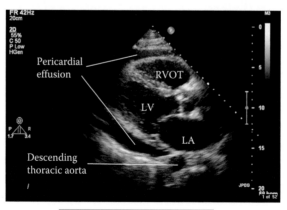

View	Parasternal long axis
Modality	2D

Figure 30.2   Pericardial effusion (anterior to descending thoracic aorta). *Abbreviations:* LA: Left atrium, LV: Left ventricle, RVOT: Right ventricular outflow tract.

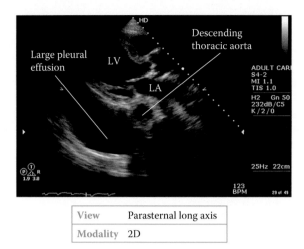

View	Parasternal long axis
Modality	2D

Figure 30.3 Pleural effusion (posterior to descending thoracic aorta). *Abbreviations:* LA: Left atrium, LV: Left ventricle.

localized effusions can sometimes be difficult to spot – for instance, if they lie within the oblique sinus – and may only be evident through the compression of adjacent structures (e.g., atria or pulmonary veins). Bear in mind that the patient's position may affect the distribution of the pericardial effusion – for instance, the effusion may localize posteriorly in a supine patient.

Assess the size of the effusion from several different views using 2D and/or M-mode echo. Record both the depth of the effusion (in cm) and the location where each measurement was taken. The size of an effusion can be gauged by its depth (**Table 30.2**). It is important to note that effusion size is not the same as clinical severity – small effusions that accumulate quickly can have a greater haemodynamic effect than large effusions that accumulate slowly.

Pericardial effusions can contain a fluid transudate or exudate, blood or pus. It can be difficult to distinguish between these on echo, and the pericardial fluid will usually look echolucent regardless of its nature. However, there may be strands of fibrin visible within the fluid, and these commonly adhere to the outside of the heart. Sometimes masses may be visible within the pericardium (**Figure 30.4**). Describe the appearance of any strands or masses, including their size and location.

Once you have assessed the appearances of the pericardial effusion, move on to assess its haemodynamic effects to look for evidence that would support a clinical diagnosis of cardiac tamponade (see below).

ESTIMATING THE VOLUME OF A PERICARDIAL EFFUSION

It's not usually necessary to estimate the volume of a pericardial effusion, but if you wish to, you can. In the apical four-chamber view, you can trace the outline of the pericardium and use the echo machine software to calculate the volume of the entire heart and pericardial effusion together. Next, trace the outline of the heart itself and calculate the heart's volume. By subtracting the latter measurement from the former, you are left with the approximate volume of the pericardial effusion.

Table 30.2 Pericardial effusion size

	Trace	Small	Moderate	Large
Depth (cm)	<0.5	0.5–1.0	1.0–2.0	>2.0
Volume (mL)	<100	100–250	250–500	>500

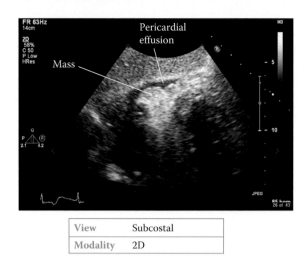

View	Subcostal
Modality	2D

Figure 30.4   Mass within a pericardial effusion.

Management of pericardial effusion

Investigate patients with pericardial effusion as appropriate to determine the underlying cause. Pericardiocentesis is indicated for

- cardiac tamponade (see below)
- suspected purulent or tuberculous effusions
- effusions measuring >2.0 cm (in diastole)

Pericardiocentesis can be performed for diagnostic purposes for effusions <2.0 cm, but this should only be done by skilled hands in an experienced centre.

CARDIAC TAMPONADE

Cardiac tamponade refers to the haemodynamic decompensation that occurs when the pressure within a pericardial effusion compresses the heart. It is a clinical diagnosis indicated by the presence of

- breathlessness (with clear lungs)
- tachycardia (>100 beats/min)
- hypotension (systolic blood pressure <100 mmHg)
- pulsus paradoxus (>10 mmHg fall in systolic blood pressure during inspiration)
- elevated jugular venous pressure
- quiet heart sounds

Echo assessment of cardiac tamponade

2D and M-mode

Use 2D and M-mode echo to confirm the presence of a pericardial effusion and to assess its extent as described above. Look carefully for signs of chamber collapse during diastole. As pressure within the pericardium rises, the right-sided chambers collapse (at least in part) during diastole (**Figure 30.5**). The first chamber to be affected is the right atrium (RA), which is seen to collapse during atrial systole, followed by the right ventricle (beginning with the right ventricular outflow tract [RVOT]). Rarely, the LA or even left ventricular (LV) collapse may be seen in severe cases.

Measure the inferior vena cava (IVC) in the subcostal view, and assess by how much its diameter reduces (if at all) during inspiration. The IVC is normally 1.5–2.5 cm in diameter and this falls by

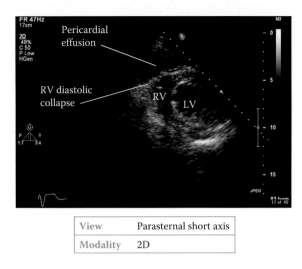

View	Parasternal short axis
Modality	2D

Figure 30.5   Cardiac tamponade (right ventricular [RV] diastolic collapse). *Abbreviation:* LV: Left ventricle.

>50% on inspiration. In the presence of tamponade, the IVC dilates and the inspiratory fall in diameter is reduced or absent.

Pulsed-wave Doppler

Use pulsed-wave (PW) Doppler to assess the right and left ventricular inflow and look for the exaggerated respiratory variation seen in tamponade. In a normal individual, inspiration increases the flow of blood returning to the right heart and decreases the flow of blood into the left heart; the opposite occurs on expiration. Cardiac tamponade exaggerates this respiratory variation.

To look for this phenomenon, use PW Doppler in the apical four-chamber view to interrogate tricuspid and mitral inflow. For both valves, measure the maximum and minimum E wave velocities seen during the cardiac cycle (for the tricuspid valve, the maximum will occur during inspiration and the minimum during expiration; vice versa for the mitral valve). The normal respiratory variation in E wave size is <25% for the tricuspid valve and <15% for the mitral valve. In the presence of cardiac tamponade, the same variation occurs but is exaggerated in extent (**Figure 30.6**). This is summarized in **Table 30.3**.

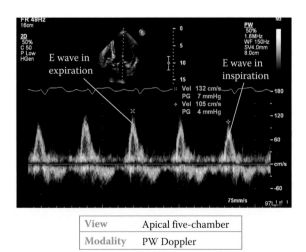

View	Apical five-chamber
Modality	PW Doppler

Figure 30.6   Cardiac tamponade (exaggerated respiratory variation in mitral inflow E wave size). *Abbreviations:* PG: Pressure gradient, Vel: Velocity.

Table 30.3 Respiratory variation in cardiac tamponade

	Normal		Cardiac tamponade	
Tricuspid E wave size				
Inspiration	$\frac{\text{Maximum}}{\text{Minimum}}$	Variation < 25%	$\frac{\text{Maximum}}{\text{Minimum}}$	Variation > 25%
Expiration				
Mitral E wave size				
Inspiration	$\frac{\text{Minimum}}{\text{Maximum}}$	Variation < 15%	$\frac{\text{Minimum}}{\text{Maximum}}$	Variation > 15%
Expiration				
RVOT V_{max} and VTI				
Inspiration	$\frac{\text{Maximum}}{\text{Minimum}}$	Variation < 10%	$\frac{\text{Maximum}}{\text{Minimum}}$	Variation > 10%
Expiration				
LVOT V_{max} and VTI				
Inspiration	$\frac{\text{Minimum}}{\text{Maximum}}$	Variation < 10%	$\frac{\text{Minimum}}{\text{Maximum}}$	Variation > 15%
Expiration				

Abbreviations: LVOT: Left ventricular outflow tract, RVOT: Right ventricular outflow tract, V_{max}: Peak velocity, VTI: Velocity time integral.

Similarly, respiratory variation in ventricular outflow can also be assessed. Use PW Doppler in the parasternal short-axis view to interrogate RVOT flow and record both the velocity time integral (VTI) and peak velocity (V_{max}); as with the RV inflow, outflow is at its maximum in inspiration and minimum in expiration. In the apical five-chamber view, make the same measurements for the LVOT; as with the LV inflow, outflow is at its minimum in inspiration and maximum in expiration. The normal respiratory variability in both parameters is <10%, but it is greater in the presence of tamponade.

Management of cardiac tamponade

Cardiac tamponade requires urgent drainage (pericardiocentesis). This is commonly performed via the subxiphisternal approach, and echo is very useful in planning the optimal route to minimize the distance from chest wall to effusion and to avoid intervening structures.

Echo guidance can help determine when the pericardiocentesis needle is correctly located within the pericardium. The needle itself is often difficult to see, and if there is doubt about the needle's position, it is possible to instil a small amount of agitated saline (9.5 mL of sterile saline agitated with 0.5 mL of air in a 10 mL syringe to create a suspension of small air bubbles) through the needle that can be detected by echo screening as bubble contrast within the effusion. If the pericardiocentesis needle has inadvertently punctured the heart, the bubbles will be seen within one of the cardiac chambers instead.

PERICARDIAL CONSTRICTION

Thickening and fibrosis of the serous pericardium can constrict the heart, like a rigid envelope, impairing filling of the ventricles in diastole and leading to equalization of the diastolic pressures in both ventricles. Filling of the heart in early diastole is rapid but then abruptly stops as the diastolic pressure plateaus. Because the heart becomes encased within a rigid 'shell', the ventricles become interdependent – in other words, the inflow of blood into one ventricle will affect the inflow into the other ventricle, as both ventricles have to function within a fixed space.

Pericardial constriction can result from pericardial inflammation, often after a long delay, and it is most common after cardiac surgery, radiotherapy and (where tuberculosis is common) tuberculous pericarditis.

Clinical features of pericardial constriction

The clinical features of pericardial constriction (**Table 30.4**) tend to be vague and the diagnosis is often delayed or missed altogether.

Table 30.4   Clinical features of pericardial constriction

Symptoms	Signs
Fatigue	Elevated JVP
Breathlessness	Rise in JVP on inspiration
Abdominal swelling and discomfort	Hypotension with low pulse pressure
	Quiet heart sounds
	Pleural effusions
	Hepatomegaly
	Ascites
	Peripheral oedema
	Muscle wasting

Abbreviation: JVP: Jugular venous pressure.

Echo assessment of pericardial constriction

2D and M-mode

Use 2D and M-mode echo to assess the structure of the pericardium in several different views:

- Is the pericardium thickened?
- Is there any calcification of the pericardium? Is this localized or generalized?

COMMON PITFALLS

- Pericardial thickness can be difficult to assess on transthoracic echo and is more reliably assessed with transoesophageal echo, which has a >90% sensitivity for detecting a pericardial thickness >3 mm.
- Cardiac computed tomography (CT) and magnetic resonance imaging (MRI) both are valuable for assessing pericardial thickness; however, echo is more useful for assessing the haemodynamics and, therefore, for making the actual diagnosis of constriction.
- In around 20% of cases of pericardial constriction, the pericardium itself appears normal. The absence of pericardial thickening (or calcification), therefore does *not* rule out the possibility of pericardial constriction.
- Conversely, the finding of a thickened pericardium does not necessarily imply the presence of pericardial constriction. A careful haemodynamic assessment is always necessary.

LV dimensions and function will usually be normal. M-mode assessment of the ventricular septum in the parasternal long-axis view may show

- abrupt posterior motion early in diastole, caused by rapid right ventricular diastolic filling, followed by
- little motion in mid-diastole, caused by equalization of right and left ventricular pressures, followed by
- abrupt anterior motion at the end of diastole (after atrial contraction) as there is further RV filling

There may also be a ventricular septal 'bounce' during inspiration. Increased filling of the RV during inspiration causes the septum to shift over to the left, due to ventricular interdependence. This can be seen as a shift in the ventricular septum towards the LV with inspiration and towards the RV with expiration.

Measure the LA in the parasternal long-axis view – it enlarges as a result of the chronically elevated LV diastolic pressure. The RA also enlarges.

Table 30.5   Pericardial constriction versus restrictive cardiomyopathy

	Pericardial constriction	Restrictive cardiomyopathy
Pericardium	Often thickened and calcified	Normal
Atrial enlargement	Mild–Moderate	Moderate–Severe
Mitral inflow	E wave respiratory variation >25%	E wave respiratory variation <15%
Tricuspid inflow	E wave respiratory variation >25%	E wave respiratory variation <15%
Ventricular septal motion	Abrupt early diastolic motion Septal 'bounce' on inspiration	Normal
Tissue Doppler imaging	Peak e' >8.0 cm/s	Peak e' <8.0 cm/s

Measure the IVC in the subcostal view, and assess how much it collapses during inspiration. The IVC is normally 1.5–2.5 cm in diameter and normally collapses by >50% on inspiration. In the presence of pericardial constriction, the IVC dilates and inspiratory collapse is reduced or absent.

Pulsed-wave Doppler

Use PW Doppler to assess right and left ventricular inflow and look for exaggerated respiratory variation, as seen in cardiac tamponade (see above).

Look particularly carefully at mitral valve inflow, as recorded by PW Doppler in the apical four-chamber view. Pericardial constriction causes

- an exaggeration of the normal E/A ratio (the E wave is larger than normal *and* the A wave is smaller)
- a rapid E wave deceleration time (<160 ms)

Pericardial constriction versus restrictive cardiomyopathy

The differentiation between pericardial constriction and restrictive cardiomyopathy can be challenging and makes a popular topic for echo accreditation examinations! Restrictive cardiomyopathy is discussed in Chapter 29. It shares many of the clinical features of pericardial constriction, so using investigations appropriately to distinguish between the two is important. **Table 30.5** lists some of the echo features that can help to distinguish constriction from restriction.

Management of pericardial constriction

Surgical intervention (pericardiectomy) is the definitive treatment for permanent pericardial constriction, with a mortality of 6%–12% and normalization of haemodynamic parameters in around 60%. The mortality after pericardiectomy tends to be worse if echo shows the presence of pericardial calcification.

OTHER PERICARDIAL ABNORMALITIES

Congenital absence of the pericardium

Congenital absence is a rare abnormality (around 1:10,000) that can affect part (left more commonly than the right) or all of the pericardium. Patients are usually asymptomatic, but it is possible for parts of the heart to become herniated or even strangulated through gaps in the pericardium. With partial absence of the pericardium, herniation of part of the heart may be apparent on 2D echo. With complete absence of the pericardium, the position of the heart as a whole may be abnormal (usually rotated posteriorly).

Pericardial cysts

Pericardial cysts are discussed on page 261. Small loculated pericardial effusions can be mistaken for congenital cysts.

Pericardial tumours

Pericardial tumours are rare. They can be primary or secondary and include such tumours as lipoma, liposarcoma, mesothelioma and lymphoma. Note the presence of any pericardial masses and describe their appearance as fully as possible.

Further reading

Adler Y et al. 2015 ESC guidelines for the diagnosis and management of pericardial diseases: the task force for the diagnosis and management of pericardial diseases of the European Society of Cardiology (ESC). Endorsed by: The European Association for Cardio-Thoracic Surgery (EACTS). *European Heart Journal* (2015). PMID 26320112.

Garcia MJ. Constrictive pericarditis versus restrictive cardiomyopathy? *Journal of the American College of Cardiology* (2016). PMID 27126534.

Klein AL et al. American Society of Echocardiography clinical recommendations for multimodality cardiovascular imaging of patients with pericardial disease. *Journal of the American Society of Echocardiography* (2013). PMID 23998693.

CHAPTER 31

The aorta

ECHO APPEARANCES OF THE NORMAL AORTA

The aorta extends all the way from the aortic valve to the point where it bifurcates into the left and right common iliac arteries. Different parts of the aorta are visible in many of the standard transthoracic echo (TTE) views (see Chapter 7):

- Left parasternal window
  - parasternal long-axis view
  - parasternal short-axis view
- Right parasternal window
- Apical window
  - apical five-chamber view
  - apical three-chamber (long-axis) view
- Subcostal window
- Suprasternal window
  - aorta view

The parasternal long-axis view is the preferred view for measuring aortic root dimensions, which are taken at four different levels. Three of these measurements should be taken at **end-diastole** (**Figure 31.1**):

- Sinuses of Valsalva
- Sinotubular junction
- Proximal ascending aorta (1 cm above the sinotubular junction)

However, measurement of the aortic annulus should be made in **mid-systole**, between the insertion points of the right coronary cusp and the non/left coronary cusp of the aortic valve.

Always measure aortic dimensions perpendicular to the axis of blood flow, at the widest diameter, from **inner edge to inner edge**. It is preferable to use 2D echo (from the parasternal long-axis window) to make measurements rather than M-mode. It is good practice to include the method of assessment in your echo report.

In 2020, the British Society of Echocardiography (BSE) updated its guidance on aortic root measurements. Aortic dimensions are now indexed for **height** (previously they were indexed for body surface area) and are now **age-independent** (previously there were different reference intervals according to age). However, there are different reference intervals for males and females.

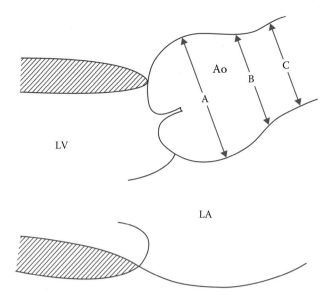

Figure 31.1 Where to measure the dimensions of the aortic root at end-diastole. *Abbreviations:* Ao: Aorta, A: Sinuses of Valsalva, B: Sinotubular junction, C: Proximal ascending aorta, LA: Left atrium, LV: Left ventricle.

For males, reference intervals for aortic root diameters, indexed for height, are as follows:

- 13.8–21.8 mm/m at the level of the sinuses of Valsalva
- 11.4–18.6 mm/m at the level of the sinotubular junction
- 11.5–19.9 mm/m at the level of the proximal ascending aorta

For females, reference intervals for aortic root diameters, indexed for height, are as follows:

- 13.1–20.7 mm/m at the level of the sinuses of Valsalva
- 11.0–17.8 mm/m at the level of the sinotubular junction
- 11.4–19.8 mm/m at the level of the proximal ascending aorta

The BSE does not quote a reference interval for aortic annulus diameter.

In addition to the aortic root, you can assess the

- aortic arch in the suprasternal window
- descending thoracic aorta (located behind the left atrium) in the parasternal long-axis view
- proximal abdominal aorta in the subcostal view

The BSE does not provide reference intervals for these measurements, but commonly quoted reference intervals (indexed for *body surface area*) at these levels are as follows:

- <1.9 cm/m² at the level of the aortic arch
- <1.6 cm/m² at the level of the descending thoracic aorta
- <1.6 cm/m² at the level of the abdominal aorta (at or above the superior mesenteric artery)

It should be noted that there are differences in methodology and in reference intervals for aortic measurements between the major international societies, so be sure to familiarize yourself with the recommendations that are applicable in the territory where you're working.

For a full echo assessment of the aorta, inspect each part of the aorta and

- describe its appearance (normal or abnormal)
- comment on any dilatation (stating location and dimensions)

Z-SCORES

Z-scores are commonly used in aortic root measurements for both paediatric and adult populations. Put simply, a Z-score shows by how many standard deviations a particular measurement deviates from a population mean. For instance, if you measure the diameter at the sinuses of Valsalva to be 42 mm, and calculate a Z-score of +2.3 for that measurement, then this means that your patient's measurement is 2.3 standard deviations above the mean. Conventionally the 'normal range' is considered to lie within ±2 standard deviations of the mean, so a Z-score greater than +2 (or less than −2) indicates that the measurement in question lies outside the normal range. Z-scores can be positive or negative, depending upon whether the measurement is larger or smaller than the population mean. In order to calculate a Z-score, you need data (mean and standard deviation) from an appropriate population to compare your measurement against. Z-score calculators can be found online, and each one is specific for a particular population in terms of age, sex and so on. When using a Z-score calculator, be sure to choose one that uses comparative data from a reference population that is applicable to your patient.

- identify any atheroma or thrombus (stating location, appearance, severity and if it is mobile)
- identify any dissection (stating the entry and exit points and whether there is any thrombus in the false lumen)
- identify any intramural haematoma (stating the location)
- identify any transection (stating the location)
- identify and characterize any coarctation of the aorta (see p. 271)

AORTIC DILATATION

Dilatation of the aorta can result from

- atherosclerosis
- hypertension
- trauma
- post-stenotic (dilatation of the ascending aorta above a stenotic aortic valve)

Aortic dilatation (and dissection) is also more likely in patients with bicuspid aortic valve (p. 270) and correlates with the degree of aortic regurgitation that may be present. Patients with bicuspid aortic valve are ten times more likely to experience an aortic dissection than those with a normal valve.

A number of connective tissue and inflammatory diseases can cause aortic dilatation:

- Marfan syndrome
- systemic lupus erythematosus
- rheumatoid arthritis
- Reiter syndrome
- syphilitic aortitis

In aortic dilatation due to Marfan syndrome, the relative proportions of the aortic root (broader at the sinuses of Valsalva, becoming narrower again at the sinotubular junction) are lost and the boundary between the sinuses of Valsalva and the ascending aorta becomes less clear – this is referred to as effacement of the sinotubular junction. Marfan syndrome is discussed on page 280. Localized dilatation of one or more sinuses of Valsalva is called sinus of Valsalva aneurysm (p. 251).

Echo assessment of aortic dilatation

Aortic dilatation can vary between cases in its extent; so, for an aortic assessment, it is important to measure the aortic dimensions at multiple levels (**Figure 31.2**):

- aortic annulus
- sinuses of Valsalva
- sinotubular junction
- ascending aorta
- aortic arch
- descending thoracic aorta
- proximal abdominal aorta

Look for, and describe any associated aortic abnormalities:

- atheroma
- thrombus
- dissection
- coarctation

In cases that involve the aortic root, look carefully for the effects on aortic valve structure and function. Dilatation of the aortic root can lead to reduced coaptation between the aortic valve cusps, so look for any distortion of the valve and use Doppler interrogation to assess aortic regurgitation. Also remember that an abnormal aortic valve can sometimes be the *cause* of aortic dilatation (e.g., bicuspid aortic valve, post-stenotic dilatation in aortic stenosis), and a full aortic valve assessment should be performed with this in mind.

Management of aortic dilatation

As the aorta dilates, a potentially catastrophic event such as dissection or rupture becomes increasingly likely. Careful monitoring with surgical intervention at an appropriate time is the key to successful management.

Patients with mild–moderate aortic root dilatation should, where possible, receive treatment with a beta-blocker and undergo echo follow-up every 6–12 months (bearing in mind that the larger an aneurysm, the more quickly it dilates). Elective surgery is usually undertaken if the

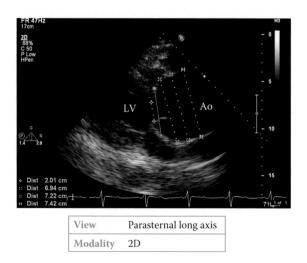

| View | Parasternal long axis |
| Modality | 2D |

Figure 31.2 Severe aortic root dilatation. *Abbreviations:* Ao: Aorta, LV: Left ventricle.

aortic diameter measures ≥5.5 cm (with lower thresholds for patients with Marfan syndrome or bicuspid aortic valve). Rapid dilatation of an aneurysm (≥0.5 cm/year) is also considered an indication for surgery.

AORTIC DISSECTION

If a tear occurs in the intimal layer of the aorta, blood flowing in the aortic lumen can penetrate through to the medial layer to create an extra channel or 'false lumen'. The blood entering the medial layer can propagate proximally or distally within the wall of the aorta. The initial tear ('entry point') can occur anywhere in the aorta, although the vast majority of aortic dissections originate either in the first few centimetres of the ascending aorta or just distal to the origin of the left subclavian artery. Blood flowing in the false lumen can re-enter the 'true' lumen of the aorta through a further intimal tear elsewhere ('exit point'). Aortic dissections are classified according to the region of aorta involved (**Table 31.1**).

Aortic dissection can occur in patients with pre-existing aortic dilatation, or conditions that place the aorta under strain or affect the strength of the wall (e.g., hypertension, pregnancy, Marfan syndrome, Ehlers–Danlos syndrome, bicuspid aortic valve, coarctation of the aorta).

Aortic dissection is a medical emergency, with 50% patients dying within the first 48 hours if left untreated. The classical presenting symptom is a sudden-onset 'tearing' interscapular pain. Patients may exhibit a difference in blood pressure (>20 mmHg) between right and left arms. A variety of other clinical features may be seen, depending on the extent of the dissection and whether it impairs the blood supply to other organs.

ACUTE AORTIC SYNDROME

Aortic dissection is one of a trio of pathological entities which can affect the wall of the aorta and cause disruption of the media layer, the others being intramural haematoma and penetrating ulcer. These are classified together under the name Acute Aortic Syndrome (AAS), of which dissection is the most common (80% of the AAS cases) and penetrating ulcer the least common (5%). Aortic dissection is diagnosed on the basis of an intimal flap dividing the aorta into true and false lumens. Intramural haematoma appears as >5 mm crescentic/circular thickening of the aortic wall, while a penetrating ulcer is characterized by a crater-like outpouching of the aortic wall, usually in association with atheroma.

Echo assessment of aortic dissection

The limited views of TTE mean that a negative study cannot exclude the diagnosis. The sensitivity of TTE is greater for dissections involving the ascending aorta than for those in the descending aorta, and the sensitivity can be improved by the use of contrast. Nonetheless, a negative TTE does not exclude a diagnosis of aortic dissection. Computed tomography (CT) is the most commonly used imaging modality for establishing the diagnosis of aortic dissection, although transoesophageal echo (TOE) and magnetic resonance imaging (MRI) can also play a role.

Table 31.1   Classification of aortic dissection

Stanford classification	DeBakey classification
Type A dissections involve the ascending aorta	Type I dissections involve the ascending aorta, arch and descending aorta
Type B dissections do not involve the ascending aorta	Type II dissections are confined to the ascending aorta
	Type III dissections originate distal to the left subclavian artery and are confined to the descending aorta

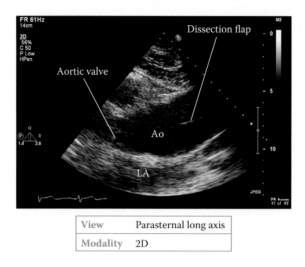

View	Parasternal long axis
Modality	2D

Figure 31.3   Aortic dissection in ascending aorta. *Abbreviations:* Ao: Aorta, LA: Left atrium.

2D and M-mode

Inspect the aorta from as many views as possible. Remember that the majority of dissections arise in the initial segment of the ascending aorta or just after the left subclavian artery. Look carefully for

- evidence of aortic dilatation
- evidence of an intimal flap

An intimal flap is a linear structure within the aorta which is mobile, but its pattern of movement is more erratic than that of the aortic wall (**Figure 31.3**). Identify the location of the dissection and try to identify the entry and exit points where possible.

Colour Doppler

Use colour Doppler to assess flow within the true and false lumens – their flow patterns are usually different. Systolic antegrade flow is usually present in the true lumen, but it may be reduced or absent in the false lumen. Colour Doppler can help to identify the entry and exit points of the false lumen, with flow being from the true lumen into the false lumen during systole. Note that there may be multiple entry/exit sites where flow between the true and false lumens can occur.

It can sometimes be difficult to decide which is the true and which is the false lumen, particularly in the descending aorta. In addition to the flow differences mentioned above, the true lumen is usually smaller in size than the false lumen, is usually more regular than the false lumen and is more likely to exhibit expansile pulsation during systole (the false lumen may show systolic compression). When echo contrast is used, contrast flow is usually early and fast in the true lumen, but delayed and slow in the false lumen.

Blood within the false lumen may start to thrombose, in which case the false lumen may show spontaneous echo contrast or absent flow. Note the presence of thrombus in the false lumen in your report.

Associated features

TTE is useful in identifying complications of aortic dissection:

- *Aortic regurgitation:* If the dissection involves the aortic root, the normal structure of the aortic valve can be distorted causing regurgitation.

- *Myocardial ischaemia/infarction:* Involvement of the coronary arteries (most commonly the right coronary artery) can lead to ischaemia/infarction, evidenced by left ventricular regional wall motion abnormalities.
- *Pericardial effusion/cardiac tamponade:* Rupture of the dissection into the pericardial space causes a haemorrhagic pericardial effusion and/or tamponade.

PITFALLS IN THE ECHO ASSESSMENT OF AORTIC DISSECTION

- *False negative diagnosis* – a normal TTE study does not exclude an aortic dissection.
- *False positive diagnosis* – echo artifact within the aortic lumen can be mistaken for dissection. Typical causes of artifact include reverberation or beam-width artifact (p. 19). Artifacts usually lack the chaotic motion seen with a dissection flap.
- In a patient with acute chest pain and left ventricular wall motion abnormality, always check for aortic dissection as a potential cause of the myocardial ischaemia/infarction.

Management of aortic dissection

Patients with aortic dissection may be critically ill and haemodynamically compromised, requiring urgent stabilization. Dissections involving the ascending aorta are managed with urgent surgical intervention. Dissections confined to the descending aorta are usually managed pharmacologically (e.g., assiduous control of hypertension), with surgery being reserved for any complications (e.g., rupture) that may occur.

INTRAMURAL HAEMATOMA

Intramural haematoma can present with similar symptoms to aortic dissection and is managed similarly. However, in intramural haematoma, there is bleeding into the aortic medial layer not from the aortic lumen but from vessels that supply the aorta itself – there is therefore no communication between the blood in the aorta and in the haematoma. Intramural haematoma can nevertheless lead to aortic dissection or rupture. On echo, an intramural haematoma appears as an echogenic circular or crescentic 'mass' within the wall of the aorta, >5 mm thick, between the intimal and adventitial layers.

SINUS OF VALSALVA ANEURYSM

Just above the level of the aortic valve lie the three sinuses of Valsalva, each one corresponding to one of the aortic valve cusps (right coronary, left coronary and non-coronary). Although any of the sinuses of Valsalva can develop aneurysmal dilatation, the right sinus is affected most commonly (around two-thirds of cases) and the non-coronary sinus in around a quarter of cases; the left sinus is seldom affected.

Sinus of Valsalva aneurysm can be congenital, occurring as a result of an abnormality of the aortic media and elastic tissue, leading to dilatation of a single sinus. Congenital aneurysms can become elongated and are classically described as having a 'windsock' appearance on echo. Acquired causes include atherosclerosis, endocarditis, cystic medial necrosis, chest trauma and syphilis. Acquired cases often affect all three sinuses. Sinus of Valsalva aneurysm is seen in around 10% of patients with Marfan syndrome.

Sinus of Valsalva aneurysm can lead to

- aortic regurgitation

- compression or distortion of local structures (e.g., coronary arteries, right ventricular outflow tract, conduction system)
- rupture of the aneurysm into an adjacent structure (most commonly the right ventricle or right atrium, or more rarely into the left heart chambers, pulmonary artery, or pericardium)

Echo assessment of sinus of Valsalva aneurysm includes

- measurement of aortic root dimensions
- description of the sinus(es) involved
- assessment of aortic valve structure and function, looking in particular for aortic regurgitation
- looking for evidence of compression or distortion of any neighbouring structures by the aneurysm
- assessment of whether rupture is present, which chamber is involved and what the haemodynamic effects are
- looking for associated abnormalities (ventricular septal defect, bicuspid aortic valve)

Repair of a ruptured sinus of Valsalva aneurysm can be performed surgically or percutaneously, using an occluder device. Unruptured aneurysms can be repaired surgically, although the optimal timing of such surgery is controversial.

AORTIC ATHEROMA

Atherosclerotic plaques can form in the aorta, particularly in patients with vascular disease elsewhere (e.g., coronary artery disease, cerebrovascular disease, peripheral vascular disease). Aortic atheroma is seen as irregular echogenic thickening of the intimal layer of the aorta, is found in the descending aorta more frequently than in the ascending aorta and is best studied with TOE (but it may be seen during TTE studies, too).

Clinical features of aortic atheroma

Aortic atheroma is commonly an incidental finding and in itself is therefore often asymptomatic. However, it can be a source for arterial emboli downstream of the plaque, causing stroke and/or peripheral emboli. Atheromatous disease of the aorta can also be a precursor to dilatation of the aorta and/or to aortic dissection (see above).

Patients with aortic atheroma may have atheromatous disease elsewhere in the arterial system, and this can cause symptoms, e.g.,

- *Coronary artery disease* – causing angina and/or acute coronary syndromes
- *Cerebrovascular disease* – causing transient ischaemic attacks and/or stroke
- *Peripheral vascular disease* – causing intermittent claudication

Review patients with aortic atheroma for symptoms and signs of vascular disease, and also for major treatable risk factors for vascular disease:

- hyperlipidaemia
- tobacco consumption
- diabetes mellitus
- hypertension

Echo assessment of aortic atheroma

Use 2D echo to examine the aorta for the presence of atheroma. If atheroma is present, describe its location:

- aortic root
- ascending aorta
- aortic arch
- descending thoracic aorta
- abdominal aorta

Describe the appearance of the atheroma:

- Is there any calcification of the atheroma?
- Is there protrusion of the atheroma into the lumen of the vessel? How thick is any protruding plaque?
- Is the atheroma mobile?
- Is the atheromatous plaque ulcerated (seen as a crater-like 'pouch')?

Finally, grade the extent of any aortic atheroma as mild, moderate or severe. Although these gradings are not clearly defined, it is reasonable to regard plaque disease that is mobile, ulcerated and/or protruding with a thickness of 5 mm or more as 'severe' or 'complex'. Plaques without any of these features are sometimes called 'simple' plaques.

SAMPLE REPORT

There is mild calcified atheromatous plaque visible in the ascending aorta, and moderate calcified plaque in the aortic arch, protruding into the aortic lumen with a thickness up to 3 mm. The atheromatous plaque is not mobile.

Management of aortic atheroma

Counsel patients with aortic atheroma about risk factor management (e.g., quitting smoking, dietary modification). Drug treatment with an antiplatelet drug (e.g., aspirin) and a statin is often appropriate. Atheroma associated with aortic dilatation or dissection may require surgical intervention.

Further reading

Curtis AE et al. The mystery of the Z-score. *Aorta* (2016). PMID 28097194.

Erbel R et al. 2014 ESC Guidelines on the diagnosis and treatment of aortic diseases: document covering acute and chronic aortic diseases of the thoracic and abdominal aorta of the adult. The Task Force for the Diagnosis and Treatment of Aortic Diseases of the European Society of Cardiology (ESC). *European Heart Journal* (2014). PMID 25173340.

Evangelista A et al. Echocardiography in aortic diseases: EAE recommendations for clinical practice. *European Journal of Echocardiography* (2010). PMID 20823280.

Evangelista A et al. The current role of echocardiography in acute aortic syndrome. *Echo Research and Practice* (2019). PMID 30921764.

Gawinecka J et al. Acute aortic dissection: pathogenesis, risk factors and diagnosis. *Swiss Medical Weekly* (2017). PMID 28871571.

Goldstein SA et al. Multimodality imaging of diseases of the thoracic aorta in adults: from the American Society of Echocardiography and the European Association of Cardiovascular Imaging: endorsed by the Society of Cardiovascular Computed Tomography and Society for Cardiovascular Magnetic Resonance. *Journal of the American Society of Echocardiography* (2015). PMID 25623219.

Harkness A et al. Normal reference intervals for cardiac dimensions and function for use in echocardiographic practice: a guideline from the British Society of Echocardiography. *Echo Research and Practice* (2020). PMID 32105051.

Loukas M et al. The anatomy of the aortic root. *Clinical Anatomy* (2014). PMID 24000000.

Spanos K et al. Guidelines on aortic disease management. *Journal of Endovascular Therapy* (2020). PMID 32813588.

Upadhyaya K et al. Echocardiographic evaluation of the thoracic aorta: tips and pitfalls. *Aorta (Stamford)* (2021). PMID 34607379.

CHAPTER 32

Cardiac masses

The finding of a cardiac mass often has significant clinical implications and therefore apparent masses need careful echo evaluation to determine, as far as possible, their likely nature. Some harmless structures, such as the right ventricular (RV) moderator band, can give the appearance of a mass, and so it is particularly important to try to distinguish a mass that is pathological from one that is a normal variant. Cardiac masses on echo can result from

- Tumours
  - primary cardiac tumours
    - benign
    - malignant
  - secondary cardiac tumours
- Thrombus
- Vegetations
- Normal variants and other conditions
  - moderator band
  - Lambl's excrescences
  - Eustachian valve
  - Chiari network
  - lipomatous hypertrophy of the interatrial septum
  - dilated vessels
  - cysts
  - implanted devices

TUMOURS

The echo assessment of a cardiac tumour should include a description of its:

- size (measure its dimensions)
- location
- shape (e.g., spherical, pedunculated, papillary, flat)
- surface appearance (e.g., regular, irregular, multilobular)
- texture (e.g., solid, layered, cystic, calcified, heterogeneous)

DOI: 10.1201/9781003304654-32

- mobility (mobile or fixed)
- associated features (local invasion, pericardial effusion)

Because echo does not allow for a *precise* diagnosis, it is generally more appropriate to report a cardiac mass as being, for example, 'suggestive of a myxoma' than as a 'definite' myxoma.

The characteristics of the commonest tumours, and the features that distinguish them from other cardiac masses, are described below.

Primary cardiac tumours

Primary cardiac tumours are those that arise from the heart itself. They are rare (1 in 2000 autopsies) and 75% are benign (**Table 32.1**).

Primary cardiac tumours can present with systemic features such as fever and weight loss, or more specifically with

- *Embolism* – either of part of the tumour itself or adherent thrombus
- *Obstruction* – usually of a valve orifice or outflow tract
- *Arrhythmias* – either tachyarrhythmias, such as ventricular tachycardia, or atrioventricular block

However, cardiac tumours are most commonly discovered incidentally during echo studies for other indications.

Myxoma

Myxoma is the commonest primary cardiac tumour, accounting for 50% of cases, and is commoner in females. It is typically diagnosed between the ages of 30 and 60 years. Myxomas are usually (but not always) solitary: 75%–80% are found in the left atrium (LA, **Figure 32.1**), 15%–20% in the right atrium (RA) and rarely in the ventricles.

Around 7% of myxomas are familial (autosomal dominant), and these are more commonly multiple and found in the ventricles. Familial myxomas tend to present at a younger age. There can be associated abnormalities such as facial freckling and endocrine tumours, and such syndromes are grouped together as a 'Carney complex'. Other myxoma syndromes include NAME syndrome and LAMB syndrome. Screening of first-degree relatives is appropriate in suspected familial cases.

Myxomas are attached to the heart by a pedunculated stalk – in the case of atrial myxomas, they attach to the interatrial septum at the fossa ovalis. The echo appearances of a myxoma are of a well-defined mass, which is often mobile, and the pedicle may be visible. The tumour itself appears heterogeneous and may contain small areas of lucency and occasionally speckles of calcium. Transthoracic echo (TTE) is usually adequate for making the diagnosis, but transoesophageal echo (TOE) has a greater sensitivity and specificity and provides a more detailed assessment of the myxoma.

Surgical resection of the myxoma is the treatment of choice. Following resection, longer-term follow-up is appropriate to monitor for tumour recurrence (particularly in familial cases, where the recurrence rate is 20%).

Table 32.1   Primary cardiac tumours

Benign (75%)	Malignant (25%)
Myxoma	Angiosarcoma
Papillary fibroelastoma	Rhabdomyosarcoma
Lipoma	
Haemangioma	
Teratoma	
Rhabdomyoma	
Fibroma	

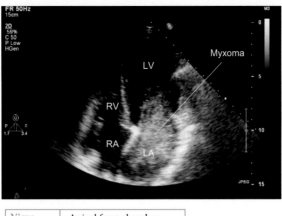

View	Apical four-chamber
Modality	2D

Figure 32.1   Large left atrial myxoma, prolapsing through the mitral valve during diastole. *Abbreviations:* LA: Left atrium, LV: Left ventricle, RA: Right atrium, RV: Right ventricle.

Other benign cardiac tumours

Papillary fibroelastoma is a small (<1.5 cm) benign tumour and is most commonly found attached to the aortic or mitral valve, although fibroelastomas can arise from any part of the endocardium. They account for 10% of primary cardiac tumours. They are usually found incidentally during echo, cardiac surgery or post mortem, and their similarity to vegetations can lead to a mistaken diagnosis of infective endocarditis. They are usually highly mobile and have been described as having a 'shimmering' appearance around the edges on echo. The tumours can be a source of thrombotic emboli, or fragments of the fibroelastoma itself can embolize, and surgical resection should therefore be considered, particularly if they are large (>1.0 cm), mobile and present in the left heart.

Lipomas are usually seen beneath the epicardium. Cardiac magnetic resonance imaging (MRI) is a useful technique to confirm the diagnosis. Lipomas are distinct from lipomatous hypertrophy of the interatrial septum (see below).

Haemangioma is a rare benign vascular tumour which can occur in any chamber.

Rhabdomyoma is the commonest cardiac tumour seen in infants and children. It is usually multiple and found in the ventricles. It is commonly associated with tuberous sclerosis.

Fibromas are also commonest in infants and children, are usually solitary, and mainly affect the interventricular septum. Fibromas are up to 10 cm in diameter and appear heterogeneous with multifocal calcification on echo. They often cause obstruction and arrhythmias.

Teratomas are germ cell tumours found in infants and children that usually affect the pericardium and are associated with a pericardial effusion. Echo shows a complex cystic mass within the pericardium and usually on the right side of the heart.

Malignant primary cardiac tumours

Malignant tumours make up 25% of primary cardiac tumours and the vast majority are sarcomas. There are various types of cardiac sarcomas, including angiosarcoma (the commonest), rhabdomyosarcoma, malignant fibrous histiocytoma and osteosarcoma.

Angiosarcomas almost always affect the RA (in contrast to the other sarcomas which can arise anywhere in the heart, but most commonly on the left) and they occur more commonly in males, usually in the age range 30–50 years. Patients often present with symptoms of right heart obstruction and, because pericardial involvement is common, cardiac tamponade. On echo the mass is broad based, often arises near the junction of the inferior cava with the RA, and may be invasive.

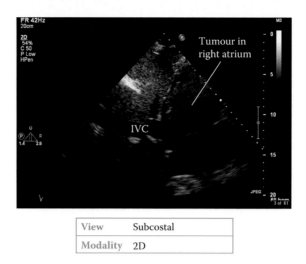

View	Subcostal
Modality	2D

Figure 32.2   Large secondary tumour within right atrium. *Abbreviation:* IVC: Inferior vena cava.

Primary cardiac lymphomas are usually non-Hodgkin lymphomas. Although it is not unusual for the heart to be affected as a consequence of lymphoma elsewhere, primary cardiac lymphoma (i.e., confined to the heart and pericardium alone) is very rare, although it is more frequent in acquired immunodeficiency syndrome and in immunosuppressed transplant recipients. Echo reveals masses, most commonly affecting the right heart, often with a pericardial effusion.

Secondary cardiac tumours

Secondary cardiac tumours are those that have arisen elsewhere in the body and have metastasized to the heart (**Figure 32.2**). They are much commoner than primary cardiac tumours (estimated to be between 30 and 1000 times commoner) but only 10% cause symptoms or signs during life. The tumours that metastasize to the heart most frequently include melanoma, breast carcinoma, bronchial carcinoma, lymphoma and leukaemia. Symptomatic patients usually present with arrhythmias or heart failure, and may have a pericardial effusion.

Echo most commonly shows epicardial thickening, although the myocardium and endocardium can also be involved, often with pericardial effusion. Tumours can also spread to the heart directly along vessels – renal cell carcinoma can invade the heart via the inferior vena cava, and bronchial carcinoma via the pulmonary veins.

THROMBUS

Cardiac thrombus is more likely to form when

1. there is stasis (or slow flow) of blood
2. there is abnormal endocardium (allowing thrombus to attach)
3. the blood is hypercoagulable (making it more likely to clot)

Thrombus formation is therefore more likely in the LA in atrial fibrillation (AF), when there is a loss of normal atrial contraction, and in the left ventricle (LV) following myocardial infarction, when reduced contractility predisposes to thrombus formation (particularly if there is aneurysm formation). The presence of an intracardiac device, such as a replacement valve or a pacing wire, can also act as a focus for thrombosis. Where there is a high risk of thrombosis (or where a thrombus has already formed), anticoagulation with a drug such as warfarin is used.

When you suspect you have found a cardiac thrombus, it is important to ask yourself, 'What is the substrate?' In other words, what is the underlying abnormality that has allowed the thrombus to form? If you cannot find a substrate, reassess whether are you observing a thrombus or a different type of cardiac mass. For instance, LV thrombus formation would be very unusual in the presence of a structurally normal LV with good function.

Echo assessment of thrombus

The echo assessment of a cardiac thrombus should include a description of its:

- size (measure its dimensions)
- location
- shape (e.g., flat, protruding, spherical)
- surface appearance (e.g., regular, irregular)
- texture (e.g., solid, layered, calcified)
- mobility (mobile or fixed)
- associated features (e.g., dilated LA, LV aneurysm)

Compared with a myxoma, a thrombus usually has a more irregular shape. Thrombus usually attaches to the endocardium via a broad base rather than a pedicle, and is consequently less mobile. A large proportion of LA thrombi are within the LA appendage, which can be difficult to inspect fully on TTE. The appendage is, however, clearly seen on TOE. It is important to try to distinguish between thrombus and the pectinate muscles, the normal muscle ridges found on the walls of both atria and the appendage. Pectinate muscles are immobile and run in bands; thrombus is usually more rounded and mobile.

Stasis of blood within the heart (and sometimes even the aorta) can be evident as 'spontaneous echo contrast'. This has the appearance of a swirling 'cloud' of tiny particles, hence it is sometimes referred to as 'smoke'. Although it is most often (and mostly clearly) seen during TOE studies, it can also be observed during TTE. Spontaneous contrast is caused by echo reflections from aggregations of red blood cells moving at low velocity, and it is most often observed in the LA in patients in AF, particularly if they also have mitral stenosis. It indicates an increased risk of thrombus formation.

Thrombus in the LV normally occurs in association with an area of wall motion abnormality and/ or aneurysm formation, commonly the apex (**Figure 32.3**). The echo texture of the thrombus is usually distinct from the adjacent myocardium. With the passage of time, the thrombus may become organized and layered, and there may be associated calcification. TTE is better than TOE for the detection of ventricular thrombus, as the ventricle is closer to the probe on TTE imaging.

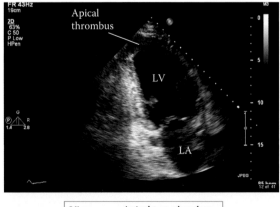

View	Apical two-chamber
Modality	2D

Figure 32.3   Left ventricular apical thrombus. *Abbreviations:* LA: Left atrium, LV: Left ventricle.

Thrombus in the right heart is less commonly found, and may represent a thromboembolism that has arisen in the peripheral veins and is 'in transit' to becoming a pulmonary embolism. Another cause of right heart thrombi is the presence of devices such as pacing/defibrillator leads or intravascular catheters, which can act as a focus for thrombus formation.

VEGETATIONS

Vegetations are discussed more fully in Chapter 28. Vegetations are usually irregular in shape, mobile and attached to valve leaflets on the upstream side (in contrast with papillary fibroelastoma, which attaches downstream). Infective endocarditis can also cause abscesses, which also have the appearance of cardiac masses. In addition to the echo features, the clinical context is important in distinguishing between vegetations and other causes of cardiac masses.

NORMAL VARIANTS AND OTHER CONDITIONS

Moderator band

The moderator band is a prominent muscular ridge of tissue that runs across the RV and is particularly well seen from the apical window. It can be mistaken for a cardiac mass. Similarly, 'false chords' in the LV (and even the papillary muscles) can inadvertently be mistaken for abnormal masses.

Lambl's excrescences

Lambl's excrescences are small filamentous strands on the ventricular side of the aortic valve. They are a normal finding in the elderly and are thought to arise from 'wear and tear' at the edges of the cusps. On echo they can be mistaken for papillary fibroelastomas, but are usually smaller.

Eustachian valve

The Eustachian valve is a membranous embryological remnant – its role in fetal life is to direct oxygenated blood towards the foramen ovale and away from the tricuspid valve. In adult life it is usually seen as a thin flap at the junction of the inferior vena cava with the RA. The size and mobility of the Eustachian valve is very much variable between individuals, but this represents normal variation.

Chiari network

A Chiari network is an embryological remnant of the sinus venosus and forms a net-like web across the RA in around 2% of the population. It has no clinical significance, although it can make passage of right heart catheters more difficult.

Lipomatous hypertrophy of the interatrial septum

Lipomatous hypertrophy of the interatrial septum is characterized by an accumulation of non-encapsulated fatty tissue within the interatrial septum. It has an incidence of 1%–8% and is commoner with obesity and increasing age. Although usually asymptomatic, associations with arrhythmias have been reported. The characteristic echo appearances are

- marked thickening of the interatrial septum (≥15 mm)
- echogenic appearance of the lipomatous tissue
- sparing of the fossa ovalis (giving a dumbbell appearance)

Dilated vessels

A **dilated coronary sinus** can give the appearance of a cystic mass behind the heart (**Figure 32.4**). Enlargement of the coronary sinus usually occurs as a result of anomalous drainage of a *left-sided* superior vena cava. This can be confirmed by an injection of agitated saline into a left arm vein – the bubbles will be seen to fill the coronary sinus, followed by the RA.

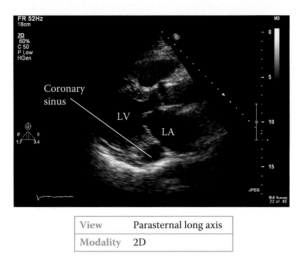

View	Parasternal long axis
Modality	2D

Figure 32.4   Dilated coronary sinus. *Abbreviations:* LA: Left atrium, LV: Left ventricle.

An **aneurysmal coronary artery** can also give the appearance of a cardiac cystic mass along the route of the coronary arteries. The right coronary artery is more commonly affected than the left coronary artery. The diagnosis can be confirmed by coronary angiography or cardiac computed tomography (CT)/magnetic resonance imaging (MRI).

Cysts

Pericardial cysts are a benign abnormality that are usually congenital but have also been reported following cardiac surgery. They are most commonly located at the right cardiophrenic angle. Most are asymptomatic and discovered incidentally, but some can present with compressive symptoms. On echo they have the appearance of an oval cavity, rather like a loculated pericardial effusion, and are commonly 1–5 cm in size. Management options include observation, percutaneous drainage and surgical resection.

Implanted devices

At first sight, implanted devices can sometimes have the appearance of a cardiac mass. The diagnosis is usually clarified simply by asking the patient about any past cardiac procedures. Devices that can cause confusion include

- pacemaker and defibrillator leads (in RV and RA)
- intravascular catheters
- replacement valves
- atrial septal occluder devices
- LV assist device

Further reading

L'Angiocola PD et al. Cardiac masses in echocardiography: a pragmatic review. *Journal of Cardiovascular Echocardiography* (2020). PMID 32766100.

Mankad R et al. Cardiac tumors: echo assessment. *Echo Research and Practice* (2016). PMID 27600455.

Tyebally S et al. Cardiac Tumors: JACC CardioOncology State-of-the-Art Review. *JACC CardioOncology* (2020). PMID 34396236.

CHAPTER 33

Congenital heart disease

This book is concerned with *adult* echocardiography, and so the congenital abnormalities described in this chapter are primarily those that may be encountered in adult patients, often following surgical or percutaneous correction. A detailed discussion of congenital heart disease is beyond the scope of this book, but a number of excellent reference works are available (see the 'Further Reading' section).

ATRIAL SEPTAL DEFECT

Atrial septal defect (ASD) is the commonest form of congenital heart disease seen in adults. The commonest form of defect is the **secundum ASD**, accounting for 80% of cases, in which the fossa ovalis is absent, leaving a defect in the centre of the interatrial septum. **Primum ASD** is less common (15% of cases) and causes a defect in the inferior interatrial septum, typically associated with abnormalities of the atrioventricular valves. **Superior sinus venosus ASD** and the rarer **inferior sinus venosus ASD** are found near to where the superior or inferior vena cava joins the right atrium (RA). They are associated with partial anomalous pulmonary venous drainage, in which one or more pulmonary veins drain directly into the RA (or one of the venae cavae) instead of the left atrium (LA).

An ASD can also be acquired as a result of deliberate puncture of the interatrial septum during balloon mitral valvuloplasty or left-sided electrophysiological procedures, or accidental puncture during the right heart catheterization or pacing.

Clinical features of atrial septal defect

ASD can remain asymptomatic for many years and may present late in adult life. It can also be an incidental finding. The clinical features are summarized in Table 33.1. ASDs cause left-to-right shunting causing right ventricular (RV) volume overload, and the resulting increase in pulmonary blood flow can eventually lead to pulmonary hypertension and, ultimately, shunt reversal (Eisenmenger physiology).

Table 33.1 Clinical features of atrial septal defect

Symptoms	Signs
May be asymptomatic	Atrial fibrillation can occur
Breathlessness	Wide fixed splitting of the second heart sound
Recurrent respiratory infections	Systolic (flow) murmur in pulmonary area
Palpitations (atrial fibrillation)	Right heart failure (advanced cases)
Paradoxical embolism	

DOI: 10.1201/9781003304654-33

SHUNT CALCULATIONS

Normally, the stroke volume of the right heart equals that of the left heart. However, the presence of a left-to-right shunt such as an ASD means that a portion of the blood that would normally leave the left heart with each heartbeat instead enters the right heart, and is pumped through the lungs before returning to the left heart again. Thus, in the presence of a left-to-right shunt, the stroke volume of the right heart is greater than that of the left, and the ratio between the two is a measure of the severity of shunting. The ratio is often referred to as Qp/Qs, where Qp is pulmonary blood flow and Qs is systemic blood flow. To calculate the shunt ratio:

- In the parasternal short-axis view (aortic valve level), measure the diameter of the right ventricular outflow tract (RVOT) in cm and then use this to calculate the cross-sectional area (CSA) of the RVOT in cm^2:

$$CSA_{RVOT} = 0.785 \times (RVOT\ Diameter)^2$$

- In the same view, measure the velocity time integral (VTI) of flow in the RVOT (using PW Doppler) to give VTI_{RVOT}, in cm.

- The stroke volume in the RVOT (SV_{RVOT}), in mL/beat, can then be calculated as follows:

$$SV_{RVOT} = CSA_{RVOT} \times VTI_{RVOT}$$

- In the parasternal long-axis view, measure the diameter of the LVOT in cm and then use this to calculate the CSA of the LVOT in cm^2:

$$CSA_{LVOT} = 0.785 \times (LVOT\ Diameter)^2$$

- In the apical five-chamber view, measure the VTI of flow in the LVOT (using PW Doppler) to give VTI_{LVOT}, in cm.

- The stroke volume in the LVOT (SV_{LVOT}), in mL/beat, can then be calculated as follows:

$$SV_{LVOT} = CSA_{LVOT} \times VTI_{LVOT}$$

The shunt ratio is the ratio of SV_{RVOT} to SV_{LVOT} which, in the presence of a left-to-right shunt, will be greater than 1. A significant limitation to shunt calculations is that they are heavily dependent on an accurate measurement of RVOT and LVOT diameter – as the calculation involves squaring these measurements, even a small inaccuracy in measurement can lead to a large error in the final result.

Echo assessment of atrial septal defect

The best transthoracic view of the interatrial septum is obtained from the **subcostal window**, although the septum can also be seen from the apical window (four-chamber view) and the parasternal window (short-axis view, at the aortic valve level). In each view, use 2D echo to assess the structure of the interatrial septum:

- Does the interatrial septum appear normal or is there any aneurysm formation (see box **Shunt Calculations**)?

- Is there any echo dropout in the septum to indicate a defect? In the apical view, it is not unusual to see areas of 'apparent' dropout in the interatrial septum, which is quite a long way from the probe, so be careful not to report dropout as an ASD unless you can also see it in other views and/or you also have further supporting evidence.

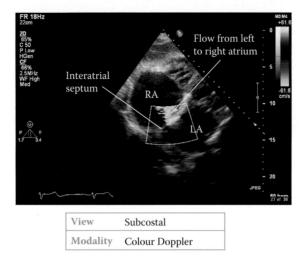

View	Subcostal
Modality	Colour Doppler

Figure 33.1   Secundum atrial septal defect. *Abbreviations:* LA: Left atrium, RA: Right atrium.

- Assess right atrial and ventricular size/function – Are they dilated as a consequence of a left-to-right shunt? Is there evidence of right heart volume overload (paradoxical motion of the inter-ventricular septum) and/or pulmonary hypertension?

Use colour Doppler to check for the presence of flow across the defect. Flow across an ASD is normally from left to right, mainly during diastole, and also in systole (**Figure 33.1**).

In the subcostal view, use pulsed-wave (PW) Doppler to assess flow across the defect.

If you identify an ASD, comment on its size and location (secundum, primum or sinus venosus), and be sure to check for any associated abnormalities (e.g., cleft anterior mitral valve leaflet). Check also for the presence of tricuspid and/or pulmonary regurgitation, and grade the likelihood of pulmonary hypertension (Chapter 26). Consider performing a shunt calculation to estimate the shunt ratio (see box Shunt Calculations), although be aware of the limitations of this – generally, RV volume overload is better than shunt ratio for gauging the haemodynamic relevance of an ASD.

If there is doubt about the presence of an ASD, it may be necessary to perform an 'agitated' saline contrast study as for patent foramen ovale (PFO). Although transthoracic echo (TTE) can often detect evidence of an ASD, transoesophageal echo (TOE) will usually be required to assess an ASD in detail (or to rule out an ASD if clinical suspicion remains after a normal TTE). Sinus venosus defects can be very difficult to visualize on TTE and usually require a TOE for diagnosis.

ATRIAL SEPTAL ANEURYSM

Atrial septal aneurysms are thought to have a prevalence of around 1%. They are defined as a bulge or deformation of the interatrial septum protruding at least 10 mm into the right or left atrium (or, if mobile, swinging by at least 10 mm from side to side) and with a diameter across their base of at least 15 mm. They have been reported to be associated with ASD and PFO (and also with mitral valve prolapse) and are also thought to be a potential cardiac source of emboli.

Management of atrial septal defect

An ASD can be closed percutaneously or surgically. Percutaneous closure is performed for secundum ASDs if there is an adequate rim of tissue around the defect to allow deployment of a septal occluder device without impinging on nearby structures. Surgical closure requires a thoracotomy to open one of the atria and suture a patch (made from Dacron or from the patient's own pericardium) over the defect.

Echo assessment following repair

Using the same views as for unrepaired ASD,

- comment on the presence of a septal occluder device or patch
- check for any residual shunt
- assess right heart size and function
- screen for evidence of pulmonary hypertension

ASD AND 3D ECHO

Three-dimensional echo can be helpful in the assessment of congenital heart disease and has been of particular value in assessing ASDs, providing information on the morphology of the interatrial septum and the surrounding structures. It has also been used to guide device closure.

PATENT FORAMEN OVALE

In utero, the foramen ovale is a flap-like structure that permits shunting of blood directly from the RA to the LA. The flap normally closes after birth, when LA pressure rises, and becomes sealed within 12 months. However, in around 25% of the general population, the foramen does not close completely and the resulting PFO is a potential conduit between right and left atria.

Clinical features of patent foramen ovale

In the majority of people, PFO causes no problems and no direct clinical findings, but in a small number, it can be a cause of stroke (allowing a clot to pass from the venous to the arterial side of the circulation – 'paradoxical embolism') and is also associated with decompression illness in scuba divers (paradoxical gas embolism). There is also a higher incidence of PFO among patients with migraines.

Echo assessment of patent foramen ovale

Echo assessment of PFO requires careful evaluation of the interatrial septum in multiple imaging views – usually the subcostal window affords the best view of the interatrial septum, as it is seen face on.

In each view, use colour Doppler to check for the presence of any flow across the interatrial septum. Asking the patient to perform and then release a Valsalva manoeuvre (deep breath in and 'bear down') can momentarily open up a PFO and reveal a brief jet of right-to-left flow.

It may be necessary to go on to perform an 'agitated' saline bubble contrast study (Chapter 10). Although TTE can sometimes detect a PFO, TOE offers greater sensitivity for PFO detection.

Management of patent foramen ovale

PFO is common and requires no treatment if it is an incidental finding. For patients who have had an embolic event as a result of paradoxical embolism, closure of a PFO may be considered. However, because PFOs are so common, closure is only recommended if there is a high probability that the PFO had a causal role in the event. Patients therefore need to be carefully selected for PFO closure, and a multidisciplinary team approach is advised.

Echo assessment following closure

Using the same views as for unrepaired PFO,

- comment on the presence of a septal occluder device or patch
- check for any residual shunt

VENTRICULAR SEPTAL DEFECT

The interventricular septum has two parts: the muscular septum and the thinner, fibrous membranous septum (which lies just below the aortic valve). A ventricular septal defect (VSD) permits flow directly between left and right ventricles, and it can be a congenital abnormality or can be acquired as a complication of myocardial infarction (p. 124).

VSDs can be categorized according to their location as follows:

- *Perimembranous VSD*: the commonest type, located in the membranous part of the septum below the aortic valve
- *Muscular VSD*: found in the muscular part of the septum. Muscular VSDs can be multiple ('Swiss cheese septum')
- *Inlet VSD*: also known as canal-type VSD, this is found immediately inferior to the atrioventricular valve apparatus and is associated with a common atrioventricular valve, typically in Down syndrome
- *Outlet VSD*: also known as supracristal, subpulmonary or doubly committed VSD, this type is uncommon, and lies just below the aortic and pulmonary valves. Outlet VSD is commonly associated with aortic regurgitation due to prolapse of the right coronary cusp of the aortic valve

A large VSD may present with heart failure in infancy; small VSDs are usually asymptomatic. VSDs cause a pansystolic murmur at the lower left sternal edge, and as a general rule, the smaller the defect, the louder the murmur. The shunting of blood causes left ventricular (LV) volume overload and the increased pulmonary flow can lead to pulmonary hypertension which can cause reversal of the shunt (see box **Eisenmenger Physiology**). Decisions on VSD closure can be complex and should take into account left ventricular volume overload, the degree of shunting and the presence of pulmonary hypertension, together with specific issues such as aortic regurgitation due to VSD-related cusp prolapse or recurrent infective endocarditis.

Echo assessment of ventricular septal defect

Inspect the interventricular septum in as many views as possible. Use 2D echo to assess the structure of the interventricular septum:

- Is there any echo dropout in the septum to indicate a defect? Describe the type of VSD according to its location (perimembranous, muscular, inlet or outlet). Assess whether multiple defects are present.
- Measure the size of the VSD.
- *Assess LV size and function* – Is there evidence of LV volume overload?

Use colour Doppler to check for the presence of flow across the interventricular septum into the RV (**Figure 33.2**). Look for aortic regurgitation with outlet and high perimembranous VSDs.

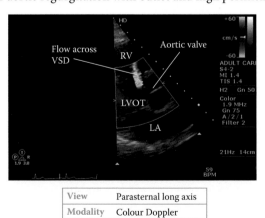

View	Parasternal long axis
Modality	Colour Doppler

Figure 33.2 Ventricular septal defect (VSD). *Abbreviations:* LA: Left atrium, LVOT: Left ventricular outflow tract, RV: Right ventricle.

In the subcostal view, use continuous wave (CW) and PW Doppler to assess flow across the defect. There is usually a high-velocity jet from left to right ventricle during systole, with lower-velocity flow during diastole.

If you identify a VSD, check for any associated abnormalities (e.g., aortic cusp prolapse, aortic regurgitation). Check also for the presence of tricuspid and/or pulmonary regurgitation and screen for pulmonary hypertension. Consider a shunt calculation to estimate the shunt ratio, while being aware of the limitations of such calculations.

Echo assessment following repair

Using the same views as for unrepaired VSD,

- comment on the presence of a septal patch
- check for any residual shunt
- check for aortic regurgitation (after closure of outflow VSD)
- assess LV size and function
- assess RV size and function
- screen for pulmonary hypertension

PERSISTENT DUCTUS ARTERIOSUS

Persistent ductus arteriosus (PDA) is also sometimes referred to as *patent* ductus arteriosus. In the fetus, the ductus arteriosus acts as a shunt connecting the pulmonary artery (at the junction of the main and left pulmonary arteries) to the aortic arch (just after the origin of the left subclavian artery). This allows most (90%) of the blood pumped by the RV to reach the systemic circulation directly, bypassing the lungs. The ductus arteriosus normally starts to close immediately after birth, and is normally fully closed within a few days, leaving behind just a cord-like remnant (the ligamentum arteriosum).

Failure of the ductus arteriosus to close means that a left-to-right shunt persists between the aortic arch and the pulmonary artery, with blood flow from the high-pressure aorta to the lower-pressure pulmonary artery. This can lead to LV volume overload and/or pulmonary hypertension (with RV pressure overload), either of which can predominate.

Clinical features of persistent ductus arteriosus

Adults with PDA can be asymptomatic if the PDA is small. Moderate PDAs can present with clinical features of either predominant LV volume overload or predominant pulmonary hypertension (with RV pressure overload). Large PDAs can lead to Eisenmenger physiology with shunt reversal and differential (lower extremity) cyanosis.

Echo assessment of persistent ductus arteriosus

With the echo probe in the **suprasternal window**, obtain an aorta view to visualize the PDA as it arises from the aortic arch.

Use colour Doppler to assess flow in the aorta, looking in particular for evidence of a PDA arising just beyond the origin of the left subclavian artery.

Next, move the probe to the left parasternal window and tilt the probe to obtain a **parasternal RVOT view**, or rotate it to obtain a **parasternal short-axis view at the aortic valve level**.

In either of these views, use colour Doppler to assess flow in the pulmonary artery, looking in particular for evidence of blood flow into the pulmonary artery via a PDA (**Figure 33.3**).

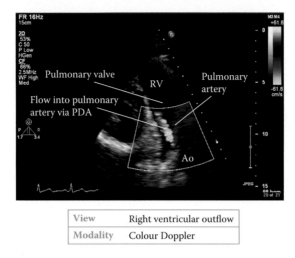

View	Right ventricular outflow
Modality	Colour Doppler

Figure 33.3 Persistent ductus arteriosus (PDA). *Abbreviations:* Ao: Aorta, RV: Right ventricle.

Look carefully for any knock-on effects of the shunt on the rest of the heart, such as the development of LV volume overload, pulmonary hypertension and RV pressure overload.

Management of persistent ductus arteriosus

Premature neonates with PDA can be treated with prostaglandin inhibitors (e.g., intravenous indometacin). Invasive techniques to close the PDA include the use of percutaneous closure devices or surgical ligation.

The presence of a PDA can sometimes be advantageous, for example in transposition of the great vessels (when it allows oxygenated blood to reach the systemic circulation), and under these circumstances, the PDA can be kept open by giving prostaglandins.

Echo assessment following repair

Using the same views as for unrepaired PDA,

- check for any residual shunt
- assess LV size and function
- assess RV size and function
- screen for pulmonary hypertension

EISENMENGER PHYSIOLOGY

The presence of a left-to-right shunt (such as an ASD, VSD or PDA) allows blood to pass directly from the left side of the circulation to the right side, increasing the volume of blood flowing through the pulmonary circulation. This leads to an increased pressure within the pulmonary vessels (pulmonary hypertension) and, over time, the vessels develop an increasing resistance to blood flow. This leads to pressure overload on the right heart and the development of right ventricular hypertrophy. Gradually, the right-sided pressures rise and begin to equal and then exceed the pressures found in the left heart. As this occurs, the left-to-right shunt reverses, causing blood to start shunting from right to left instead. At this point, the patient is said to have developed Eisenmenger physiology. This means that a portion of the venous (deoxygenated) blood entering the right heart starts crossing directly into the left heart or arterial circulation, bypassing the lungs, and reducing the overall oxygen content in the arterial circulation. Clinically, the patient develops cyanosis, a blue discoloration of the skin and tongue, together with breathlessness and a fall in exercise capacity.

BICUSPID AORTIC VALVE

A bicuspid aortic valve has two functioning cusps, usually of unequal size, with just a single line of coaptation. Pseudobicuspid valves have three cusps, but fusion of two of the cusps ('functionally' bicuspid). There is a strong association with coarctation of the aorta (CoA, p. 271), a bicuspid aortic valve being present in at least 50% of cases.

The prevalence of bicuspid aortic valve is 1%–2% of the population, and it is thought to be responsible for around half of the cases of severe aortic stenosis in adults. It is the commonest congenital aortic valve abnormality. The stenotic process is similar to that seen in calcific degeneration, but occurs at a younger age. Fibrosis typically starts in a patient's teens, with gradual calcification from their 30s onwards. Patients who require surgery for stenosis of a bicuspid aortic valve do so on average 5 years earlier than those with calcific degeneration of a tricuspid aortic valve.

Bicuspid aortic valve is often asymptomatic, but with the onset of valve dysfunction patients may develop clinical features of aortic stenosis or regurgitation. Patients are also at significant risk of aortic root dilatation (up to 80% of patients will develop ascending aortic dilatation) and infective endocarditis. Clinical examination often reveals a systolic ejection click, and features of aortic stenosis or regurgitation may be present.

Once a bicuspid aortic valve has been diagnosed, serial follow-up echo is required to monitor for the onset of aortic valve dysfunction and/or aortic root dilatation, which should be managed as appropriate.

Echo assessment of bicuspid aortic valve

In the parasternal long- and short-axis (at the aortic valve level) views, use 2D echo to

- assess the appearances and dimensions of the aortic valve (**Figure 33.4**). Fibrosis and calcification of a bicuspid aortic valve can distort the valve, making recognition of its bicuspid nature difficult on echocardiography
- look for evidence of cusp fusion (pseudobicuspid valve) – the line where the cusps are fused is called a raphe. Describe which cusps are fused
- look at the closure line of the aortic valve in the parasternal long-axis view – M-mode imaging is best for this. A bicuspid valve will usually have an eccentric closure line (i.e., no longer in the middle of the aortic annulus)
- assess aortic root dimensions

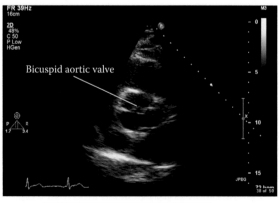

View	Parasternal short axis (aortic valve level)
Modality	2D

Figure 33.4   Bicuspid aortic valve.

Use colour Doppler to look for evidence of aortic regurgitation.

Use CW and PW Doppler to assess flow through the aortic valve and assess the severity of any aortic stenosis or regurgitation (Chapter 20).

Perform a complete echo study, looking in particular for evidence of associated CoA.

SUBVALVAR AND SUPRAVALVAR AORTIC STENOSIS

The echo assessment of aortic stenosis is discussed in Chapter 20, p. 139.

Coarctation of the aorta

CoA is a narrowing of the aorta that most commonly occurs just distal to the origin of the left subclavian artery, at the insertion of the ductus arteriosus. The narrowing can be discrete or can extend over a long hypoplastic segment. It occurs in 1 in 3000 live births (more commonly in males). There is more to CoA than just a narrowing of the aorta however, and the condition should be considered to be part of a more generalized arteriopathy.

Clinical features of coarctation of the aorta

Children with CoA may present with heart failure or problems resulting from reduced arterial perfusion to the lower half of the body. Adults with CoA are often asymptomatic and the diagnosis is made during assessment of hypertension or as an incidental finding (**Table 33.2**). Patients may have the clinical features of an associated condition such as bicuspid aortic valve or Turner syndrome. It is also associated with subvalvar, valvular and supravalvar aortic stenosis and with parachute mitral valve.

Echo assessment of coarctation of the aorta

With the echo probe in the **suprasternal window**, obtain an aorta view to visualize the aortic arch:

- use 2D echo to assess the appearances and dimensions of the aortic arch. CoA is seen most commonly just distal to the origin of the left subclavian artery. There may be dilatation of the aorta on either side of the coarctation
- use colour Doppler to assess flow in the aorta, looking in particular for evidence of high-velocity or turbulent flow in the region of a suspected CoA
- use CW Doppler to assess flow in the descending aorta, looking for evidence of increased flow velocity through the CoA. However, be aware that high flow velocities measured with CW Doppler are *not* a reliable guide to CoA severity. A better guide is the presence of sustained anterograde diastolic flow in the aorta (diastolic 'tail' or 'run-off'), the presence of which suggests a significant coarctation (**Figure 33.5**)

Perform a complete echo study to look carefully for any other abnormalities that can be associated with, or result from, CoA, including

- bicuspid aortic valve (present in up to 85% of cases)
- subvalvar or supravalvar aortic stenosis
- VSD
- LV hypertrophy (LVH) or dysfunction (as a consequence of hypertension)

Table 33.2   Clinical features of coarctation of the aorta

Symptoms	Signs
Often asymptomatic	Hypertension
Headache	Systolic murmur
Abdominal angina	Weak femoral pulse
Claudication/cold feet	Radio-femoral delay (femoral pulse occurs after radial)

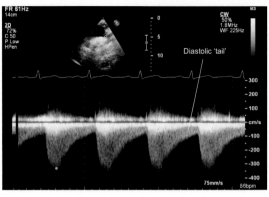

View	Suprasternal
Modality	CW Doppler

Figure 33.5 Coarctation of the aorta – continuous wave (CW) Doppler study from suprasternal window showing diastolic 'tail' and a peak velocity of 3.5 m/s in the descending thoracic aorta.

Management of coarctation of the aorta

CoA can be managed by surgical excision of the area of coarctation (followed either by end-to-end anastomosis of the aorta or with the use of a graft to bridge the resulting gap). It can also be managed percutaneously by stenting of the coarctation.

Echo assessment following repair

Following correction, patients with CoA require lifelong follow-up with annual echo studies. Using the same views as for unrepaired CoA,

- measure any residual gradient
- check for the development of any dilatation of the aorta

In addition,

- assess any LVH (patients may remain hypertensive)
- assess any associated abnormalities such as bicuspid aortic valve

Recoarctation is commoner in those who underwent repair as a neonate (recoarctation incidence 2.4%–5.5%) than later in life (incidence <1%). It can be challenging to assess recoarctation (and residual coarctation) using echo, as the repaired area can be difficult to visualize and Doppler gradients tend to be overestimated. As described above, look for sustained anterograde diastolic flow in the aorta as an indicator of a significant recoarctation.

SUBVALVAR, VALVAR AND SUPRAVALVAR PULMONARY STENOSIS

The echo assessment of pulmonary stenosis is discussed in Chapter 25, p. 195.

EBSTEIN'S ANOMALY

In Ebstein's anomaly, the tricuspid valve (specifically the septal and posterior leaflets) is displaced towards the RV apex. As a result, part of the RV becomes 'atrialized' – although it becomes part of the RA, it still contracts with the RV, which impairs the haemodynamic function of the right heart and tends to exacerbate the tricuspid regurgitation that is usually present (and ranges in severity from mild to severe). There are several associated conditions:

- secundum ASD or PFO
- accessory pathways in the conduction system

When Ebstein's anomaly presents in adult life, it can be with

- breathlessness and fatigue
- tricuspid regurgitation
- right heart failure
- cyanosis
- palpitations

Echo assessment of Ebstein's anomaly

The tricuspid valve can be studied in

- Left parasternal window
  - parasternal right ventricular inflow view
  - parasternal short-axis view
- Apical window
  - apical four-chamber view
  - subcostal window
  - subcostal long-axis view

2D

Use 2D echo to assess the structure of the tricuspid valve:

- Is the tricuspid valve position normal or is it displaced apically? In Ebstein's anomaly, the septal or posterior tricuspid leaflet is displaced towards the RV apex by at least 0.8 cm/m^2 (in adults, the displacement should be indexed for body surface area), in comparison with the mitral valve plane.
- Are the tricuspid valve leaflets morphologically normal or abnormal? Do the leaflets coapt normally or eccentrically?
- Is the RA dilated?
- Is the RV dilated? Is RV function impaired?

Colour Doppler

Use colour Doppler to

- assess the severity of tricuspid regurgitation
- look for shunts (see the 'Associated Features' section)

CW and PW Doppler

Use CW Doppler to obtain a trace of regurgitant flow through the tricuspid valve. Obtain traces from the apex and from at least one other position, such as the parasternal short-axis or RV inflow views. Assess the severity of tricuspid regurgitation and screen for pulmonary hypertension.

Associated features

A number of conditions can be associated with Ebstein's anomaly, so perform a complete echo study to look for them:

- ASD
- PFO (as a consequence of RA dilatation)
- VSD
- pulmonary stenosis

Management of Ebstein's anomaly

The management of Ebstein's anomaly includes the treatment of any RV failure and arrhythmias. Surgical options include tricuspid valve repair (or sometimes replacement), resection of the atrialized portion of the RV and correction of any shunts.

TETRALOGY OF FALLOT

Tetralogy of Fallot (ToF) accounts for 3.5% of cases of congenital heart disease and, as the word 'tetralogy' suggests, consists of four key abnormalities (**Figure 33.6**):

- VSD
- Overriding aorta
- RVOT obstruction
- RV hypertrophy

The RVOT obstruction can be due to narrowing of

- the muscular part (infundibulum) of the RVOT that leads into the pulmonary artery
- the pulmonary valve itself (where there can be a degree of cusp tethering)
- the supravalvular region
- the branch pulmonary arteries

RV hypertrophy develops in response to the pressure overload that results from the RVOT obstruction.

In some cases, ToF may be diagnosed in utero with fetal ultrasound scanning. After birth, the clinical severity depends primarily upon how severe the RVOT obstruction is. Neonates may present with failure to thrive and/or cyanosis, although cyanotic episodes may not appear until later. The clinical features include a harsh ejection systolic murmur in the pulmonary area, cyanosis and clubbing.

Management and echo follow-up in tetralogy of Fallot

It's very rare to see adults with untreated ToF, as fewer than 10% of patients with untreated ToF survive to the age of 20 years. As a result, almost all the adults seen with a history of ToF will have

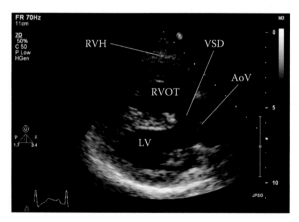

View	Parasternal long axis
Modality	2D

Figure 33.6 Tetralogy of Fallot. *Abbreviations:* AoV: Aortic valve, LV: Left ventricle, RVH: Right ventricular hypertrophy, RVOT: Right ventricular outflow tract, VSD: Ventricular septal defect.

undergone surgical correction. ToF is usually treated with primary repair (closing the VSD and relieving the RVOT obstruction) before the age of 1 year. However, where necessary, it is possible to perform a modified Blalock–Taussig shunt procedure (placing a graft between the subclavian artery and the pulmonary artery) as a palliative measure – this does not fully correct the ToF, but it does increase blood flow to the pulmonary circulation.

Following primary ToF repair in childhood, survival at 30 years is over 90%. As a result, there are now many adults with previous ToF repair who need follow-up. The key problems to assess during echo follow-up include

- pulmonary regurgitation
- severity of any residual RVOT obstruction
- any shunting across a residual VSD
- RV dysfunction (from residual PR and/or RVOT obstruction)
- tricuspid regurgitation (from RV dilatation)
- LV dysfunction (from arterial shunts and/or residual VSD)
- infective endocarditis
- aortic regurgitation and aortic dilatation (mechanisms uncertain)

Pulmonary regurgitation is common following repair and this can lead to RV dilatation and dysfunction (and a risk of ventricular tachycardia). It is therefore important to assess the degree of any pulmonary regurgitation, in addition to assessing the impact of this on RV dimensions and function (Chapter 22). Quantify any residual RVOT obstruction with Doppler studies. Use colour Doppler to detect any shunting across a residual VSD and then go on to assess the degree of shunting.

Note that although echo plays an important role in follow-up after ToF repair, cardiac magnetic resonance imaging can provide more detailed information about residual right heart abnormalities.

Further reading

Baumgartner H et al. 2020 ESC guidelines for the management of adult congenital heart disease. *European Heart Journal* (2021). PMID 32860028.

Pristipino C et al. European position paper on the management of patients with patent foramen ovale. General approach and left circulation thromboembolism. *European Heart Journal* (2019). PMID 30358849.

Simpson J et al. Three-dimensional echocardiography in congenital heart disease: an expert consensus document from the European Association of Cardiovascular Imaging and the American Society of Echocardiography. *Journal of the American Society of Echocardiography* (2017). PMID 27838227.

Stout KK et al. 2018 AHA/ACC guideline for the management of adults with congenital heart disease: a report of the American College of Cardiology/American Heart Association task force on clinical practice guidelines. *Journal of the American College of Cardiology* (2019). PMID 30121240.

CHAPTER 34

Common echo requests

A number of echo requests crop up commonly, such as 'Breathlessness? cause' and 'Stroke? cardiac source of emboli'. This chapter considers some of the requests you will see most often and discusses the key points that you need to consider in each case.

BREATHLESSNESS

Breathlessness is a common symptom that has a multitude of possible causes. In many cases, the clinician will want the sonographer to look for evidence of heart failure (systolic or diastolic), but it is important to be alert to a broad range of possible diagnoses as you perform the echo study. Even if you do find evidence of left ventricular (LV) dysfunction, remember that an individual patient can have more than one contributing factor for their symptoms. Common causes of breathlessness are listed below:

- Heart failure
  - measure left and right ventricular dimensions
  - assess left and right ventricular systolic function
  - check for LV diastolic dysfunction
  - describe any regional wall motion abnormalities
  - check for associated valvular disease
- Valvular disease
  - assess valvular structure and function
  - assess chamber dimensions and function
  - screen for pulmonary hypertension
- Ischaemic heart disease
  - are there any regional wall motion abnormalities?
  - consider stress echo
- Lung disease
  - assess right ventricular (RV) dimensions and function
  - screen for pulmonary hypertension
  - is there any evidence of pulmonary embolism?

Remain alert to non-cardiac causes of breathlessness that might nonetheless be detected on echo, such as a pleural effusion (**Figure 30.3**, p. 237).

DOI: 10.1201/9781003304654-34

ARRHYTHMIAS

Echo is frequently requested in patients with arrhythmias to check for associated structural heart disease. Although the heart will often prove to be structurally normal, it is nonetheless important to perform a full echo study as there are several possible abnormalities that may be found. It is helpful to have as much detail as possible about the nature of the arrhythmia to help guide the echo study. An echo is part of the assessment of patients with sustained (or non-sustained) supraventricular or ventricular tachyarrhythmias. It is not usually helpful in those with isolated supraventricular or ventricular ectopic beats, in the absence of any other features.

Atrial fibrillation

Atrial fibrillation (AF) is the commonest sustained arrhythmia, affecting 0.5% of the adult population (and 10% of those aged over 75 years). Many conditions can cause AF (**Table 34.1**), and an echo may reveal evidence of these, in particular

- ischaemic heart disease
- valvular heart disease
- cardiomyopathy
- LV hypertrophy (LVH) in hypertension
- right heart abnormalities in pulmonary disease or pulmonary embolism

Long-standing AF leads to dilatation of the left and right atria (**Figure 34.1**), but be sure to check for other causes of atrial enlargement, such as mitral/tricuspid valve disease or restrictive cardiomyopathy. Atrial enlargement indicates a lower success rate for cardioversion (see below).

Table 34.1   Causes of atrial fibrillation

Ischaemic heart disease	Pulmonary disease
Valvular heart disease	Pulmonary embolism
Hypertension	Pneumonia
Cardiomyopathy	Pericarditis
Myocarditis	'Lone' atrial fibrillation (no identified cause)
Alcohol	
Thyrotoxicosis	

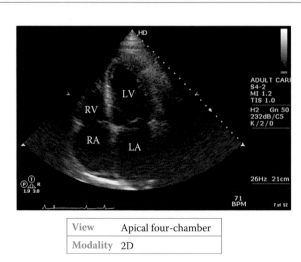

View	Apical four-chamber
Modality	2D

Figure 34.1   Dilated atria in long-standing atrial fibrillation. *Abbreviations:* LA: Left atrium, LV: Left ventricle, RA: Right atrium, RV: Right ventricle.

AF is a risk factor for embolic stroke and patients at high risk should be considered for anticoagulation with warfarin. Echo can identify indicators of increased stroke risk, including the presence of valve disease or impaired LV function (clinical indicators include age, sex, heart failure, previous stroke/transient ischaemic attack (TIA) or peripheral embolic events, hypertension, diabetes or vascular disease).

Cardioversion of persistent AF back to sinus rhythm should be considered in patients where the procedure is likely to succeed (and sinus rhythm maintained in the longer term). The presence of structural heart disease on echo (such as dilated atria) suggests a lower likelihood of successful cardioversion.

If cardioversion is going to be undertaken for a patient who has been in AF for longer than 48 hours, it is important to minimize the risk of embolism either by arranging therapeutic anticoagulation for at least 3 weeks prior to the cardioversion or by performing a transoesophageal echo (TOE) to rule out intracardiac thrombus – this is called TOE-guided cardioversion.

Ventricular arrhythmias

Ventricular tachycardia and/or fibrillation commonly result from underlying structural heart disease. Echo is therefore part of the assessment of patients who have had, or are regarded as being at high risk of, ventricular arrhythmias, looking in particular for evidence of

- myocardial infarction/ischaemia
- cardiomyopathy (e.g., hypertrophic cardiomyopathy, dilated cardiomyopathy, arrhythmogenic RV cardiomyopathy)

A full assessment of both LV and RV dimensions, morphology and function is required. If myocardial ischaemia is suspected, a stress echo study may be required (Chapter 9).

One treatment option for patients at risk of ventricular arrhythmias is an implantable cardioverter defibrillator (ICD) device, and the accurate measurement of LV ejection fraction plays a key role in identifying patients most likely to benefit from ICD implantation.

EJECTION SYSTOLIC MURMUR

An ejection systolic murmur begins after the first heart sound, rises in intensity to reach a peak during systole and then falls in intensity to end before the second heart sound (**Figure 34.2**). The murmur is also described as 'diamond-shaped' or 'crescendo-decrescendo'.

Causes of an ejection systolic murmur include

- aortic stenosis
- bicuspid aortic valve
- hypertrophic obstructive cardiomyopathy
- pulmonary stenosis

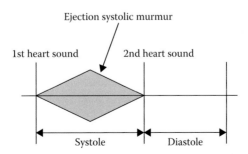

Figure 34.2   Ejection systolic murmur.

Remember that aortic and pulmonary stenosis can occur not just at the valve but also with obstruction to outflow at a subvalvular or supravalvular level.

'Ejection systolic murmur? cause' is a common echo request and must include a search for all these structural abnormalities. If no structural heart disease is found, the murmur is likely to be a result of increased flow across a normal aortic or pulmonary valve, as seen in hyperdynamic flow states (e.g., exercise, anaemia, pregnancy, thyrotoxicosis).

HYPERTENSION

Hypertension is a major risk factor for cardiovascular disease. In 95% of cases, hypertension is idiopathic, but in 5% there is an identifiable underlying cause such as renal disease, metabolic/endocrine abnormalities or coarctation of the aorta.

Echo assessment is appropriate for patients with suspected hypertensive heart disease, but not as a routine screening tool in uncomplicated hypertension. When performing an echo in hypertension, look for coarctation of the aorta (Chapter 33) and for end-organ damage as a consequence of the hypertension:

- LVH and diastolic dysfunction
- LV dilatation and systolic dysfunction
- aortic root dilatation and aortic regurgitation

COLLAGEN ABNORMALITIES

Marfan syndrome is a genetic condition with an autosomal dominant pattern of inheritance (although in a quarter of cases there is no family history, i.e., a new mutation) and an incidence of 2–3 per 10,000 population. Patients with Marfan syndrome have an abnormality of fibrillin, a constituent of connective tissue, and this can cause abnormalities affecting the musculoskeletal and cardiovascular systems, and also the skin and eyes.

The diagnosis of Marfan syndrome is based on the revised Ghent nosology, which incorporates a multifactorial scoring system. Cardiovascular criteria include

- aortic root dilatation
- dissection of the ascending aorta
- mitral valve prolapse

Echo therefore plays an important role in the diagnosis of Marfan syndrome. It is also essential in follow-up; patients with Marfan syndrome require regular echo monitoring with particular attention to the aortic root, measured at the level of the aortic annulus, the sinuses of Valsalva (which is where dilatation usually begins), the sinotubular junction and the ascending aorta (proximal, mid and distal).

Also measure the aorta at the arch, in the descending thoracic aorta and in the abdominal aorta (at or above the level of the superior mesenteric artery). Make measurements from inner edge to inner edge, taking the widest diameter at each level, as described in Chapter 31.

The echo study in Marfan syndrome also includes:

- inspection of the morphology of the sinotubular junction
- inspection of the mitral valve for prolapse, calcification and regurgitation
- measurement of pulmonary artery diameter

It is recommended that an echo be performed at the time of diagnosis of Marfan syndrome, and 6 months later, to assess aortic root dimensions and the rate of progression of any dilatation. For follow-up studies, it is important to ensure that the measurements are reproducible and therefore can be compared from one study to the next. Longer-term echo follow-up should occur at least annually in adults (and every 6–12 months in children) if the aortic dimensions are stable, or more frequently, if the maximum aortic diameter is ≥4.5 cm or there is a significant increase in size compared to baseline.

The risk of aortic dissection is related to the aortic diameter, and the risk of rupture is particularly high if the aortic root diameter exceeds 5.5 cm. Treatment with beta-blockers should be considered if any degree of aortic dilatation is present, and surgical referral should be made if the aortic root diameter is ≥5.0 cm, or considered at a threshold of 4.5 cm if additional risk factors are present, including

- family history of aortic dissection
- rate of increase >3 mm/year
- severe aortic regurgitation
- planning for pregnancy

For details on the risks of pregnancy in Marfan syndrome, see below.

Ehlers–Danlos syndrome is a group of genetic disorders, classified into six subgroups, characterized by collagen abnormalities. Some patients develop mitral valve prolapse and echo assessment is important if this is suspected. Patients with the Ehlers–Danlos vascular subtype (type IV) are prone to develop arterial aneurysms that can include the aorta, and a screening echo to assess the aortic root and arch is appropriate.

RENAL FAILURE

The echo assessment of patients with chronic renal failure includes a full assessment of LV dimensions and systolic and diastolic function. Hypertension is common in chronic renal failure and may be associated with LVH. Both systolic and diastolic dysfunction may be impaired.

Amyloidosis refers to a group of conditions in which amyloid protein builds up in tissues, including the kidney and the heart. Patients with amyloid-related renal failure may therefore show signs of cardiac amyloid on echo (p. 232).

Mitral annular calcification is a frequent finding in chronic renal failure, and its presence is associated with a poor prognosis. It is recognized as a calcified (echodense) area at the junction of the posterior mitral valve leaflet and atrioventricular groove (**Figure 34.3**).

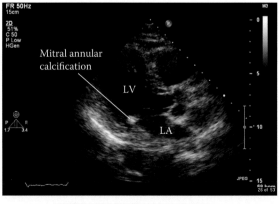

View	Parasternal long axis
Modality	2D

Figure 34.3   Mitral annular calcification. *Abbreviations:* LA: Left atrium, LV: Left ventricle.

Uraemia is a consequence of renal failure and can cause uraemic pericarditis, in which pericardial effusion (and possibly cardiac tamponade) may occur.

Coronary artery disease (CAD) is the commonest cause of death in patients with chronic renal failure, and its detection (and treatment) prior to renal transplantation is important. Dobutamine stress echo (DSE; Chapter 9) has proven a valuable technique for detecting CAD in these patients (and is superior to exercise treadmill testing). It also provides information on prognosis – the greater the extent of myocardial ischaemia (percentage of ischaemic segments) during DSE, the greater the risk of premature death.

STROKE

Cardiac emboli account for 15%–40% of embolic strokes. In patients who have had a TIA, embolic stroke or peripheral arterial embolism, an echo is commonly requested to check whether there is a cardiac source of emboli. However, the yield of such studies tends to be low, particularly in the absence of any other features in the history, examination or ECG that point towards a cardiac abnormality. The use of echo to assess for an embolic source varies from centre to centre, but a transthoracic echo (TTE) is often requested in patients who are younger than 50 years of age or if clinical evaluation is suggestive of an underlying cardiac abnormality. The diagnostic yield of transoesophageal echo (TOE) is better than that of TTE, and TOE is often considered in younger patients (<50 years), or if there is ongoing clinical suspicion of a cardiac source of emboli after a normal TTE, or if an abnormality found on TTE requires more detailed evaluation.

Echo may identify a direct source of emboli:

- LV thrombus
- LA thrombus (especially LA appendage)
- Left heart tumour (e.g., myxoma)
- infective endocarditis
- aortic atheroma

Alternatively, echo may find a condition associated with an increased risk of emboli:

- atrial septal aneurysm
- patent foramen ovale/atrial septal defect (paradoxical embolism)
- ventricular septal defect (with pulmonary hypertension)
- acute myocardial infarction
- dilated cardiomyopathy
- mitral stenosis
- replacement heart valve

One of the commonest cardiac causes of emboli is AF. Although this is diagnosed with an ECG rather than an echo, an echo is nonetheless important in the assessment of patients with this condition (see above).

PREGNANCY

Echo provides a safe and effective means of assessing the heart during pregnancy. Pregnant patients may require an echo to assess known pre-existing cardiac problems (maternal cardiac disease is seen in 2% of pregnancies, of which adult congenital heart disease is the commonest), or as a diagnostic investigation in the case of new symptoms (e.g., breathlessness) or signs (e.g., murmurs). It is important to be aware of the normal cardiovascular changes in pregnancy and the effect that these changes can have on those with prior cardiac conditions.

During a normal pregnancy, cardiac output increases by around 40%, because of a rise in both heart rate and stroke volume, reaching a peak towards the end of the second trimester. Cardiac output then remains on a plateau until the time of delivery, at which point there is a further increase (due to an increase in venous return to the heart, relief of pressure on the inferior vena cava and the return of blood from the contracted uterus to the circulation) before gradually returning to normal over the next 2 weeks (although this can sometimes take longer).

The 'volume overload' of pregnancy leads to an increase in LV end-diastolic volume (which may be detectable by 10 weeks' gestation) and also an increase in LV mass. There is also an increase in the dimensions of the right ventricle and of both atria. Valvular annular dimensions increase, and it is common to see tricuspid and pulmonary regurgitation. Despite the volume overload, cardiac filling pressures remain largely unchanged during pregnancy as the normal heart usually adapts well to the hypervolaemic state.

Afterload falls in line with a fall in systemic vascular resistance, which is at its lowest around the end of the second trimester before increasing again during the third trimester. Preload depends upon maternal position, falling when the mother is supine (as the inferior vena cava is compressed by the uterus and venous return is reduced). The effects of vena caval compression are more marked in twin pregnancies. To mitigate the effects of venal caval compression, it is usually better to perform echo with the mother in the left lateral decubitus position rather than supine. LV ejection fraction is influenced by preload and afterload conditions, and overall there is no significant change.

Average systolic strain rate remains unchanged during pregnancy, as do the peak myocardial systolic velocity and E/E' ratio. Right ventricular systolic pressure also remains unchanged.

Pre-existing dilated cardiomyopathy is poorly tolerated during pregnancy, with a high maternal mortality rate, particularly if the patient has an LV ejection fraction <30%. A cardiomyopathy can also develop as a consequence of pregnancy (**peripartum cardiomyopathy**, defined as an ejection fraction <45% occurring in the last months of pregnancy or within 5 months of delivery). The left ventricle is usually dilated (although not always), and left ventricular thrombus may be present. The right ventricle may also show evidence of dilatation and impairment, and significant mitral and tricuspid regurgitation can occur. Although fetal outcome is generally good, maternal mortality can be high.

Following delivery, LV function returns to normal in a quarter to a half of patients. Patients with an LV end-diastolic diameter >60 mm or an LV ejection fraction <30% have a poor likelihood of normalization of LV function. However, even if LV function does normalize, there is always a risk of recurrence in future pregnancies. For all patients, it is important to assess the risk of recurrence – persistently abnormal LV function 1 year after pregnancy predicts a high (20%) risk of mortality in a subsequent pregnancy.

'Innocent' flow-related heart murmurs are common in pregnancy, and they are a frequent reason for echo referrals. However, not all murmurs in pregnancy are benign, and structural valvular disease must be identified and assessed carefully. Obstructive cardiac lesions such as mitral stenosis and aortic stenosis (and also hypertrophic obstructive cardiomyopathy) can be very poorly tolerated and require careful clinical and echo assessment.

Patients with Marfan syndrome (see above) have a 1% risk of aortic dissection during pregnancy, even if the aortic dimensions are initially normal. This risk is much higher if the aortic root is dilated >4.0 cm (or is rapidly dilating), or if there is cardiac involvement or a poor family history. Monthly clinical assessment and echo are appropriate, with the full involvement of a multidisciplinary specialist team (particularly at the time of delivery). Beta-blockers should be continued throughout pregnancy. For women with Marfan syndrome who are contemplating pregnancy, prophylactic replacement of the aortic root and ascending aorta can be considered if the diameter is >4.0 cm.

Patients with pre-existing congenital heart disease should receive appropriate assessment and counselling before planning a pregnancy. Some conditions are very high risk – patients with

Eisenmenger syndrome, for example, have a maternal mortality of around 40% and are advised to avoid pregnancy (and indeed pulmonary hypertension, whatever the cause, generally presents a high risk in pregnancy). A detailed discussion of the risks of pregnancy in different congenital heart problems is beyond the scope of this book, but helpful guidance is available (see the 'Further Reading' section).

CARDIO-ONCOLOGY

Echo has an important role to play in cardio-oncology, the provision of cardiovascular care for patients with cancer. Cancer therapy-related cardiac dysfunction (CTRCD) is a commonly encountered problem, particularly in patients receiving anthracyclines (e.g., doxorubicin, epirubicin) and/or trastuzumab (Herceptin), drugs that are potentially cardiotoxic and can affect LV function.

These patients require accurate assessment of LV systolic function at baseline and at appropriate intervals during and after treatment, including an assessment, wherever possible, of LVEF using both 2D and 3D echo, together with the global longitudinal strain (GLS, Chapter 12) and right ventricular assessment (Chapter 22). Contrast echocardiography may be required when endocardial border definition is suboptimal for the accurate assessment of LVEF (e.g., when a minimum of two contiguous LV segments from any apical view cannot be reliably assessed).

The British Society of Echocardiography's definition of cardiotoxicity is a decline in LVEF by >10% (absolute percentage points) to an LVEF <50%. Probable subclinical cardiotoxicity is defined by a decline in LVEF by >10% (absolute percentage points) to an LVEF ≥50% with an accompanying fall in GLS >15% (where measured). Possible subclinical cardiotoxicity is defined by a decline in LVEF by <10% (absolute percentage points) to an LVEF <50%, or by a relative reduction in GLS >15% from the baseline value.

Treatment-related factors that indicate an increased risk of cardiotoxicity include

- increased lifetime dose of anthracycline:
  - >Doxorubicin 250 mg/m^2 or equivalent = high risk
  - >Doxorubicin 400 mg/m^2 or equivalent = very high risk
- prior anthracycline/trastuzumab-related cardiotoxicity
- sequential anthracycline and trastuzumab therapy
- high-dose radiotherapy to central chest, including the heart in the radiation field ≥30 Gy

Patient-related factors that indicate an increased risk of cardiotoxicity include

- female sex
- age:
  - 50–64 years = high risk
  - ≥65 years = highest risk
- presence of hypertension, smoking, obesity, dyslipidaemia, insulin resistance
- reduced or borderline low LVEF prior to treatment
- pre-existing cardiovascular disease (e.g., coronary artery disease, peripheral arterial disease, cardiomyopathy, heart failure, severe valvular disease, diabetes)
- chronic kidney disease (stage 2+)
- elevated troponin and/or NT-pro-BNP at baseline or during treatment

Assessment of risk helps to inform decisions about the frequency of echo surveillance and the need to involve a cardio-oncology team in the patient's care.

ECHO IN CRITICAL CARE

Echo (both TTE and TOE) can be an invaluable tool in the assessment of many conditions commonly encountered in the intensive care unit (ICU) setting. A number of 'focused' echo protocols, aimed at answering key questions in the critically ill, have been developed over recent years, including

- FEEL (Focused Echo in Emergency Life Support), which uses the parasternal long-axis, parasternal short-axis, apical four-chamber and subcostal views to identify potentially treatable problems in the cardiac arrest/peri-arrest setting
- FATE (Focused Assessed Transthoracic Echo), which uses the parasternal long-axis, parasternal short-axis, apical four-chamber and subcostal views (together with a pleural assessment) to assess critically ill patients in the ICU setting
- FAST (Focused Assessed Sonography in Trauma), which uses a subcostal view (to exclude cardiac tamponade) together with abdominal and pelvic views in trauma patients

TTE can prove challenging on the intensive care unit, as patients may have had recent chest surgery or have sustained chest trauma. In ventilated patients, lung inflation and the use of positive end-expiratory pressure (PEEP) can interfere with transthoracic imaging. It may be possible to reduce PEEP (if clinically safe to do so) during the TTE study, but TOE may be preferable in these situations.

In the **hypotensive patient**, echo helps to distinguish between cardiac and non-cardiac causes of hypotension. Echo will help identify left or right ventricular dysfunction (and may show an ischaemic aetiology), valvular dysfunction, ventricular septal rupture following acute myocardial infarction, obstructive cardiac lesions (valvular stenosis and hypertrophic obstructive cardiomyopathy), acute pulmonary embolism, aortic dissection or cardiac tamponade.

Besides cardiac causes, hypotension may also result from **hypovolaemia**, as seen in acute haemorrhage. Echo reveals a small (underfilled) left ventricular cavity with hyperdynamic function, leading to 'cavity obliteration' at end-systole. Sometimes dynamic LV outflow tract obstruction is seen as a result of this, and strikingly high obstructive gradients can occur (which resolve as the hypovolaemia is corrected).

Echo should not generally be regarded as diagnostic in **pulmonary embolism**, but may reveal clues to the diagnosis. In massive pulmonary embolism, the obstruction to blood flow from the embolism leads to an acute rise in systolic pressure upstream, causing dilatation of the pulmonary artery, RV dilatation and tricuspid regurgitation. RA pressure rises, leading to a dilated (and fixed) inferior vena cava.

Echo shows a dilated RV with hypokinesia which typically affects the RV wall but not the apex (an echo finding known as the McConnell sign). A ratio of RV to LV end diastolic diameter >0.6 is consistent with massive pulmonary embolism. The interventricular septum bulges towards the left in systole as a result of RV pressure overload, giving the LV myocardium a 'D-shaped' appearance on short-axis views. Sometimes, a thrombus may be seen in the right heart (or occasionally straddling a patent foramen ovale between right and left atria, known as 'thrombus in transit', which can lead to an arterial or 'paradoxical' embolism).

The recognition and management of **aortic dissection** is discussed on page 249, and of **cardiac tamponade** on page 238.

Further reading

Afari HA et al. Echocardiography for the pregnant heart. *Current Treatment Options in Cardiovascular Medicine* (2021). PMID 34075291.

Dabbouseh NM et al. Role of echocardiography in managing acute pulmonary embolism. *Heart* (2019). PMID 31439657.

Dobson R et al. British Society for Echocardiography and British Cardio-Oncology Society guideline for transthoracic echocardiographic assessment of adult cancer patients receiving anthracyclines and/or trastuzumab. *Echo Research and Practice* (2021). PMID 34106116.

Regitz-Zagrosek V et al. 2018 ESC Guidelines for the management of cardiovascular diseases during pregnancy: the task force for the management of cardiovascular diseases during pregnancy of the European Society of Cardiology (ESC). *European Heart Journal* (2018). PMID 30165544.

Saric M et al. Guidelines for the use of echocardiography in the evaluation of a cardiac source of embolism. *Journal of the American Society of Echocardiography* (2016). PMID 26765302.

APPENDIX: Echo resources

TEXTBOOKS

Introductory handbooks

Chambers J et al. *Echocardiography: A Practical Guide for Reporting and Interpretation*, 3rd ed. Boca Raton: CRC Press, 2023. ISBN-13: 978-1032151601.

Kaddoura S. *Echo Made Easy*, 3rd ed. Edinburgh: Elsevier, 2016. ISBN-13: 978-0702066566.

Leeson P et al. *Echocardiography (Oxford Specialist Handbooks in Cardiology)*, 3rd ed. Oxford: Oxford University Press, 2020. ISBN-13: 978-0198804161.

COMPREHENSIVE REFERENCE BOOKS

Armstrong WF et al. *Feigenbaum's Echocardiography*, 8th ed. Philadelphia: Lippincott Williams & Wilkins, 2018. ISBN-13: 978-1451194272.

Lang RM et al. *ASE's Comprehensive Echocardiography*, 3rd ed. Philadelphia: Elsevier, 2022. ISBN-13: 978-0323698306.

Otto CM. *The Practice of Clinical Echocardiography*, 6th ed. Philadelphia: Elsevier, 2022. ISBN-13: 978-0323697286.

JOURNALS

Cardiovascular Ultrasound:

cardiovascularultrasound.biomedcentral.com

Echo – Journal of the British Society of Echocardiography:

www.bsecho.org

Echo Research & Practice

echo.biomedcentral.com

European Heart Journal – Cardiovascular Imaging:

academic.oup.com/ehjcimaging

Journal of the American Society of Echocardiography:

www.onlinejase.com

KEY GUIDELINES

The British Society of Echocardiography (BSE) has several key guidelines and protocols available via its website (www.bsecho.org):

- A practical guideline for performing a comprehensive transthoracic echocardiogram in adults: the British Society of Echocardiography minimum dataset
- Normal reference intervals for cardiac dimensions and function for use in echocardiographic practice
- The assessment of mitral valve disease: a guideline from the British Society of Echocardiography

- Echocardiographic assessment of aortic stenosis: a practical guideline from the British Society of Echocardiography
- Echocardiographic assessment of the right heart in adults: a practical guideline from the British Society of Echocardiography
- Echocardiographic assessment of the tricuspid and pulmonary valves: a practical guideline from the British Society of Echocardiography
- Echocardiographic assessment of pulmonary hypertension: a guideline protocol from the British Society of Echocardiography
- A minimum dataset for a standard transoesophageal echocardiogram: a guideline protocol from the British Society of Echocardiography
- A safety checklist for transoesophageal echocardiography from the British Society of Echocardiography and the Association of Cardiothoracic Anaesthetists

Posters published by the BSE (can be obtained from the BSE website):

- Echocardiography: Reference Intervals & Functional Assessment
- Echocardiography: Valve Disease Assessment
- Clinical Indications & Triage of Echocardiography:
  - Emergency Inpatient and Critical Care
  - Out-Patient Requests (excluding the follow-up of established valve disease)
  - Heart Valve Disease
- Lancellotti P et al. Recommendations for the echocardiographic assessment of native valvular regurgitation: an executive summary from the European Association of Cardiovascular Imaging. *European Heart Journal – Cardiovascular Imaging* (2013). PMID 23733442.
- Lang RM et al. Recommendations for cardiac chamber quantification by echocardiography in adults: an update from the American Society of Echocardiography and the European Association of Cardiovascular Imaging. *Journal of the American Society of Echocardiography* (2015). PMID 25559473.
- Zoghbi WA et al. Recommendations for noninvasive evaluation of native valvular regurgitation: a report from the American Society of Echocardiography developed in collaboration with the Society for Cardiovascular Magnetic Resonance. *Journal of the American Society of Echocardiography* (2017). PMID 28314623.

SOCIETIES

British Society of Echocardiography (BSE)

Address:	Unit 204
	The Print Rooms
	164-180 Union Street
	London SE1 0LH
	United Kingdom
Tel:	0208 065 5794
Website:	www.bsecho.org

European Association of Cardiovascular Imaging (EACVI)

Address:	European Society of Cardiology
	European Heart House
	Les Templiers
	2035, Route des Colles
	CS 80179 Biot

	06903, Sophia Antipolis
	France
Tel:	+33.4.92.94.76.00
Fax:	+33.4.92.94.76.01
Website:	www.escardio.org/Sub-specialty-communities/ European-Association-of-Cardiovascular-Imaging-(EACVI)

American Society of Echocardiography (ASE)

Address:	2530 Meridian Parkway
	Suite 450
	Durham
	NC 27713
	United States of America
Tel:	+919 861 5574
Website:	www.asecho.org

WEBSITES

In addition to the websites already listed above, the following sites contain material of interest to anyone learning or practising echocardiography:

- *Medmastery*: www.medmastery.com
- *e-Echocardiography*: e-echocardiography.com
- *123sonography*: 123sonography.com
- *ASE live & virtual courses*: www.asecho.org/courses/

Index